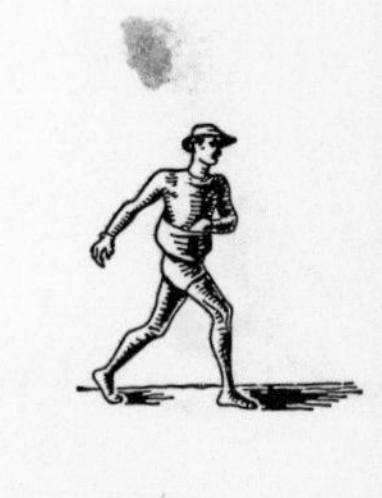

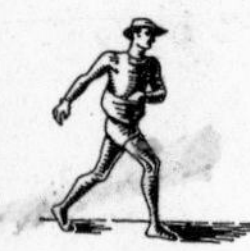

SIMON AND SCHUSTER · *New York*

THE COMPLETE ALLERGY GUIDE

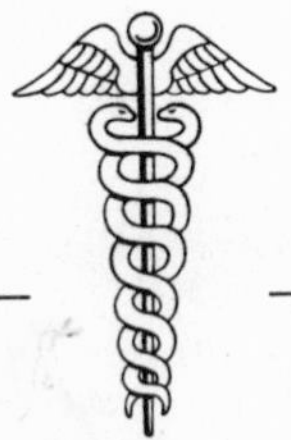

by

HOWARD G. RAPAPORT, M.D.

and

SHIRLEY MOTTER LINDE, M.S.

PUBLISHED BY SIMON AND SCHUSTER
ROCKEFELLER CENTER, 630 FIFTH AVENUE
NEW YORK, NEW YORK 10020

FIRST PRINTING

SBN 671-20667-2
LIBRARY OF CONGRESS CATALOG CARD NUMBER: 77-132775
DESIGNED BY CARL WEISS
MANUFACTURED IN THE UNITED STATES OF AMERICA

ACKNOWLEDGMENTS

This book is addressed to the millions of people suffering from allergies—to both those who know they have allergy and those who have untold symptoms of every system in the body that they don't realize are due to allergies. It is also hoped that physicians will find the book broad enough in scope and filled with enough practical details that they—no matter whether allergists, general practitioners, internists, psychiatrists, or pediatricians—will be able to use it in their practice as a means of instructing their allergy patients.

We wish to express thanks and appreciation to the following people for their help as we prepared this book on allergy: Dr. Theodore Haywood, Evelyn Singer, John Dolkart, Dr. Stephen D. Lockey, Dr. John H. Epstein, Dr. William Wilson, Dr. Bernard Fein, Mildred Bellomy, J. B. Kahn, Dr. W. Sawyer Eisenstadt, Dr. Irvin Caplin, Roy Keaton, Thelma Heatwole, Dr. A. Ford Wolf, Dr. Claude Frazier, Dr. William Schorr, Dr. Ben Feingold, Dr. Merle Scherr, Dr. Mason Lowance, Dr. Bernard A. Berman, Dr. Frederic Speer, Dr. Franklin Pass, Dominic Crolla, Scott Linde and Bob Linde.

We wish especially to thank Dr. John P. McGovern, professor of allergy at the University of Texas, clinical professor of pediatric allergy and microbiology at Baylor College of Medicine, and director of McGovern Allergy Clinic in Houston, for his early encouragement and guidance.

Also of great help to us were the following organizations: the American College of Allergists, the American Academy of Allergy, the Allergy Foundation of America, the American Academy of Dermatology, the National Tuberculosis and Respiratory Disease Association, the American Medical Association, the National Institute of Allergy and Infectious Diseases, the Allergy Rehabilitation Foundation, the U.S. Department of Health, Education, and Welfare, the National Clearinghouse for Smoking and Health, the American Cancer Society, the National Air Pollution Control Administration, the National Jewish Hospital and Research Center, the Asthmatic Children's Foundation of New York, the National Foundation for Asthmatic Children at Tucson, the Texas Allergy Research Foundation, Abbott Laboratories, Winthrop Laboratories, Dome Laboratories, Ar-Ex Products Co., Hollister-Stier Laboratories, Schieffelin and Co., Texas Pharmacal Co., Riker Laboratories, Borden Company, Neutrogena Corp., Westwood Pharmaceuticals, Rye-Krisp, USV Pharmaceutical Corp., Schering Laboratories, A. H. Robins and Co., Center Laboratories, and Ross Laboratories.

The assistance of these and many others helped make the writing of this book possible.

HOWARD G. RAPAPORT
SHIRLEY LINDE

CONTENTS

ACKNOWLEDGMENTS 5
PREFACE 9
CHAPTER 1 *The Tragedy of Allergy* 13
CHAPTER 2 *The Many Faces of Allergy* 17
CHAPTER 3 *The Allergic Infant* 24
CHAPTER 4 *Allergies of Childhood* 44
CHAPTER 5 *Hayfever* 87
CHAPTER 6 *Asthma* 118
CHAPTER 7 *Emphysema and Chronic Bronchitis* 159
CHAPTER 8 *Cigarette Smoking and How to Conquer It* 177
CHAPTER 9 *Food Allergies* 197
CHAPTER 10 *Skin Allergies* 217
CHAPTER 11 *Allergies to Insects* 258
CHAPTER 12 *Allergies to Drugs* 278
CHAPTER 13 *Allergic Headache, Earache, Sinus Trouble and Other Allergic Symptoms* 311
CHAPTER 14 *Physical Allergies: Cold, Heat and Light* 325
CHAPTER 15 *Going to the Doctor* 331
CHAPTER 16 *Research and the Future* 353

APPENDIX A *Some of the Things You Can Be Allergic To* 381
APPENDIX B *Instructions for Giving Self-Injections* 384
APPENDIX C *Antihistamine Preparations* 386
APPENDIX D *Manufacturers of Other Allergy Products* 393
APPENDIX E *Where to Go to Escape Ragweed* 396
APPENDIX F *Glossary of Terms* 417

INDEX 427

PREFACE

There are many ways to prevent and treat allergies today that are not being used. The public does not have the facts about allergy relief that are known to allergists.

We wrote this book to bring these facts to you.

The Complete Allergy Guide is designed to bridge the gap in knowledge that is keeping the millions of allergy sufferers from receiving the help that they could have. It brings to you all of the most up-to-the-minute information about allergy from the best-known allergy specialists and researchers in the world.

It is written to show you as an allergy sufferer specifically what can be done to help your particular condition. We also give you needed facts to help any members of your family who have allergies.

Whether you have a newborn baby with a rash or a grandfather with chronic bronchitis; whether you yourself have hayfever, asthma, emphysema, hives or eczema; whether you are allergic to foods, bee stings, drugs, heat, cold or light, you will find valuable information in these pages.

We will tell you how allergies are caused and the many factors that can add to or subtract from the symptoms. We will give you advice on feeding allergic infants and dealing with allergic children and their accompanying emotional problems. We will tell you about hayfever, asthma and bronchitis and the many startling new things that have been found to cause them. There are charts of foods and recipes to help you with food allergies, and helpful advice about skin allergies and what you can most effectively do about them. We tell you what to do in the precious first few minutes of an allergic attack from insect stings or drugs. We tell about other problems that often can be caused by allergies but are not recognized as such—like headaches, ear infections, deafness, visual problems, heart conditions. We discuss emotional factors and the role they may play. We tell you how to allergy-condition your home, where to get professional help, when to send your asthmatic child to camp, where to go to live or vacation to be free of pollen, what products to try if you are sensitive to cosmetics or soaps. We tell you how to cooperate with your doctor to discover the basis of your allergy, and how to work with him to treat it.

THE COMPLETE ALLERGY GUIDE

Chapter 1

THE TRAGEDY OF ALLERGY

If you have an allergy, you are not alone. Millions of people in the world today suffer from allergies.

Their allergies taunt them and cripple them—both physically and psychologically. Allergies can ruin health, shorten lives, produce sick personalities, cause accidents, lose jobs, separate lovers, and break up marriages. Allergies can change normal youngsters to overly sensitive lonely outcasts, change normally pleasant men and women to hypochondriacs or irritating whiners. Allergies kill many thousands of people every year, put many others in hospitals, and destroy the happiness and productivity of millions.

In fact, it is estimated that *at least one half of the entire world population* suffers some type of allergy, mild or serious. One out of every five or ten persons has a really major allergy of serious crippling proportions and consequences. The others have less crippling but still debilitating problems.

Consider these statistics showing the seriousness of the problem:

In the United States some 100 million persons are said to have allergies.

Asthma and hayfever together rank third in prevalence among all chronic diseases. Thousands die of asthma alone, and hundreds of thousands are disabled by it. Millions have hayfever at certain seasons or year round.

One third of *all* chronic diseases in children under age seventeen are caused by hayfever, asthma or other allergic disorders. This makes allergies the most common cause of disability among schoolchildren.

Some 5 percent of the population is said to be allergic to penicillin alone, while an increasing number are becoming allergic to detergents, cosmetics, plastics and other new drugs and products.

Some 600,000 workers are victims of occupational dermatitis.

■ THE COST OF ALLERGIES

These same allergies account for more than 36 million days lost by children from school and play each year.

Of men rejected from military service, more than one out of every sixteen with medical disqualifications were rejected because of allergy. It ranks seventh among medical reasons for draft rejection.

Industry loses a staggering 184 million days of work because of employees who have allergies. The number of people home from work or school and restricted in activity just today—right now—is probably 500,000.

Allergy victims spend an estimated $135 million for medicines and another $100 million for injections. Allergic patients require an average of *three times* as many medical visits as those with other types of illnesses.

The price for allergy is high—enormously high in dollars and cents, and even higher yet when you consider the losses in education, career fulfillment, happiness, and lives not lived as fully as possible.

■ MUCH OF THE TRAGEDY IS NEEDLESS

Many of these people do not need to suffer from their allergies. They can be helped. Many facts are known to allergists about the prevention and treatment of various kinds of allergies, and research is turning up new helpful facts each day. But the paradox is that these facts and these principles of prevention and treatment are not reaching the public.

It is not necessarily the fault of the family physician trying to treat the allergic patient, because many facts are not reaching the doctor either.

Over and over we have seen people suffering needlessly, wasting years of their lives in discomfort, misery and poor health—unnecessarily. Allergists discuss these problems in their scientific meetings and in their journals.

Charles Marph, a New York doctor, said at one meeting:

"These people go from doctor to doctor, seeking a cure for their disease, but finding that the average physician is unable to give them more than temporary relief despite his years of clinical training and experience."

Dr. Samuel Feinberg, an allergist at Northwestern University, wrote in the *Journal of the American Medical Association:*

"The diagnosis and treatment of allergies have been greatly facilitated by the discoveries of the past 50 years, but much of the available knowledge of the subject is not being applied. . . . In spite of the advances in our knowledge of allergy, only a small part of the population with allergies is receiving maximal benefits."

So we doctors know about the problem, but somehow the knowledge fails to reach the public and unfortunately many doctors themselves.

■ THE REASONS FOR THE PARADOX

Why are these techniques of prevention and treatment known by allergists, and yet not known to the vast majority of people?

There are several reasons, and the major ones are these:

1. There are not enough allergists in this country to go around. Only 1,300 allergists take care of the 100 million people with allergies. Of these 1,300 allergists, only 625 have received board certification.

2. Many other physicians who do not specialize in allergy have inadequate knowledge about it. Some even feel, mistakenly, that all allergies are due to emotions, or they wishfully believe children will eventually outgrow their allergies.

3. There is very little training concerning the prevention and treatment of allergies given either in medical school or in internship. In

fact, of the seventy medical school administrators replying to a questionnaire, many said their schools gave a total of only four or five hours of allergy training in four years, and some schools gave no training in allergy at all.

4. Students graduating from medical school appear to be more interested in other aspects of medicine. Nearly half of the residency training programs now available for young physicians to become allergy specialists are remaining unfilled. In fact, a recent survey showed only forty-six allergy residents in training in the entire United States.

5. Many patients have misconceptions about their allergies, and therefore do not go to a doctor to get the help that is available. They feel nothing can be done, when actually there is much that can help.

6. Many patients go to the doctor, get advice on how to handle their problem, and then ignore that advice. They do not follow their diets or do not take the medicines that the doctor prescribes, continuing to suffer needlessly. Often children with allergy symptoms do poorly in school and have permanent physical handicaps because their parents fail to carry out the doctor's recommendations.

These are the reasons that many people are suffering needlessly. Now let's see if there is something we can *do* about it.

But before we go into the details on the prevention and treatment of your allergy, let's look at just how your allergy is caused.

Chapter **2**

THE MANY FACES OF ALLERGY

At the moment you are born you are exposed to an entirely new environment. You leave your mother's dark, quiet, soft, wet, warm womb where you floated in weightlessness. You are suddenly startled by light and noises. You take in your first deep breath of the strange new stuff called air. You get chemicals put in your eyes, have your temperature taken, are weighed, get a vitamin shot, then are wrapped in a warm blanket and shipped off to mother or the nursery. You are now on your own, breathing in air and all that's in it, touching things against your skin, and you soon will be taking food into your new body.

From those first moments of birth on, through the rest of our lives, we are exposed to many things in our environment—things in the air that we breathe, things that we eat and drink, things that we touch. And the way we react to these things we breathe, eat and touch is the story of allergy. Different people react differently. If your reactions to the things you come in contact with are normal, there is no problem. If your body is sensitive to them, you become allergic.

Allergists see people with many different allergies, with many different causes.

A thirty-four-year-old housewife in Monterey, California, eats a bag of peanuts. Thirty minutes later her eyes swell nearly shut, red blotches cover her skin, and hives break out in irregular lumps all over her body. The itching is intense, and she digs into her eyes and makes deep scratches in her skin. By the time she reaches a doctor, she can barely breathe.

A thirteen-year-old boy in Chicago is scrawny and has a rather sunken chest and a pale face. He doesn't go out much for sports, too weak. The other kids ignore him, call him a sissy. He is unhappy and mopey. Sometimes in the middle of the night he wakes with a spasm of coughing and ends up gasping for breath.

Every August and September a man in Kansas feels like crawling into a hole and dying for eight weeks. He sneezes, his nose drips, his eyes water and itch and puff up and look baggy. His ears and throat itch inside. He digs deeply with his finger in his ear and vainly scrapes his tongue against his throat, but the itch goes on. The symptoms are even worse when he goes to bed, and he struggles to get a few hours of sleep each night. By the end of the first week of misery he scarcely has the energy to drag out of bed to go to work. He has suffered this way for two months out of every year since he was ten. He is now forty-two.

A teen-age girl starts for a walk through a meadow on a balmy day in spring. She climbs over a fence, brushes against a hornet, is stung. In a few seconds her face swells. In three minutes she is unconscious. In fifteen minutes she is dead.

A ten-year-old boy constantly sniffs and snorts and hawks and coughs. He rubs his nose frequently—his parents say constantly—and he usually has his mouth hanging open because he can't breathe through his nose.

A bank clerk in Des Moines gets a scaly red rash every time he handles money, and is forced to quit his job.

A woman gets blisters on her lips every time she uses lipstick.

A three-month-old baby doubles up his tiny body and screams in anguish with the pains of colic.

A grandmother suffers severe diarrhea every time she eats a box of chocolates.

A girl swells up over her entire body after she spends an hour in the hot sun of summer.

A boy has an ear infection every two months or so.

A woman has frequent pounding headaches.

A girl gets hives the night before her wedding.

A man collapses after getting a penicillin injection. His life is barely saved.

Their troubles were all caused by allergies.

■ CAUSES OF ALLERGIES

You may be allergic to one thing. You may be allergic to dozens, or hundreds.

The many things you may be allergic to—doctors call these things "allergens"—break down into seven major categories. The categories are based mostly on the avenues by which the troublemaking allergens reach your body and cause the turmoil.

Here are the categories of things that can cause allergies:

1. Things you breathe (dust, particles, chemical vapors, animal danders, feathers, pollen, molds, cosmetics)
2. Things you eat or drink (foods, drinks, medicines)
3. Things you touch (fabrics, poison plants, metals, woods, plastics, medicines, cosmetics, soaps)
4. Things you are injected with (vaccines or drugs, venom from insect stings or snakebites)
5. Things you are infected with (bacteria, fungi, molds)
6. Physical factors (heat, cold, light, sun)
7. Emotional factors (conscious or unconscious feelings)

■ EFFECTS CAUSED IN YOUR BODY

There are many allergens in the environment that can cause allergies; and as the foregoing list shows, there are many avenues by which these troublemakers can reach your body. Once they reach your body, they can act on different parts of the body. The identical troublemaking allergen can affect different organs in different people and can cause entirely different symptoms. One person who eats chocolate, for example, may have swollen eyes the next morning; another person may get hives; another might have diarrhea, and another a severe headache.

And there is no relationship between how the troublemaker gets into your body and what symptoms it causes. Something you breathe may cause a skin rash, whereas something you eat may cause breathing difficulties and not even affect your digestive system at all.

Nearly any organ in the body can be hit as the target organ. Allergies can affect your eyes and nose as in hayfever. They can affect your lungs and bronchial tubes as in asthma. They can affect your skin, causing hives and itching or a scaly rash. They can affect the digestive system, causing everything from canker sores to diarrhea or constipation. They can give you headaches, earaches, slight hearing loss or even total deafness, heart and blood vessel conditions, and visual problems. They can affect your entire body all at once and kill you.

New evidence points to the possibility that allergies may also be involved in causing major chronic diseases like arthritis and rheumatic fever and other infectious diseases. Other new evidence indicates that even aging may be due in great part to allergic reactions.

■ THE MYSTERIOUS H SUBSTANCE

How are these various symptoms actually caused?

All the details are not yet known. This is one of the major research problems that allergists are working on right now in many laboratories throughout the world. They have come up with some evidence, and have several different theories as to what underlies the allergic reaction. In the final analysis, the mechanism is not clearly understood. What really happens in allergy remains one of the mysteries of medicine that must still be solved.

But here in general is what happens.

For an allergy to develop, you must first be exposed to an allergen and develop a sensitivity to it. The first exposure produces the sensitization; the second or third exposure produces the reaction. Sometimes it seems an individual reacts upon a first exposure, but there must have been either an unrecognized exposure to the substance or to something closely related to it. In some instances sensitization occurs before birth. Sensitization can also occur to substances within a person's own body.

The body's basic mechanism of defense is the ability to recognize something that is foreign. Then it produces antibodies to neutralize the foreign substances, which are known as antigens. This is the basis of all immunization and the basis of all allergy. When this mechanism produces immunity to germs it is desirable. When it means an allergy to some substance that produces sneezing or hives, then it is undesirable.

Let's say that you are allergic to strawberries. It's spring. The strawberries are lush and beautiful and you gorge yourself on them. When the strawberries reach your stomach and intestines, they are digested and broken down to simpler substances called polypeptides. As polypeptides, the troublemaking molecules of the strawberries enter the bloodstream. What happens next—how these molecules interact in your body and with what substances they interact—is not completely understood. Some scientists think an enzyme is involved. Others have different theories. But no matter what the mechanism is, antibodies are formed. Antibodies are the protective substances manufactured by the defense system of the body. Then a substance—the "mysterious H substance"—is released from your body cells. Several substances have been incriminated, but most often the substance is a compound called histamine. This mysterious H substance, histamine, is a chemical always present in your body. In fact it is normally present in all plants and animals. But during an allergy attack, a great deal of it is produced, and it causes symptoms.

As a result of the presence of large quantities of histamine, smooth muscles surrounding the large bronchi, or air tubes, go into spasm. This narrows the air tubes, and restricts the amount of air inhaled and exhaled. In addition, many glands are stimulated. They pour out large quantities of mucus in the walls of the large air tubes, compounding the problems of breathing.

The mysterious H substance also acts on the tiny capillary blood vessels in your body, causing them to open and expand. More blood comes to the stretched vessels. The thin capillary wall is usually only one cell thick, and with the dilatation, the fluid of the blood easily leaks through the wall into the nearby tissues and makes them swell. The presence of this fluid—no matter what tissue it's in—is the source of most allergy symptoms. What symptoms occur and how severe they are will depend on where the swelling occurs from the fluid, and how severe the swelling is. If the excess fluid occurs in the skin, you will have hives. If the fluid causes swelling in the lining tissue of the nose, your nose will be stuffed and you will not be able to breathe. If the swelling occurs in the tissue that lines the bronchial tubes in the lungs, the airways may be blocked, and you get the coughing and wheezing of asthma.

■ WHY ALLERGIC REACTIONS CAN VARY FROM TIME TO TIME

An allergic person has a level of resistance—or threshold—against the substances that produce allergy. (Again, we call these substances that produce allergies "allergens.") Let's take an example. If only a few of those strawberries had been eaten, they might not have exceeded the threshold of your body, so might not have bothered you. But when the threshold was breached, then trouble began. It's like when water builds up behind a dike, reaches the critical level, then spills over and breaks through in a roaring surge.

Thresholds vary from person to person, just as symptoms do, and thresholds of any one person also vary under different circumstances. Many outside factors can contribute by raising or lowering your threshold, too, and so change your reactions.

OUTSIDE INFLUENCES

Major influencing factors that may cause a threshold to be lowered and so increase symptoms are these: degree of exposure, infection, changes of climate or temperature, emotional upset, exertion, fatigue, hormone upsets, poor nutritional status, lack of enough sleep, strong odors or fumes that irritate the mucous membranes.

These changing factors can explain why you react at one time to a particular allergen, but not at another time. Ten strawberries might not go over your threshold level under ordinary conditions. But on a day when you are tired and upset or haven't been eating or had a fight with your wife or kids—they could cause a walloping reaction.

ALLERGIES CAN ADD TOGETHER

Another important thing about the threshold concept is that if you have two or more allergies—as most allergic people do—one allergy can add on to the other and reinforce it. Perhaps you did not eat enough strawberries to produce symptoms, but at the same time you were petting a cat. If you are allergic to cat dandruff, the two together could exceed your threshold and set off your symptoms.

BIOLOGICAL RHYTHM IN EVERYDAY LIVING

Allergies can even vary with time. You may have noticed a rhythmic pattern in the symptoms of your allergy. In a large number of asthmatic patients, for example, attacks repeatedly recur or become worse at night, generally between 11:00 P.M. and 4:00 A.M. This is exactly the same time that your adrenal hormone production is down.

All living organisms, plants and animals, have a built-in biological rhythm—a coming and going of high activity and low activity. And the interesting thing is that allergy attacks happen most often at the times when your blood pressure, your lung function, your hormone production are all reduced. Many allergists believe these twenty-four-hour rhythms may make your resistance to allergies lower at certain times.

So because of the many factors that cause allergies, because of the many symptoms that can be caused and because of the many influencing factors that affect each allergy and each exposure to that allergy, your allergy may become very complex. Because of its complexity, prevention and treatment are not always simple.

But even though the total problem is difficult and complicated, we believe you can be helped. We will look at all phases—and faces—of allergy with you, and we will help you with ways to look at your entire way of life to really understand your problem. Then by carefully reading the book and being guided by our suggestions, and by cooperating with your own physician, you can find the particular methods of prevention and treatment that are best for you to meet your particular problem.

We will review some of these particular problems in the next chapters.

Chapter **3**

THE ALLERGIC INFANT

Allergies are more common in infants than is usually believed. The allergic signs may be mild in infants or they may be serious enough to make his little life, as well as that of his parents, utterly miserable. They may range from skin rashes to respiratory problems to digestive upsets.

In coping with allergic problems, a physician must truly be a Sherlock Holmes to determine what specific factor or factors are causing any one person's allergy. He must sift through many bits of evidence of what the person comes into contact with in his everyday life. When the patient is an infant, the problem is even more difficult. The physician must be a very special supersleuth, and the mother a female Doctor Watson. The infant cannot talk, so the mother must be ever alert for unspoken clues.

As the detective searches for leads at the scene of the crime, you and your doctor must search for clues in each day of living. You must work with your physician painstakingly and methodically, investigating tiny details and being on the alert for unusual signs. Sometimes it's easy to find the solution to the problem; at other times it takes a good deal of effort on the part of both physician and parents to narrow the list of suspected factors and point the diagnostic finger at the guilty troublemaker.

Your doctor will want to know how often your baby's allergy attacks occur and exactly when. He will want to know what your baby was doing in the time leading up to the attack. He will ask about places visited, foods eaten, pets in the house, and many details about your home. It's a good idea for you to keep a notebook of the circumstances surrounding each allergy attack so that a more complete picture may be presented to the physician.

■ HOW TO TELL IF YOUR BABY HAS AN ALLERGY

It is not always easy to tell whether a baby is allergic because many allergies masquerade as other illnesses. However, there are some symptoms that you can be on the lookout for. Sometimes they are continual; sometimes they come and go. If they occur frequently, the chances are strong that your baby is starting early in life with an allergy.

Here are the clues to watch for:

His formula does not seem to agree with him and needs to be changed frequently.
He has much gas and colic often and continues to scream and double up with pain even after he has been thoroughly burped.
He has other vague and unexplained abdominal pain.
He has unexplained diarrhea or constipation.
He spits up large amounts of formula or other food.
He has extreme likes and dislikes in foods.
He has frequent canker sores or fever blisters on the lips or in the mouth.
He has persistent sniffles or a constantly running nose.
He has unexplained skin rashes.
He is unusually cranky or irritable.
He has a persistent night cough.
He has rapid breathing or shortness of breath.
He rubs or scratches his face or arms or legs or the creases of his body frequently.

■ THE ROLE OF HEREDITY

There is still a good deal of controversy among allergists as to the role that heredity plays in the cause of allergies. Most believe that children do not inherit their specific allergies, but they do inherit the tendency—the soil—to develop allergies.

In some allergic diseases heredity plays an essential part, but in others it plays practically none. It plays an important role in bronchial asthma, seasonal and year-round hayfever, and hives. In other allergic diseases, such as contact eczema, gastrointestinal allergy and some forms of migraine headache, the hereditary factor apparently has no influence at all.

In the transmission of the allergies in which heredity does play a part, the outlook is as follows. When *one* parent suffers from the allergy while the other does not, 50 percent of their children will carry the gene causing the allergy, but only 30 to 40 percent of the children will actually show clinical allergic symptoms. When *both* parents have asthma, 75 to 100 percent of the children will carry the gene causing the allergy, and about 60 percent will actually have the clinical allergic condition.

■ WHAT HAPPENS TO INFANT ALLERGIES?

One physician found in his practice that *four out of every five children who had a skin allergy subsequently developed a disorder of the upper or lower respiratory tract or both.* In fact, when the past health history of a long-standing allergic pattient is reviewed carefully, it will almost always reveal that the allergic patient, when he was less than six months old, had a skin rash that often lasted several weeks. Some of these infants, at about four weeks, manifested colic which lasted several months or more. Between three months and six years, as he began eating other foods, he developed eczema or hives. As he grew older in childhood, allergies of the respiratory tract appeared, either as nasal stuffiness or as dripping or frequent colds, or hayfever or asthma.

Not every older allergy patient has shown all of these problems in his babyhood, but the larger number have shown this typical pattern of allergies right from the beginning of their life.

This seems to be the universal pattern and the one you should watch for: (1) simple skin rashes, (2) then colic, (3) then eczemas due to foods, (4) then nasal allergy generally due to inhalant substances and (5) in some instances, chest involvement. One symptom disappears only to be replaced by another.

It is important to treat these allergies adequately initially, not only to make the baby's life and yours more pleasant now, but because the mild allergies as they change their patterns also become much more serious as the years pass if they are neglected.

The chain can be broken only by proper treatment.

Children almost never outgrow their allergies. This is one of the major myths about allergy. Not only do many parents believe this myth about children outgrowing their allergies, but amazingly many physicians do too. The only allergies that usually are outgrown are the very mild food allergies of infancy. Other allergies almost never get better without specific treatment, and usually continue to get worse and worse as they follow the typical pattern. Finally they can become severely crippling. So, get your child to a doctor so that his particular allergies can be identified early and treated adequately.

If your doctor says, "Oh, don't worry about his allergy, Mrs. Smith, he'll outgrow it," then he does not have enough background in allergy. Despite the fact that he may be an excellent doctor in other respects, we suggest that you find yourself another physician to treat your baby's allergy problem.

■ FOOD ALLERGIES IN INFANTS

Food is the major cause of allergy in children under the age of one. After that, other factors, principally environmental ones, become more important.

FOOD ALLERGY VERSUS FOOD TOLERANCE

First we would like to point out that there is a difference between food allergy and food intolerance. Intolerance simply means that the baby's digestive system will not tolerate a food because of physical reasons. The food may be too hot, too cold, too fatty, or may have some substance in it that the child's stomach will not accept. Food allergy, on the other hand, is a specific allergic reaction, with the body being immunologically sensitive to a particular food.

An example of food intolerance: a child could develop colic from drinking hot milk, not because he was allergic to the milk, but because his digestive system would not tolerate the excess heat. Many times we have found that children who kept their parents awake for hours every night with colic have become contented and quiet infants after their mothers began giving them cold milk directly from the refrigerator instead of heating the bottle. But a child with an *allergy* to milk has a different problem.

SYMPTOMS OF FOOD ALLERGY

Signs that especially point toward a food allergy rather than another cause are loss of appetite, canker sores, a deeply fissured tongue, spitting up, vomiting, colic, distention of the stomach, excessive gas, diarrhea, mucus or blood in the stools. *These almost always suggest a food allergy.*

Other clues that *sometimes* indicate food as being responsible for the allergy, but can also mean other problems, are migraine headache, severe behavior disturbances, persistent crying, irritability, restlessness, fatigue, lack of energy and sweating, especially of the head.

Dr. Frederic Speer, from the pediatric allergy clinic at the University of Kansas Medical Center, studied several hundred children under age two who were allergic to foods. *The symptoms of food allergy found most often were runny nose and coughing.* They occurred in more than half of the food-allergic infants. Other symptoms found in these food-allergic infants (in the order of their frequency) were as follows: wheezing, diarrhea, abdominal pain, excessive sweating, mucus in the chest, eczema, constipation, vomiting and hives. Other symptoms that were considered important, but which occurred in less than 5 percent of the children, were sneezing, nosebleeds, ear infections, croup, abdominal distention, geographic tongue (where the tongue is marked like a map), blood in the stools, itching around the anus and genitals, purple patches on the skin, tension, fatigue, headache, paleness, and redness and irritation of the eyes. Some infants even went into collapse or shock.

Food allergy in infants can be mild or it can be very serious and a real problem. When it is mild, you can often make the diagnosis and eliminate the offending food yourself, but when the cause is hidden or the symptoms are severe, then a physician must be consulted.

OTHER CAUSES THAT MASQUERADE AS FOOD ALLERGY

These leads are valuable, but have to be considered in the light of the entire picture of a baby's life. Sometimes a food allergy appears to be the cause of an infant's problems when actually an entirely unrelated disorder is causing the trouble. For example, an infant may have a watery, runny nose for weeks without a fever, and both parents and physician label it an allergy. However, that runny nose could be caused by a streptococcal infection. If a specific food cannot be found causing an allergy, a culture needs to be taken to see if any such bacteria are present. Sometimes poor nutrition, especially a deficiency of certain vitamins (vitamin A, C and B_6) or minerals, can cause allergiclike symptoms. In some instances symptoms may be caused by an allergy other than to food (remember what you breathe can cause gastrointestinal upsets and what you eat can cause asthma). Emotional factors can be involved. Sometimes the mother has emotional reactions to certain foods that have affected the baby. Occasionally the tense and disturbed infant may be helped by sedatives, antispasmodics, tranquilizers or a warm comforting nurse, a rocking chair and a pacifier.

Vitamins, laxatives and other medicines can also be a cause of allergies in infants. Eczema caused by taking cod liver oil has been reported. Some laxatives can also cause allergies because of their action on the digestive tract, causing rapid absorption of proteins that are generally not absorbed.

Drugs commonly used in infants that are capable of causing allergic problems are aspirin, opium and its relatives, barbiturates, mercury, insulin, sulfa drugs and antibiotics. If you believe that your baby is allergic to any medicines, tell your doctor of your suspicions immediately, and if at any time you consult a different doctor, be sure to tell him also. Drugs should be prescribed only when there are clear indications for their use.

SPECIFIC FOODS THAT OFTEN CAUSE TROUBLE

What foods can a baby be allergic to? An infant may develop sensitivity to any food, really. Even foods generally considered completely safe like special nonallergenic milk formulas, lamb, pear, rice and white potato can cause problems. An infant's first food—cow's milk—has been a major troublemaker. The cow is only the foster mother of the human race, and its secretion is sometimes not acceptable to highly allergic infants. It may precipitate a considerable degree of allergy in infants.

One doctor studied a large group of infants to determine their particular trouble-causing foods and found that citrus fruits caused allergies in 41 percent of the children; foods of the pea family, including beans, soybeans, peanuts and peas, caused allergies in 30 percent of the children; eggs caused allergies in 28 percent; and chocolate in 27 percent. The astute mathematicians among you may have noticed these figures add up to more than 100 percent. This is because many of the infants were allergic to more than one food. A number of children have also been found to be allergic to corn, wheat, tomato, rice, oats, beef, barley, chicken, apple, pork, banana, plums, grape, sweet potato, carrots, turkey, spinach, beets, onions, mint, cinnamon, tea, strawberries, potatoes, fish, squash, artificial food coloring, and vitamin drops.

SEARCHING OUT YOUR CHILD'S TROUBLEMAKERS

How do you find what *your* child is allergic to? The painstaking search for food allergens will depend a good deal on you. When you visit the doctor, he will ask you what foods you suspect are causing the symptoms or are making the child not feel well after eating. You will have to keep careful track of possible suspect foods, often to the point of writing down every single food that is eaten during every day and then noting the occurrence of any allergy symptoms. Skin tests are helpful in detecting food allergies but have some limitations. As a final test, when you think you know the guilty food, you remove it from the diet to see whether the symptoms stop. If they do, then you give a small amount of the food again to see whether the symptoms reappear. If they do appear, then this is your "guilty" food, and you eliminate it from the baby's diet.

When a baby is being breast-fed, the survey of diet must also include the mother's diet, since some of the antigens from allergy-causing foods can pass from the mother's digestive system into the breast milk, thereby sensitizing the infant.

Many doctors have different systems for working out the trial-and-error testing of various foods. One popular method is to eliminate *all* of the foods that are suspected, feeding the baby only those foods that are considered safe. The mother keeps a diary, writing down each item of food she gives the baby, even if in small amounts. After a week, or preferably two weeks, one of the suspected foods is added back into the diet. If the child has a return of its allergic symptoms, then this food is the troublemaker. If after two or three days of getting this food the child does *not* have a return of his allergic symptoms, then this food is not a troublemaker, but is safe to have. Every three or four days one of the suspected foods is added back into the diet until the guilty food (or foods) is found.

The biggest mistake made with this plan is that the suspected foods are not omitted from the diet for a long enough period of time, since mothers are generally very impatient. The suspected foods must be kept out until the original symptoms disappear. If milk is the troublemaker, it will usually have to be withheld for a minimum of three weeks, sometimes as long as two months before the symptoms clear. Peanuts or chocolate usually needs to be withheld about five to seven days.

Confusion can also arise at times because allergy to foods can vary. For example, a child may be more allergic to a food if he has a concurrent infection or diarrhea or if he eats an excessive amount of the food. He can also become more sensitive to it when the weather becomes colder or if he is excessively fatigued or upset.

HIDDEN FORMS OF TROUBLE

Another reason for failure in determining causes of food allergies, and also for failure in treating them, is that often parents do not realize that the problem food may occur in disguised form in other foods. For example, *if your child is allergic to milk,* you must eliminate regular milk, dried milk, evaporated milk, skim milk, buttermilk, ice cream, sherbet, frozen dairy products, creamed foods, cheese and custard. They all contain milk in one form or another.

If your child is allergic to corn, he must not have candy, cookies, most breads, buns, canned fruit, jams, jellies, chewing gum, peanut butter, hot dogs, lunch meat or ice cream. They all contain corn syrup. He must not have baked goods or fish sticks because they contain cornmeal. He should not have oils, margarines, mayonnaise or salad dressings because they contain corn oil. He must not have gravies, soups or powdered sugars. They contain cornstarch. He must not have any corn cereals or corn products like hominy grits. We assume because of his age you would not be giving him Fritos, Corn Curls, popcorn, tacos, tamales, bourbon or beer anyway.

If your child is allergic to eggs, he cannot have any baked goods except the simplest breads, cookies and crackers. He cannot have noodles, mayonnaise, many salad dressings, meat loaf, breaded foods, meringue, custard, french toast, divinity or icings. In egg sensitivity, albumin is more important than the yolk. Sometimes it appears that a child is sensitive to egg yolk when actually the cause of his allergy is the infinitesimally small quantity of the white part of the egg that sticks to the yolk. Babies should never be given any form of egg until they are ten to twelve months old and have built up some protection against egg white allergy.

If your child is allergic to wheat or other cereals, he may not have any flour products, any breads, cakes, crackers, donuts, cookies, waffles, pancakes, pretzels, ice-cream cones, pie crust, macaroons, rolls, cereals, macaroni, spaghetti or gravy.

If your child is allergic to cinnamon, he must not have spice cakes, cookies, rolls, pies, cinnamon-flavored chewing gum or candy, chili, wieners, lunch meat or catsup.

If your child is allergic to artificial food coloring, he must not have colored drinks, medicine, soda pop, bubble gum, artificially colored wieners, Jello or popsicles.

You must learn to read and study labels on every package, bottle, and can of food when your child is allergic in order to find all these hidden sources of danger.

Once you know with some certainty which foods your baby can and cannot eat, your doctor will work with you to find a nourishing and suitably attractive diet for your baby. It is not only necessary to eliminate all the foods that are causing your baby's allergy, but also necessary that your baby get a balanced diet with the proper amount of calories, proteins, minerals and vitamins.

LOOK OUT FOR RELATED FOODS

Children who are sensitive to one food are especially likely to be allergically sensitive to other foods that are in the same plant family. For example, there is a cross-relation and cross-reactivity between peanuts and peas, apples and pears, chocolates and cola.

Study the list of related foods on page 205. If your child is allergic to one of the items on the list, you should not feed him the other foods in that category of foods either. For instance, if your child is allergic to apples, don't feed him pears either; if he is allergic to orange juice, beware of lemons and grapefruits.

MILK ALLERGY

One thing you can do to help keep your child from getting allergies is to nurse him from the breast for as long as possible. Breast milk will not produce allergies as cow's milk will, and it also gives the new infant immunity against infections because he gets antibodies against the infections directly from his mother's milk. We hope that the apparent trend toward increased breast-feeding will continue. If it does, a lot fewer infants will have allergies. Milk is one of the biggest causes of allergies that we know. Babies given bottle milk instead of breast milk have eight times more eczema.

The worst case we know was a baby boy who went home from the hospital on the usual evaporated milk formula with sugar added. Shortly after leaving the hospital he developed severe diarrhea and became so dehydrated he had to be sent back to the hospital. His formula was changed several times, but the diarrhea continued so severely he had to be given intravenous feedings. He improved on a nonmilk substitute and cortisone. But when a little cow's milk was added to his formula again, he vomited, became pale and listless, developed more diarrhea with blood and appeared acutely ill. He was put back on the nonmilk formula. At fifteen months, he was given a few teaspoons of homogenized cow's milk. Within two hours he began to vomit. He was returned to his nonmilk formula. Seldom is a baby found this sensitive to milk.

Usually if a baby is allergic to milk, he will refuse to nurse, will spit up a great deal, vomit or have diarrhea. A typical reaction is that he comes hungry to the bottle, grasps the nipple eagerly, takes a suck or two, then turns away with distaste. With urging, he takes an ounce or so, then spits up or vomits, but sometimes finishes the bottle. For an hour or two, he then has pain, gas and frequent gassy stools. Sometimes instead of showing distaste, the baby will gulp irregularly with much thrashing about and irritability while nursing.

There is often a family history of intolerance to milk, with one of the parents admitting they never did like milk or they get diarrhea from it.

If your child is allergic to milk, try boiling the milk. This sometimes breaks down the protein sufficiently to prevent the allergic symptoms. Also try using evaporated milk or powdered milk. If these measures fail, then try one of the milk substitutes such as

Mull-soy, Sobee, Nutramigen or Isomil. Keep your child on evaporated milk diluted with water for as long as possible, even past age two if you can. Even if a child is not allergic to milk, he should not be rushed in changing from evaporated milk to whole milk.

BREAST-FEEDING YOUR BABY

Illinois pediatrician Dr. E. Robbins Kimball says that babies who have been breast-fed get sick less often than nonbreast-feeders, and when they are sick their symptoms are less severe. In a study in Evanston Hospital in Illinois he found that children who had *not* been breast-fed had 4 times the respiratory infections, 20 times more diarrhea, 22 times more miscellaneous infections, 8 times the rate of eczema, 21 times more asthma, 27 times more hayfever, 11 times more surgery for tonsils and adenoids, 4 times the rate of ear problems, 11 times more hospital admissions and 8 times more physician house calls.

Mothers should try to breast-feed their new babies when possible, says Dr. Kimball, because of the benefits.

Here are some tips on successful nursing. Keep from being overly nervous, anxious, angry or tired. Learn to hand-express your milk for a few seconds before the baby nurses so that the milk is ready at your nipples when the baby starts suckling. To get him to take the nipple, stroke his cheek and mouth, which will stimulate him to open his mouth. After he has been nursing long enough, if you hold his nose about thirty seconds it will make him let go. To prevent sore or cracked nipples, during the first few days, limit nursing to one minute for each breast at any one time, but twice from each breast during the feeding if necessary. Cleanse your breasts with clear water or a mild soap and water. Toughen up your breasts before you begin to nurse to keep them from being sensitive. Expose them a bit to sunlight or sun lamp irradiation and to fresh air, and dry them vigorously with a towel after bathing. In the first few days and even later allow the baby to control the number of daily feedings, even though they come every two or three hours instead of the artificially specified four hours. Make sure you get sufficient rest and a nap each day. Don't worry if your baby doesn't seem to be satisfied at first. Milk always comes slowly in the beginning. Relax. The amount of milk will increase as your baby needs more. Dr. Kimball's "booze and snooze" method works well. If the baby is crying and you can't seem to relax enough to let the milk flow or the baby is too upset to nurse properly, change his diapers then settle in a bed or lounge chair, have your husband pour you a glass of wine, a highball or a glass of beer. Let him take the baby and cuddle it while you have a drink. Take a short nap, and when you wake up, chances are both you and the baby will be relaxed enough for nursing. Or try a hot cup of tea.

A NEW TREATMENT FOR CEREAL ALLERGY

If your child's major problem is cereals, try—with your physician if possible—to establish whether your child can tolerate some cereal other than one with wheat. Rice, corn and barley cereal are all available. In addition you might want to try giving your child poi, a popular Polynesian food that looks about like wallpaper paste. It tastes like wallpaper paste, too, but children seem to like it.

Poi is prepared from the taro root and has been the staple carbohydrate food of Hawaiians and other Polynesian people for centuries. It has been highly successful in treating infants allergic to cereals and will be accepted by infants as young as three days of age according to recent research.

GENERAL PRINCIPLES OF PREVENTION AND TREATMENT

Find the troublemakers and eliminate them. Those are the major principles for helping your child with food allergy. Look out for related foods and hidden sources of danger in seemingly innocent preparations. Be sure he gets a balanced diet despite the foods he cannot eat.

One of the elements of prevention is to never force your baby to take foods he doesn't want. If he gets a well-balanced diet, one food more or less won't make any difference. He may know that certain foods upset him. Forcing can precipitate psychological problems as well.

If you are pregnant or apt to be soon again, remember that preventive measures against a baby getting allergy can and should begin right from the time of conception. Pregnant women should not eat highly allergenic foods because the troublemaking parts of the foods can pass right through the linings of the stomach and intestines into the bloodstream and then through the placenta to the developing embryo.

■ ALLERGENS IN THE AIR

After foods, another major cause of allergies in infants is what they breathe from the air. The things in the air that can cause trouble include animal dandruff, ragweed, all types of feathers, grass pollens, tree pollens, molds and dust. The sensitivity to these substances can occur at amazingly young ages.

YOUR PETS MAY BE CAUSING THE TROUBLE

One of the biggest causes of allergic diseases in humans is dander and hairs from cats, dogs and other animals. In fact some of our leading allergists call cats and dogs the single most important cause of allergies in children under age two.

Dogs and cats are not the only animals that can cause allergy. Monkeys, guinea pigs, hamsters, gerbils and birds can do it. Some people even get hives from a dog's saliva. Even when the pet is kept in a box or cage in another room, the particles from their hairs or feathers will penetrate every corner of every room. Short hair, long hair, fuzz or feathers make no difference. The smallest bird or chihuahua can cause an allergy. And the myth that asthma will leave a child and go to a chihuahua is completely false.

If your baby has eczema or asthma or a runny nose and you have an animal in the house, it should be the first thing you consider as a cause of the allergy.

No matter how much you love your pet, you must consider getting rid of him. First, however, as a test, put your dog or cat in a kennel or with friends for several weeks. Clean the house thoroughly, vacuuming rugs, drapes and furniture, washing down hard surfaces to get rid of all traces of dog hairs and dander. If your baby stops sniffing and sneezing or if his skin rash goes away, you can be almost sure it was the dog or cat that was causing it. Then no matter how much you love the pet, you must get rid of it. Get your child a snake or turtle or chameleon. They don't cause allergies. If after this time, your child still has his symptoms, then something other than your pet is causing the trouble, and you and your physician must carefully and repetitively review the whole situation.

DETERMINING THE CAUSE OF AIRBORNE ALLERGIES

The first thing you will need to determine is when your baby has the symptoms. Your physician will ask you when and where and how the symptoms occurred. Are they in the spring, summer or the fall? Or year round? Does he have the symptoms more during one time of the day or night than any other? Does he have the symptoms only in certain rooms, or when he visits certain people? Or after he has done certain things?

If his sneezing and runny nose come in August and September, he is probably allergic to ragweed. If he sneezes in the spring, he is probably allergic to the tree pollens. If he sneezes in the summer, it may be grass pollens causing the trouble. Sometimes the baby's source of trouble is connected with his father's occupation. He may be bringing wheat dust home from the bakery, horse dander from the race track or orris root from the barber shop. Or it may be connected to a family hobby. Do you or your older children horseback ride?

One baby was fine except when he crawled around on the floor. Every time he spent a few minutes on the carpeting, his nose would start dripping and he would begin to cough. The cause—the jute rug pad under the living room carpeting. Carpeting itself can do it, too, especially if it is wool.

Another baby had his major trouble when he was in bed. His troublemaker—the luxurious comforter his grandmother had bought him as his first present. Every time his mother tucked the comforter around him, she set off another allergy attack. Feather pillows and feather-filled furniture can do the same thing. The baby's bedroom deserves special consideration, since the infant spends at least half his time there. His bedding, his pillows, his toys or even things stored in the closet in his room may be the cause of his allergy.

After you have carefully watched your baby and have come up with a few suspect substances, your doctor can do skin-testing of the suspected substances. The doctor makes a tiny scratch in the baby's skin and rubs a drop of the suspect substance into the scratch. If the baby is allergic to the substance, a red spot will raise on the skin. If he is not allergic to the substance, there will be no reaction.

GETTING RID OF THE CAUSE

Once you find what the cause of your baby's allergy is, you must take proper steps to remove the cause from his environment. It is not inexpensive to replace furnishings, but if it means the health of your child, it is necessary. Get rid of kapok or moss-stuffed mattresses. If the troublemaker is something simple like wool carpeting or a rug pad, get rid of it and get a different kind that will not cause trouble. If feathers are the cause, dispose of all feathered pillows, feather-filled furniture and feather comforters. If ragweed or other pollen is the cause, you will have to keep the baby in during the season involved and install an air conditioner in the rooms that he occupies, leaving windows in those rooms closed. Also—and this is more significant—have him tested to see what pollen is the troublemaker and have him treated by hyposensitization to the pollen. If dust is causing the trouble, you will have to dust-proof his room and other rooms in the house that he occupies, getting rid of all drapes, bedding, pillows, carpeting or dust-collecting toys. Some people do not realize how much environmental dust gets around. If your child is sensitive to feathers, just eliminating a feather pillow from his bed is not sufficient. You must take the feather pillows away from the beds in *all* the rooms. We give you more details on how to allergy-proof your house in a later chapter in this book.

There are other irritants that do not cause allergy themselves, but may aggravate allergy. Such irritants include dampness, paint, tobacco smoke, strong fumes and all pungent odors, including perfume. Eliminate them also.

■ ASTHMA IN INFANCY

Can an infant have asthma?

It certainly can. Asthma in infancy is much more frequent than generally believed. Both physicians and patients have believed that asthma seldom occurs in babies, but now we know better.

The problem has been that it is somewhat difficult to make a conclusive diagnosis of asthma during the baby's first year. It often occurs without wheezing, and though skin tests are valuable for allergies under age one, they are difficult to interpret. However, recently Dr. Bernard A. Berman and his associate Dr. James Cavanaugh of St. Elizabeth Hospital of Boston have diagnosed asthma in an average of two infants every week. They found that skin tests used to diagnose asthma in infants often did not show a positive reaction until 24 to 48 hours after the skin test was given, so they had parents bring the babies back for reexamination at that time. They tell of one child who had been hospitalized four times with various kinds of pneumonia before he was even one year old. He had no wheezing, but skin tests showed that he was sensitive to dog and cat hairs and to dust. The house was made as allergy-proof as possible, the bedroom was humidified, and the family dog and cat were taken away. His condition cleared up quickly.

However, other conditions can sometimes masquerade as asthma. Both the parent and the physician may think the baby has asthma when he really has some other problem, such as an infection, an obstruction of the respiratory tract, or a congenital heart disease. Sometimes there is also a condition called congenital laryngeal stridor, in which babies have wheezing breathing because of an obstruction of the throat present from birth. Usually the first episode of allergic asthma in a baby lasts only a short time. If the baby has an attack of wheezing that persists for several days, it is probably a foreign body that he has choked on.

One little girl, fourteen months old, had had frequent colds. One day she was sitting on her potty chair. Her mother said she suddenly turned blue and started to choke and wheeze. The doctor was called. Both he and the mother thought the child was having a severe asthma attack. He gave the girl epinephrine, which resulted in some relief, but the cough and wheezing persisted. She was taken to the hospital where she was examined thoroughly. Finally, an x-ray of the chest revealed a screw sitting on a ridge of tissue at the top of the bronchial tubes. The screw was removed and returned to its proper place on the potty seat, and the child made an uneventful recovery.

■ ECZEMA AND OTHER RASHES

Skin rashes are one of the most common symptoms of allergy in infants. But not all skin rashes are caused by allergies.

SKIN RASHES THAT ARE NOT ALLERGIES

In the first few months, babies sometimes get tiny shiny white pimples on their cheeks. Sometimes they are raised and pearly, sometimes flat and red. They are not important and eventually go away.

Cradle cap often occurs on the scalp in the early months. More frequent washing helps get rid of the scaly crust, or sometimes cleaning the scalp with baby oil is better. There are also commercial preparations that will help clear it up.

Cold weather can sometimes cause rough skin. If so, find a more sheltered place for your baby to get his fresh air. Keep him inside when the weather is cold and windy.

Irritation can be caused by things rubbing on the skin. See if there is a wool sweater rubbing where he is getting the rash, or perhaps rubber pants are too tight or have rough edges.

Prickly heat appears during hot weather, especially around the shoulders and neck. It is made up of patches of tiny pinkish-tan pimples that have blisters on them. It does not bother the baby too much and you can treat it simply by patting a solution of bicarbonate of soda or cornstarch powder on the rash. When the weather is hot, take the baby's clothes off and keep him cooler. Do not use boric acid on prickly heat or on any other rash on a baby, since it can be absorbed into the skin and is very toxic. Large doses of vitamin C have been reported effective in treating difficult cases of prickly heat.

Diaper rash may appear in the areas that are wet with urine. The rash may be made up of pink or red pimples or patches of rough red skin or may be smooth and pink, almost like a burn. It is generally caused by irritation from ammonia formed in the urine. When the baby has a diaper rash, take off his waterproof pants so that the urine will not be held against his skin. Use an antiseptic when you wash the diapers or some preparation, such as Diaparene chloride, made to counteract the bacteria that act on the urine to produce the ammonia. If the rash is really bad—and it can become bad enough to cause large open raw sores—it is best to expose the whole diaper area to the air all day. If your infant is a boy, we suggest that you drape some sheets around the crib to protect the walls.

If your baby has an attack of diarrhea, he sometimes will get a very sore rash around his anus. Try Diaparene Peri-anal or a zinc ointment.

ALLERGIC RASHES

The important thing is to distinguish all these simple rashes from eczema—the rough, red scaly rash caused by allergy. It appears in patches and usually comes and goes. In a tiny baby it is apt to start on the cheeks or forehead as a bright red or tannish-pink patch. If it is not treated, it may spread from the cheeks and forehead to the ears and neck. As it gets more severe, it may change from light pink to deep red and become scaly and itchy. If the baby scratches or rubs it, it may begin to ooze, then become crusty.

Toward the end of the first year, the eczema is apt to appear on the trunk of the body instead of his cheeks. After the first year, it is more apt to appear behind the knees and in the folds of the elbows.

Eczemas can be caused by allergens that the baby breathes in from the air as well as by foods, so you and your doctor must check foods, pets, bedding, drapes, rugs, pollens and other things that we mentioned before as possible causes.

TREATMENT OF ECZEMA

What can you do to help the allergic eczema?

Don't use regular soaps on it, but use a soap with sulfur, or castor oil with sulfur, or warm olive oil or baby oil to clean the baby's skin. Wash his clothes and bed covers in a mild detergent and make sure they are rinsed thoroughly.

There are several lotions and ointments on the market to try. If you use any, check the label to see if they contain coal tar or coal tar derivatives. These can cause sensitivity to the sun. If there is any form of coal tar, then do not expose your baby to direct sunlight.

Keep your baby from becoming too warm. Perspiration is irritating to a skin rash, so keep clothing and blankets lightweight.

Changing the baby's diet is sometimes of benefit. Fat babies tend to be bothered more by eczema than skinny babies, so check with your doctor about eliminating sugar from the milk formula so that your baby does not gain weight so rapidly.

One group of researchers reports that adding unsaturated fatty acids to the diet sometimes helps. Try giving your baby a teaspoon or two of lard or linseed oil each day.

In extremely severe cases of eczema, cortisone and its related compounds can give relief, but these hormones can have serious side effects and should be used only when nothing else will work.

To keep the infant from scratching so much, keep his fingernails cut short. Turn the cuff on his gown over his hands, or dress him in a gown that is too big and pin the cuffs shut over the hands. For an older baby, you may need to use elbow restraints which can be made from sturdy cotton cloth and tongue depressors and pinned to his sleeves. Or put a paper cup over the elbow so he cannot bend his arm to reach the rash. Restraints should be removed several times a day so that the child's arms will be properly exercised. You should also take them off when the child is being held because you can watch his hands then.

Cuddling is important, by the way, even more than usual for a child sick with an allergy. Sometimes a mother hesitates to cuddle a child if his skin is all broken out with a rash, especially if it's covered with a greasy medicine. But he needs closeness and love *now more than ever*. Allergy rashes are not contagious and medicine will wash off, so give him the extra cuddling he needs.

On the other hand, if your child is sick for a long time, make a point of getting away for at least part of the day each week. Get a baby-sitter and get out for a few hours to avoid the resentment that might otherwise build up. Then you can return relaxed, to continue your role as a loving mother.

Whether your baby has eczema or asthma or some other allergy, the important thing is to find out what is causing the symptoms and to remove the cause and treat the allergy. Allergies of all types tend to get worse and to become chronic, especially in infants and children. It is important for parents and physicians to recognize allergies as early as possible and to get medical attention started.

■ VACCINATIONS AND THE ALLERGIC CHILD

Allergic children should receive the same immunizations as non-allergic children against diphtheria, tetanus, smallpox, pertussis (whooping cough), measles and polio. The injections are usually well-tolerated. If a reaction is feared because of extreme sensitivity, a fraction of the dosage may be injected and the rest of the vaccine given in several small doses later.

SMALLPOX

If your baby has active eczema, he *must not* have a vaccination against smallpox. If you are taking your baby in for a regular check-up, be sure to tell your doctor about the eczema so he may postpone any vaccinations until the skin has completely cleared up. In fact if a child has eczema, no one in the household should receive a smallpox vaccination. He must not be exposed to other children who have recently been vaccinated, and he must not be exposed to people with fever blisters, chickenpox or shingles.

Smallpox vaccination should not be performed on a child taking cortisone or related drugs, nor should children exposed to or having chickenpox receive cortisone.

DIPHTHERIA AND TETANUS

Immunization against diphtheria and tetanus by means of toxoid is particularly important for allergic infants, so that the child will never have to be given antitoxins prepared from horse serum, to which sensitivity is very common. For this reason, too, boosters of tetanus toxoid should be kept up-to-date. Parents should keep a careful record of tetanus immunization and volunteer this information to any new doctor called on to treat an injury. If the immunization has been kept up-to-date, then only a booster of tetanus toxoid need be given and the injection of horse serum avoided.

WHOOPING COUGH, POLIO, INFLUENZA AND MEASLES

Protection against whooping cough is especially important because of the tendency of this disease to aggravate bronchial asthma.

Oral polio vaccine is safer for allergic children than injected polio vaccine.

Polyvalent influenza vaccine may prevent viral infections of the respiratory tract and may therefore be an aid in the control of asthma. However, since this vaccine contains egg protein, caution is required in cases of sensitivity to egg.

The measles vaccine also contains egg protein and precautions should therefore be taken. It should not be administered to persons highly sensitive to egg or chicken. It should not be given to patients who are taking cortisone or related drugs.

Parents of allergic children should keep especially accurate records of immunization procedures.

Chapter **4**

ALLERGIES OF CHILDHOOD

Allergy in children is an unbelievably widespread and significant problem. More than three fourths of all allergy appears first in childhood.

The most recent and extensive surveys of children in the United States and Canada show that the incidence of allergy in children is much higher than was previously suspected. The studies show that anywhere from *one fifth to one third of all children have a major allergy*. And only *one fourth to one third* of these had received treatment for their illness. If minor allergies were included, the number of known allergic children would be even higher.

The medical profession and the public must come to grips with the problem.

Allergy is *the* major chronic illness of childhood. In fact, the Department of Health, Education, and Welfare reports that allergic illness accounts for one third of *all* chronic conditions in children under seventeen. Asthma alone is responsible for nearly one fourth of all days reported lost from school because of chronic disease. In the words of the report: ". . . the prevalence of chronic conditions among children represents a public health problem of staggering proportions."

There are probably twelve million children in this country with allergic problems requiring medical supervision, and the problem is compounded by the fact that there are only a few hundred certified pediatric allergists to take care of them.

These are underprivileged children—the big losers. Many miss a good part of their education either through absenteeism, poor physical condition, or because of hearing loss and associated learning difficulties. Many are unable to participate in group activities or sports, or else they learn to fear any endeavor that involves physical effort. They become afraid to venture into any new situation where the risk of discovering new trauma awaits them. Their schooling suffers, their physical development and mental health suffer, and their families suffer. Their life is sometimes a constant struggle, emotional as well as financial, against chronic illness. Millions of these children are handicapped by poor appetite, poor sleep, inability to compete with other children in play and at school, often with resulting frustration and personality changes. Their allergic conditions may produce malnutrition and mental and physical retardation. They can become disabled with permanent lung changes that handicap their entire life.

Allergies cause immeasurable and irreplaceable loss of school time, play time and growth time. Asthma alone accounted for more than seven and a half million days lost from school last year, and hayfever and other allergies cost another one and a half million. Allergy-caused sinus trouble, bronchitis and hearing impairments lost additional days. Besides the days lost from school, activity was restricted on many days for many children. Asthma accounted for twenty-four million restricted activity days, hayfever caused more than four million restricted days, and other allergies seven million days.

Often the true nature of their disorder is never learned. Their parents never realize their children's problems are due to hidden allergy.

Allergies not only cripple this way—they also kill. Few people know that allergic illness kills more children each year than poliomyelitis, rheumatic fever or pneumonia. In fact, asthma alone kills more children under the age of fifteen than any other disease except tuberculosis. And the problems of allergic disease in childhood, the crippling and the death rates, unfortunately are increasing each year.

The information about personal attitudes of parents shown by surveys is astounding. There often is a negative or fatalistic attitude toward allergy. Time and time again we hear comments: "You can't do anything about allergy," or "You're born with it, you die with it."

Some people feel allergy is a visitation from on high, something that must be endured without much hope of relief.

This is not true. Children are simply not being adequately diagnosed and treated.

The fact that what is known about allergy is not being utilized is true with all age groups, but is especially true with children. Few physicians start practice today with any actual experience in practical day-to-day diagnosis and treatment of allergy. They often do not recognize or consider significant the individual signs and symptoms of allergic illness and the part they play in health and disease. They treat the allergy symptoms, but not the cause. The parents are reassured that these are the so-called normal troubles of childhood, that the child will outgrow them and that nothing further need be done. The physician is all too apt to treat and forget these "minor illnesses," and the allergy goes on untreated, causing more severe problems with added years. As a former pediatrician before I became an allergist, I can recall many children whom I treated symptomatically for colic, or eczema, or winter-long colds without any realization that these illnesses were probably part of a more significant problem of allergy. The baby who has colic, then eczema, grows up to be the child who has frequent colds or chronically stuffed nose, or asthma.

Pills have been dispensed by the millions: antihistamines, aspirins, antibiotics, corticosteroids, sprays, chest rubs, cough medicines, inhalations, nose drops, sedatives and tranquilizers. *Temporary relief is not enough. The basic allergy must be recognized, studied and attacked.*

■ CHILDHOOD ALLERGY PATTERNS

In many ways the allergies of infants, the allergies of children, and the allergies of adults are the same. But in many other ways they are different.

CHILDREN VS. ADULTS

Allergies have different patterns in children, and they pose different problems in management. Children are not simply little adults; they differ from adults in anatomy, in physiology and in their body responses.

Symptoms can be different. Children often have fever and vomiting with asthma, and often have warnings—"prodromal symptoms"—that come before an attack. All of these occur rarely in adults.

In hayfever the symptoms for most children are like those for adults: sneezing, coughing, dripping nose, itching of the palate and ear passages, and red, itchy and weeping eyes. However, in infants and very young children the symptoms of hayfever are usually atypical and sometimes masked. Children may simply have ear stuffiness and hearing impairment with none of the other adult symptoms, or they may have only prolonged nasal stuffiness or mild "pinkeye," only later developing adult-type symptoms.

Diagnosis can be different. Skin tests supply more information in children than in adults, but respiratory allergies can be harder to pin down because of a child's frequent colds.

Causes are usually the same, but can be different. An acute infection, for example, can precipitate an allergy attack in children.

And most important—the outcome in children is different. Allergies of all kinds, if they are adequately treated, have a much better prognosis in childhood than they do in adulthood. In most people allergic symptoms first appear before age five and, if left untreated, will continue to cause progressively more severe, and harder to treat, illness throughout life. The sooner allergic sensitivity is diagnosed and treated, the greater are the chances of a successful result. So early treatment is essential.

CHANGES FROM INFANCY

The pattern of allergies changes as your youngster grows from infancy to childhood. In infancy the two most common forms of allergy are disorders of the skin and disorders of the respiratory tract, and the two most common causes are foods and animals. Now as your child grows older, skin disorders and foods become less of a problem. Now allergies to things in the air become more and more important. In fact about 90 percent of allergic manifestations in children result from inhalation of pollen, dust, animal dander, molds and other substances. Pollen sensitivities, especially, start appearing around the age of five, and hayfever and asthma become more prevalent.

As the child grows into puberty, the change in hormones often has an effect. One recent survey showed that 40 percent of girls who had asthma lost it when they became old enough to have menstrual periods. Boys also showed an inexplicably high rate of recovery during adolescence.

PRESENT PATTERNS

Several studies have shown that as age increases, the number of children developing allergies increases tremendously.

One study done by Dr. Herbert Arbeiter on schoolchildren in Munster, Indiana, showed that hayfever—including both the seasonal and year-round kind—was by far the most common allergy in children aged 5 to 15, and the incidence of hayfever increased with age, with 12 percent of children aged 5 to 8 having hayfever and 17 percent of children 9 to 15 having it. More boys were bothered than girls. (In most studies twice as many boys as girls have allergies.)

Asthma occurred most often in the fall. Hayfever occurred most in the fall and summer, least in the winter.

As to the cause of the allergies in these children, one third were allergic to pollen and house dust and one fifth were allergic to feathers, animal hair, food, and molds. More than 2 percent of all children in the school were sensitive to penicillin.

■ ASSESSING YOUR CHILD'S ALLERGY

Allergy in children can take the form of eczema, hives, asthma, hayfever and perennial rhinitis, and can be involved in such common problems as colic, sinus trouble, bronchitis, nosebleed, recurrent ear infections, or hearing impairments. Allergies have also been suspected in the causation of less familiar problems such as enlarged thymus gland, celiac disease, ulcerative colitis, various eye disorders and connective tissue diseases, headache, convulsions and neuritis. Many physicians strongly urge that allergy be considered in the differential diagnosis of *any* child with generalized body symptoms of undetermined cause. These allergies develop in a variety of ways, often insidiously. You must maintain an attitude of suspicion, particularly when symptoms of the respiratory tract or skin predominate.

A child who has many colds during the year—a child who used to be labeled "susceptible" to colds—is more than likely a child with respiratory allergy. Allergy may be easier to treat in childhood, but it is also more difficult to detect and diagnose because of the confusion with normal childhood illnesses. Croup, colic, head colds, hives, coughing bouts, sneezing, bronchitis, stomachache—both parents and physicians come in contact with these complaints frequently. They *may* stem from simple infections. But also any one of these common childhood complaints can be the first clinical manifestation of what could become a chronic lifelong problem of allergy.

Think back over your child's history. Think of it in the new light of the possibilities of allergy. How many of his "colds" and other seemingly unconnected illness were really allergies?

Does he have a hereditary background with parents or grandparents having allergies? Did he have colic? Does he have stomachaches now? Headaches? Canker sores? Hives? Rashes? Eye irritations?

THE ALLERGIC LOOK

Many times a doctor knows the minute a child walks into his office that he is allergic. There is often—not always—but often an "allergic look" that is unmistakable.

"Facies" is the medical term indicating a particular appearance of the face. An allergic child may be pale and sallow and have dark circles under the eyes and puffiness around them. The shadows and the swelling, especially of the lower eyelid, produce what allergists call "the allergic shiner." Frequently his face is elongated. The cheekbones may be high and flattened out with depressions below each eye, and the tip of the nose is elevated and often has a crease across it from the constant pushing against it. His mouth sometimes hangs open, persistently agape from habitual mouth breathing. Because of the constant mouth breathing the teeth may be deformed. In fact, deformities of the teeth and jaw occur in 60 to 75 percent of all allergic children. There is often crowding of the front teeth of both upper and lower jaws, enlargement of the lower lip, and shortening of the upper lip with marked overbite.

How much change occurs in facial structure depends on the severity of the respiratory allergies and on the age at which they begin. If year-round hayfever begins in early infancy, the face may be retarded in all three dimensions. If it begins in the second year, less pronounced deformities occur. When symptoms begin at five or six years, only a slight decrease in forward or downward growth occurs.

The allergy can affect the rest of the body too. Many children with chronic respiratory allergy have a pigeon breast and slumped shoulders and humped-over back. They often have long silky eyelashes that

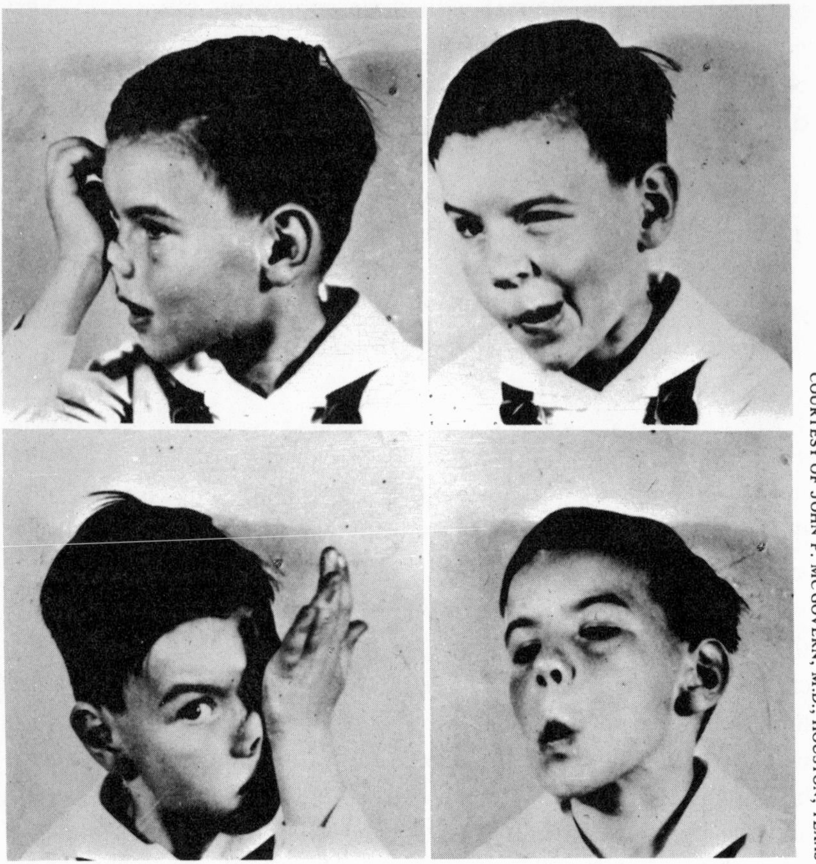

COURTESY OF JOHN P. MC GOVERN, M.D., HOUSTON, TEXAS

The "allergic salute" and other characteristic grimaces of a child with nasal allergy as he tries to open nasal passages and get more air.

are an indication that mucous membranes have thickened. Sometimes the white parts of the eyes have a muddy appearance, or sometimes inflammation makes the eyelids resemble cobblestones.

Dr. Meyer B. Marks, a pediatric allergist of Miami Beach, Florida, says that with early treatment many of these facial deformities can be made to disappear. He recommends elevation of the foot of the bed on blocks, beginning with a height of six inches and increasing by three inches every three months until a height of eighteen inches, which is then maintained. This will aid considerably in improving venous drainage of the congested eye areas during sleeping hours. Remarkable improvement was also found in allergic shiners when children attended yoga classes or performed headstands once or twice daily for several minutes. Use of an oral nasal decongestant often helps these signs also.

Dr. Marks has issued a plea for parents and physicians to be alert for mouth breathing and other deformities caused by chronic nasal allergy, so that modern allergic treatment can be instituted early to stop further development of the deformities.

■ TAKING YOUR CHILD TO THE DOCTOR

There are several questions you can think through before taking your child to a physician. Knowing these answers ahead of time will save you time in the doctor's office and will help him do a more effective job of finding the particular cause of your child's problem.

Ask yourself these questions to help pinpoint the source of trouble. Has there been any seasonal pattern in the appearance of symptoms —can they be related to a pollen season or to spring housecleaning? Is there a geographic pattern—do the symptoms appear only when the child is at summer camp, or when he is at home but not away at the seashore? Does he have any strong food dislikes? Can specific foods be associated with diarrhea, heartburn or gastrointestinal distress, or with rash or edema? Is there anything unusual in the child's sleeping habits—does he need to be propped up with pillows to avoid coughing, sneezing, wheezing or heavy chest? Does he get shortwinded? Does he have a rash? Does he scratch? Does he breathe through his mouth? Does he constantly clear his throat, have dry lips, or red eyes? Do these symptoms persist for long periods or do they occur over and over?

For example, wheezing should always be investigated fully for allergy even if it's associated with a cold. Today most allergists believe that wheezing, no matter what its cause, is a manifestation of allergy. Also if any symptoms persist for long periods or if they occur over and over despite attempts at treatment, they usually are caused by an allergy.

We have prepared a questionnaire for you to help you think in helpful areas. Fill it in before you go to your doctor and give it to him at the beginning of the examination.

ALLERGY SURVEY QUESTIONNAIRE

Indicate "Yes" answers with a "√" on line.

1. Are there any allergic illnesses (asthma, hayfever, food allergies) in family? . . . .

		Age at First Allergic Symptom	*Age at First Diagnosis*
2. How many people in family?			
Mother		. . . .	. . . .
Father		. . . .	. . . .
Children	1. sex	. . . .	. . . .
	2. sex	. . . .	. . . .
	3. sex	. . . .	. . . .

3. Did allergic patient have difficulty with infant feeding? . . . .
   Milk used: breast . . . . evaporated . . . . homogenized . . . .
   milk substitute . . . .
4. Did allergic patient have colic . . . . rash . . . . vomiting . . . .?
   Age of onset . . . .?
5. Did allergic patient have croup . . . . croupy cough . . . .
   frequent colds . . . . with fever . . . . without fever . . . .?
   Age of onset . . . . which months . . . .
   all year . . . .?
6. Attacks of sinusitis? . . . . frequency . . . .
7. Were tonsils and adenoids removed? . . . . age . . . .
   month . . . . year . . . .
8. Did allergic patient have prolonged nasal stuffiness . . . . . wheezing . . . . .
   eye tearing . . . . sneezing . . . . skin rashes . . . .?
   Age of onset . . . . which months . . . . all year . . . .?
   Was the diagnosis made by a doctor? . . . . Yes . . . . .No.
9. Was a diagnosis of asthmatic bronchitis made? . . . . . . Age of onset . . . . . .
   which months . . . . all year . . . .?
   Was the diagnosis made by a doctor? . . . . Yes . . . . .No.
10. Was a diagnosis of asthma ever made? . . . . Age of onset . . . .
    which months . . . . all year . . . .?
    Was the diagnosis made by a doctor? . . . . Yes . . . . .No.
11. Was a diagnosis of hayfever made? . . . . Age of onset . . . .
    which months . . . . all year . . . .?
    Was the diagnosis made by a doctor? . . . . Yes . . . . .No.
12. Are symptoms associated with dust . . . . foods . . . .
    animal pets . . . . plants . . . . furs . . . .
    cosmetics . . . . nervousness . . . . dampness . . . .
    medicines . . . .?
13. Treatment: Medicine by mouth? . . . . Injections? . . . .
    Treatment series? . . . . How long? . . . . Result? . . . .

Let your child help play detective, too. Explain to him that you are trying to find out what is bothering him and causing his itching or sneezing. Ask him if *he* has any ideas when it is worst or what might cause it. He may astonish you with some very observant remarks and good clues.

THE FIRST VISIT

No matter how young your child is, explain to him in simple terms why you are taking him to the doctor. Tell him what is going to happen. Tell him that the doctor is going to try to find out what's causing all the itching or sneezing and that you and he are going to have to work hard, too, to help the doctor. When he is going to have skin tests, explain to him how they will be given and what the reasons for them are.

A competent physician will know how to build rapport with your child and how to explain scratch tests to him so he will not be afraid. As I make a scratch in the skin and mix the drop of solution into the scratch, I tell my young patients that I am making mud pies on their skin. They are delighted with the concept of a grown man in a white coat playing with mud pies.

Include your child in the situation. If the doctor suggests eliminating certain foods or keeping track of foods that are eaten, stress to your child how important it is for him to stick to the rules and not to sneak any of the food without telling you.

If he is to get injections, explain to him why they are necessary. For the preschool child this may mean saying, "They will help you feel better." Give the child a chance to express his feelings about the injections. If he is afraid, let him handle the injection equipment and see how it works. Include him in any conversations with the doctor or nurse and let him ask any questions he wishes. Don't tell the child that the shot won't hurt. Let him know that it probably will hurt a little bit, but that it will hurt only a short time and that it will make him feel better. Never threaten the child with "shots" as a punishment.

After an injection a child should stay in the doctor's office for ten to twenty minutes to make sure no untoward reactions occur.

Because treatment of an allergy is a long-term affair and because your child has so many insecurities intertwined with his illness, it is important to choose a doctor whom your child likes and who is willing to spend enough time to establish a warm personal rapport. If you do not feel there is the proper rapport between your physician and your child, feel free to discuss it with the doctor or to change to another physician.

And please, despite the discouraging long time necessary to treat allergy problems, you should continue to bring your child in for periodic follow-up review with your physician. How often you take him to see your physician will depend on what progress he makes, but close follow-up is necessary, if for no other reason than the fact that periodic careful observation permits the physician to modify the treatment program as necessary as the years go by.

The important thing to remember in treating any allergy of childhood is that the treatment must begin early. And treatment should not be just management of the symptoms, but should also be aimed at the cause of allergy. Treating only the symptoms leaves unresolved, deeper, more important problems of chronic illness—which in most cases sooner or later will have to be faced.

■ PERENNIAL ALLERGIC RHINITIS

Doctors call the condition perennial allergic rhinitis—and parents call it one of the most bothersome, worrisome, debilitating energy-sapping, confusing conditions they must cope with. It is the persistent all-year-round kind of nasal allergy, probably the most common allergy of children. The nose is sometimes normal, sometimes runny and dripping and sometimes stuffy. The condition comes and it goes, and because children have so many colds, parents often figure the child is just having another cold when it is really an allergy.

Typical signs are that your child sniffs and snorts and hawks and coughs off and on. He doesn't usually blow his nose; he rubs it until it's red and raw. He breathes through his mouth.

He typically shows what is called an allergic salute. He pushes his hand or his sleeve upward against his nose, moving the tip of the nose in an attempt to get more air. This repeated upward rubbing can actually cause permanent changes, with a definite crease developing across the bridge of the nose. Allergists look for the crease whenever a patient comes into their office.

There are several ways to tell whether your child has a cold or year-round nasal allergy. Colds usually only last a few days. If the sniffing and stuffiness linger for a longer time, or if your child seems overly subject to colds, getting them more than six times a year, then you probably are dealing with an allergy, and you should take your child to an allergist for a complete evaluation.

Sometimes parents see thick mucus and so believe there is an infection. Sometimes there *is* an infection, but sometimes it is an allergy complicated by an infection. Children with allergies do seem to get more respiratory infections. The allergy provides the soil that permits infections to flourish again and again, so that many times the problem is a joint one. Only a physician can tell whether it is an allergy, an infection, or both.

THE CAUSES OF YEAR-ROUND ALLERGY

Perennial nasal allergy is caused mostly by substances breathed in from the air: house dust, animal dander, mold spores and pollens from trees, grasses and weeds. Recently it has been discovered that dust from insect wings and tiny microscopic algae floating in the air can also cause trouble. Food can be a cause, but not as frequently.

The snorting and rubbing occur because of the persistent irritation, itching and blockage of the nose. Mucus accumulates, but blowing usually doesn't help much. The major difficulty in breathing is due to swelling of the membranes inside the nasal air passages. They become swollen and pale, sometimes even bluish or violet from the allergic changes.

Swollen membranes also extend like a blanket into the upper back part of the throat, into the openings of the sinuses, and into the openings of the eustachian tubes that lead to the middle ears. This is why complications can occur. Because of the obstruction from the swelling, for example, the protection the membranes ordinarily afford is diminished and infection can more easily get in. This is why allergy and infections often occur together.

EFFECT ON THE HEARING

Because of the swelling and because the persistent nasal allergy can cause inflammation of the ear, hearing can be affected, especially in babies and small children. There may be repetitive severe earache or intermittent or long-term hearing impairment or even rupture of the eardrum. There is a real possibility of prolonged or permanent hearing loss.

One allergist tells of an unfortunate patient of his, a sweet five-year-old who had his eardrum pierced ninety-seven times in only four years before he was finally brought to an allergist for treatment to cure the problem and relieve the bouts of inflammation of the ear. The amount of physical and psychological distress for this child and his parents was enormous.

Ear problems, like those of the nose, are often mistakenly attributed to colds in the head. You should be suspicious of ear complications if your child persists in using a louder voice than usual, indicating he may have a partial hearing loss. Or a child will sometimes say his head feels heavy, blocked or full. Or he may feel or hear fluid in his ear when he turns his head.

Sometimes neither parent nor child realizes there is a hearing loss, so that the child may be thought inattentive or slow in understanding or even disobedient. If you notice any of these signs in your child, take him to a physician for a thorough examination and discuss the problems and your theories with the doctor.

MOUTH BREATHING

Because of the obstructed airways, the child with year-round nasal allergy becomes accustomed to breathing through his mouth. In some children the habit becomes so firmly established that even after the allergy has been "cured," mouth breathing persists. They forget how to breathe through the nose. For most children, retraining is possible once the allergic condition has been brought under control.

Mouth breathing can also cause the teeth to protrude. An orthodontist can frequently do much to correct the "buck" teeth. However, if the mouth breathing continues into adulthood, it is much harder to retrain to nose breathing and much more difficult to correct the alignment of the teeth.

OTHER COMPLICATIONS

There are five other major complications that can be caused by perennial allergic rhinitis: sinus trouble, asthma, chronic cough, loss of the sense of smell, and an outgrowing of little protuberances from the lining of the nose called nasal polyps.

Sinus trouble is one of the most common problems that bring the patient to the allergist. The sinuses are actually cavities, hollow areas, in the bones of the forehead and bones of the cheeks. Small openings join some of them together and also join them to the upper air passages of the nose. When the membranes are swollen, they obstruct these openings, closing them off so that mucus and infection are trapped within them. This can lead to acute or chronic sinusitis.

Polyps inside the nose are another complication, but usually only as a result of serious long-term nasal allergy. Grapelike clusters grow out of the nasal mucous membranes as small saclike protrusions that are clear and translucent. These block the airways still further. The polyps are usually removed by operation. Some investigators, however, have found success in shrinking them by giving steroid hormones by pill or injection or by applying steroid hormones directly to the polyps. If polyps occur in very young children they are sometimes a sign of cystic fibrosis. Eventually all polyps should be removed.

Loss of sense of smell is a common complication in children with allergic rhinitis if the allergy has been present for a long time. Sometimes the child completely loses the ability to smell. Sometimes he may still be able to recognize an odor, but loses some acuity. Sometimes not only the sense of smell but even the sense of taste can be modified. Usually the senses can be regained after proper treatment, but if the condition is allowed to persist, if the child should go untreated month after month with the airways partially blocked, smell and taste can sometimes be lost forever.

Nasal allergy is also often accompanied by the so-called allergic-cough syndrome—a persistent, repetitive and all-but-uncontrollable cough that is believed to be caused by irritation of the membranes that line the trachea or windpipe. Then it is made worse by post-nasal drip, that constant dripping of mucus down the back of the throat.

Perennial allergic rhinitis can also lead to asthma. Sometimes asthma will develop gradually, sometimes suddenly, and strangely enough it sometimes follows the removal of tonsils and adenoids. Because of the serious long-term crippling effects that asthma can cause, it is especially important to treat an allergic child promptly. Only by correcting the primary allergy, the underlying basis for the disease, can complications be prevented.

In fact, to avoid all of these complications it is vital to have early, vigorous and correct treatment of the nasal allergies. Fortunately, the allergist can help if he is given a chance. He can be most helpful if the child is brought to him before the condition has been allowed to endure for years.

TREATING THE YEAR-ROUND ALLERGY

The treatment program for year-round nasal allergy is similar to that for most allergic conditions. The allergist will try to find the things to which the child is sensitive by asking questions or by doing skin tests. He will give medicines for relief. He will give injections to desensitize the child, to lower his sensitivity to the things to which he is allergic. He will have you try to eliminate as many allergens from the environment as possible by cutting down the dust in the house, using nonallergic bedding, etc.

A word about nose drops. They should be used with the greatest discretion, if at all, because following prolonged use they often have been noted to cause permanent damage to the already injured membranes. They also sometimes have a rebound effect, so that when the short-term helpful effect wears off, the nose tissue swells again all the more and stays that way. We frequently tell mothers, "Don't put anything into your child's nose or ear smaller than your elbow."

Watch paper facial tissues also. Some tissues contain formaldehyde that can occasionally increase irritation. Try using handkerchiefs to see if there is less reaction.

Should tonsils and adenoids be removed in these allergic children? Although the tonsils and adenoids are often enlarged in children with perennial allergic rhinitis, they are frequently only the innocent bystanders and may cause only a very small part of the blockage. Often when a physician hears that the child has frequent sore throats or colds he will recommend taking out the tonsils and adenoids, especially if he sees little cobblestonelike plaques at the back of the throat. But since the tonsils and adenoids are not usually the cause of the child's problem, their removal usually fails to bring about any improvement. It is the swelling of the lining membranes that is at fault, and those lining membranes cannot be cut away. Basically the indications for the removal of the tonsils and adenoids are the same for the child with allergy as for the child without. However, in any allergic child an attempt should be made to control the allergy for a minimum of one year of treatment; then if there is no improvement, removing the tonsils and adenoids may be suggested.

There will be other suggestions from the allergist as he learns more of your child's disease and of his environment. The important thing is that he have the opportunity to find out what's wrong, that you get your child to an allergist or pediatrician if you think he has allergic problems. What happens then may determine the course and consequence of his illness throughout the rest of his life.

■ THE ASTHMATIC CHILD

Asthma, with its frightening wheezing, coughing and air hunger, is the most dreaded of all the chronic allergic conditions. Alarmingly, about one out of every three of all allergic children do eventually develop asthma.

There are now approximately six million chronic asthmatics in this country. Some three million of them are children under age sixteen.

The attack itself is frightening. The child wheezes and gasps for breath, his face turns bluish. Sometimes in panic he cries out for help. Other times he slumps silently to the floor. The attack is panic-producing, frightening to himself, his family and indeed, at times, his physician. The attack can be severely serious—5,000 asthmatics died in the paroxysms of their attacks last year.

WHAT CAUSES ASTHMA

Asthma is caused by the same kind of things that other allergies are caused by: foods, feathers, furs, animal danders, pollens. And once the pattern of wheezing is established, the asthma may also be triggered by other things such as infection, psychological upset, barometric changes or weather changes.

One never knows when an asthmatic child is in danger, about to develop an attack of asthma. A few grains of pollen, a bite of chocolate, a peanut or two, a romp with the dog, running through the field—any of these may precipitate an attack.

Some asthma patients suffer acute attacks after exposure to excess air pollution, and doctors find that asthmatic patients who live in heavily air-polluted communities generally are in poorer health than those whose community air is cleaner.

A few doctors believe that almost all asthma, especially the kind that doesn't respond to treatment, is due to food allergy. Others are positive that asthma is *never* caused by food. Both of these convictions represent extreme viewpoints and give us constant conversational material at our annual meetings. It's the same with emotional factors. Some doctors feel that emotional tensions between parents and child are the primary cause of asthma. Others believe it is completely physical in cause, and emotional tensions arise simply because the disease causes so much worry.

Actually in different children there can be different causes, and in some children all of the factors are interrelated.

The symptoms themselves are caused, as are other allergy symptoms, by histamine and other H substances that induce muscle spasms, swelling of tissues or mucus. The small bronchial tubes in the lungs suddenly narrow and the asthmatic child cannot get enough air, wheezing or gasping as he develops varying degrees of air hunger.

DIAGNOSIS OF ALLERGY

If you think your child has symptoms of bronchial asthma, a complete allergy evaluation is necessary, because many other diseases mimic asthma, such as heart disease and cystic fibrosis, or simply some obstruction in the bronchial tubes.

For example, Dr. Roy F. Goddard, of Albuquerque, New Mexico, says, "In too many instances a child has been followed for many years as a severe asthmatic without having had a complete respiratory-allergy evaluation. When an examination is complete and includes sweat and other diagnostic tests for cystic fibrosis, we often find that the patient has cystic fibrosis rather than intractable asthma."

You need a doctor to determine whether your child has asthma or one of these other diseases.

TREATMENT OF THE ASTHMATIC CHILD

The treatment goal for the asthmatic child should be a well-planned combination including avoidance of the troublemaking allergens, hyposensitization injections when necessary, drug therapy, physiotherapy, psychotherapy and other supportive measures. The aim is to have the child engage in normal activities as much as possible and avoid the feeling of being different and feeling incapacitated because of his disease.

Many times a child or his parents can recognize impending attacks of asthma. The child's feelings are almost analogous to the aura of an impending epileptic seizure.

A parent can also learn to be on the lookout for certain specific factors that tend to precipitate asthma in the child, such as sudden changes in climate or temperature, marked overexertion, colds, emotional trauma. Then treatment can be started in the very early phase of an attack—in fact, almost before it begins. This early stage is when the attack is most easily and effectively blocked. So at the first sign or even premonition that an attack is on the way, give your child his prescribed medication, generally a mild dose of a bronchodilating medicine.

Cold or hot steam works very well to thin out mucus and affords general relief in opening airways. The child should also drink a great deal of warm fluid to keep the mucus loose and also to keep the child himself from becoming dried out. Any time a child is dehydrated, his symptoms are intensified; so always make sure he gets plenty to drink.

Mild sedation may be extremely helpful when given in the early phase of an attack of asthma before it builds up. When all other methods of control have failed, the use of cortisone substances called corticosteroids can be used by your physician. But injections of adrenaline and the use of corticosteroid hormones should be limited and, of course, should be supervised by a competent physician. Prolonged use of cortisone hormones, especially in large amounts for long periods, may retard a young child's growth, may produce a disease called Cushing's syndrome, may cause physical or psychological addiction and may cause sleep disturbances, depression or euphoria. Infections may be reactivated and other hormones of the body may be affected, such as those from the adrenal gland. If your child must have corticosteroids, the physician should control the dose to the lowest level. And when he decides to stop the medicine, which should be as soon as he has achieved the benefits of this medication for the patient, he should wean your child gradually from the medicine, not stop the drug suddenly.

For some unknown reason childhood deaths from asthma are increasing markedly. Paradoxically this is the period in which steroids and antibiotics became more widely used for asthmatic children. Some physicians believe that the steroids reduced resistance to infection and that the indiscriminate use of antibiotics permitted the emergence of resistant strains of germs, the two factors together possibly causing the increase in the deaths from asthma.

In addition to drugs and injections, there are other steps you can take to help your child.

Dr. Elliott Ellis, chief of pediatrics at National Jewish Hospital in Denver, recommends a strong exercise program for nearly all asthmatic children. The Denver hospital studied patients who had failed to respond to other forms of treatment for their severe asthma. They performed two hours of physical exercise a day—one hour of calisthenics and one hour of sports. After three months, he reported three out of four were able to breathe more efficiently as measured by lung function tests, and none showed any harmful effects from this exercise program.

What about emotional support?

Dr. Jerome Glaser, clinical professor of pediatrics at the Rochester School of Medicine, suggests this advice to parents on how to help manage the lives of their asthmatic children. Parents should strike a balance between sympathetic affection and discipline. Quarreling between husband and wife in the child's presence should be avoided, since it adds to his insecurity. The asthmatic child should not be made to feel inferior to his brothers and sisters or playmates because of his asthma, because it saps his self-confidence. Brothers and sisters should be taught to cooperate and not make the asthmatic child hated because, for example, the family cannot have a dog or a cat. Special effort should be made to determine his talents, his good features and strong points, and to help him develop them so that he may have some point of superiority to bolster his own ego structure. He must never be permitted to use his asthma as a device for getting his own way.

■ ALLERGY AND INFECTION

Allergies often follow infections.

Infections often follow allergies.

Infections can often trigger allergic reactions.

And some children are even allergic to certain bacteria or viruses themselves.

The interactions between infection and allergy can occur both in respiratory allergies and in skin allergies. The child who scratches and itches in allergic dermatitis, for example, is likely to develop a secondary infection from the scratching. In hayfever, excessive mucus may lead to blocking of the respiratory passages and cause impaired drainage so that the child readily develops a complicating secondary respiratory infection.

Many hayfever patients say that they generally get a respiratory infection at the end of the pollen season, after the hayfever symptoms have cleared. This could be due to the weakness of the respiratory system at this time as well as to the general weakness and susceptibility of the person himself.

When a child has a pattern of allergy and repeated infections that keep occurring for several years, many physicians prescribe daily antibiotics and chemotherapy just as they do with some other chronic diseases, such as rheumatic fever. They avoid giving penicillin, however, since it is a more sensitizing drug and more people are allergic to it.

Some physicians also use injectable bacterial and viral vaccines to try to break the pattern of allergy and infection, since they believe this may tend to build up the level of immunity to infection.

Usually total treatment of the child's allergy will also tend to lessen the number of infections and so tend to influence favorably the patient's overall condition.

One pattern of relationship between allergy and an infection occurs when a child gets a contagious disease such as whooping cough, measles, chickenpox, mumps or various viral diseases. In these diseases the symptoms of allergy are aggravated during the onset. The child with hayfever will have severe asthma; the eczematous child will have a worse rash. Then as the infectious disease nears its peak, the allergy symptoms become less severe, even less than he ordinarily experiences, and he may actually be entirely free of any allergic signs. With convalescence, the allergy signs again occur with great severity. After the infection the allergy may become so aggravated that the child may have his initial attack of asthma, or a previously mild eczema may become more pronounced and may spread.

A different pattern commonly occurs with bacterial infections involving the upper respiratory tract. In these infections there is no apparent change in the allergy during the start of the infection, but at the peak of the infection the allergy becomes worse, exactly opposite of the first type of pattern with the other childhood infections. Often the allergy that is associated with the second type of infection does not respond to the usual medical management for allergy.

One of the important things to realize about allergies, whether they involve coughing and sneezing or eczema of the skin or asthma, is that they are not in any way catching. The allergy is a chronic illness and a serious one which demands attention, but it is not infectious or contagious in any way. Many parents needlessly worry about this.

BACTERIAL ALLERGY

Among the many forms of allergy, one that is often not easily recognized is bacterial allergy; that is, just as a child can be sensitive to strawberries or ragweed, he can become allergic to bacteria, usually the ones that cause upper respiratory infections. There is an incubation period just like in infectious diseases. Generally seven to ten days after the child gets a "cold," the allergic reaction becomes evident. The next time he is exposed to the germ, he will have an allergic response with coughing or wheezing. Sometimes these episodes of allergy will be a year or more apart.

The typical history is that a young child has a cold and suddenly develops a choky spasmodic cough and may experience some difficulty in breathing, or may make strange noises. Prescription drugs, fluids and steam usually tend to relieve the symptoms and the episode runs its course within two tc five days. In a few instances one or two episodes of asthma are all that ever occur. However, in most instances the condition recurs anywhere from once or twice a winter to once every two or three weeks for several years. Unless allergy to bacteria is thought of, the child continues to be ill, and he usually goes on to develop bronchial asthma.

■ HEARING DISTURBANCES DUE TO ALLERGY

More and more in recent years physicians have been noting a new pattern of illness in children that they have termed "allergic paracusis." It is a hearing disturbance due to allergy. Dr. Victor Szanton, a pediatric allergist of Derby, Connecticut, studied the hearing acuity in a random number of allergic patients who came to his office. None of them had any complaints of hearing difficulties, but he found that of the first 120 patients studied 50 had some degree of hearing loss. Some of the hearing loss was persistent, some was intermittent.

The hearing losses were much more common in children than in adults. In fact, of the patients under age nine, he found that *56 percent* showed a hearing loss. Of those older than nine years, 22 percent had a hearing loss.

These findings, plus those of other doctors interested in this problem, indicate that most of these hearing disturbances disappear as children grow older. However, not always.

And while the child does have the hearing loss, it can take a heavy toll on his young life, especially when it is unsuspected. The behavioral disturbances that it causes are often falsely attributed to immaturity, inattentiveness, stupidity or emotional insecurity.

A young child learns through sight and hearing, and his behavior reflects the degree of accuracy with which his eyes and ears convey the outside world to him. If he does not hear well, his speech development may be slow or abnormal. A hearing loss will affect not only the quality of his speech, but also the amount of attention he will give and how much he can learn. In kindergarten or school he is often considered dull or stupid, or even retarded.

Tens of thousands of these children are going unrecognized.

Allergy can affect hearing in the following way: The eustachian tubes normally open periodically to maintain an equal pressure on each side of the eardrum. When the eustachian tube is obstructed because of the swollen tissue present in allergic illness, the equal pressure is not maintained and the eardrum is drawn inward. The result is a hearing loss, usually with no pain. Later, serum and mucus exude into the ear cavity, and the child may hear ringing or buzzing in his ear and have a still greater loss in hearing ability. Doctors call this everything from secretory otitis media, serous otitis media, otitis media ex vacuo, otitis media with effusion, nonsuppurative otitis media, indolent otitis media, hydrops of the middle ear to tubotympanic catarrh. No matter what it's called, it can be a major cause of learning difficulties in children.

■ CROUP

Sometimes doctors treat croup as an infection and sometimes as an allergy. Here is one simple treatment. Wrap the child in a blanket and place a towel over his shoulders. Soak a washcloth in ice cold water (with ice cubes in it) and apply the cloth to the child's neck. This will often clear croup in five to ten minutes even without steam.

■ GASTROINTESTINAL ALLERGIES IN CHILDREN

Allergic reactions may occur anywhere along the gastrointestinal tract, and the symptoms depend on the location and intensity of the reaction. The food allergy often causes pain and tenderness that may mimic the pain of inflammation of the gallbladder, peptic ulcer or appendicitis. The allergy can cause retention of food in the stomach, spasm or swelling of the stomach and the intestines, increased or decreased motility of the intestines that would in turn cause either diarrhea or constipation.

Attacks of abdominal pain, abdominal cramps sometimes lasting for one or two hours, are the most common complaint associated with food allergy in children. This may or may not be associated with vomiting or diarrhea. Canker sores which may have an allergic basis are frequently seen in the older child.

The same guides for testing for food allergies, both by skin test and by elimination of suspected foods from the diet, are used in the older child as were used in the infant.

■ ALLERGY AND BED-WETTING

Bladder tissue can be affected by allergy, too. A study of 100 children who were chronic bed-wetters and who had failed to respond to conventional treatment was made. None of the children had any anatomical deformities that might have caused the problem. Suspecting that an allergic reaction in the bladder might cause an irritation and a feeling of fullness that would lead to bed-wetting, some of the foods that commonly cause allergies were removed, and the children were started on antiallergy medication. Bed-wetting was eliminated in 87 of the 100 children within six days! When the offending foods were reintroduced to the diet, the bed-wetting started up again.

Similar results were found in a follow-up study in Canada. One fourth to one third of bed-wetters stayed dry through the night within two to four weeks after problem foods were identified and removed from their diets.

One twelve-year-old girl persisted in wetting her bed despite a variety of therapeutic approaches. When dairy products were removed from her diet, in two weeks her bed-wetting stopped completely. A month later she ate some ice cream, and again began to wet the bed. Put back on a diet that was free of dairy products, she once more became continent.

Some of the possible dietary causes to check for if your child is a bed-wetter are milk and dairy products, eggs, citrus fruits and juices, tomatoes, soft drinks with coloring agents, Kool-Aid and Coca-Cola.

When dietary restrictions do not produce improvement, there are drugs on the market that may be used, such as imipramine. Others are helped by programs to stretch the capacity of the bladder, with the child trying to hold his urine a bit longer each day.

■ ALLERGIC TENSION-FATIGUE IN CHILDREN

Physicians have long sought evidence that allergy directly affects the nervous system. Now they know of the syndrome called "allergic tension-fatigue." This is a very specific set of symptoms that often occur in children, but are easily and often overlooked. The symptoms: the child is restless, but languid, and has the appearance of being vaguely ill without any clear-cut evidence of real disease.

Such children are often subjected to long and costly diagnostic studies that reveal nothing. However, when a physician or parent is alerted for the condition, it is readily recognizable. There are five symptoms that are basic to the syndrome: (1) fatigue, (2) irritability and other emotional symptoms, (3) paleness even without any demonstrable evidence of anemia, (4) dark circles under the eyes, and (5) nasal congestion.

Two general patterns appear. In the first, the child suffers from lethargy and sluggishness. He often has difficulty waking up and sometimes after getting up reacts slowly and sluggishly. He often suffers from school problems because he is unable to keep up with other children. He is always tired, no matter how little or much he does; and the tiredness is not relieved by rest, but is often made worse. Sometimes his response may be so sluggish that he appears to be drugged.

In the second pattern, which can exist separately or appear concurrently, the child is excessively irritable and tense, with increased motor activity, restlessness and inability to relax. He is constantly on the move, opening and closing doors, going from one thing to another, interrupting conversations, creating commotions. There would appear to be an increased sensory activity also, with fretfulness and insomnia. The nervous, high-strung personality leads to tantrums and tyrannical behavior on the child's part. He is displeased often with trivial matters and persists in crying for long periods for the slightest reason. He may end up in the long run as a maladjusted, resentful, aggressive, badly "spoiled" child.

So the child is divided between the extremes of feeling irritable and tense and of feeling extreme fatigue and listlessness.

He may also complain of abdominal pain and headaches and vague muscle aches. Sometimes there is also bed-wetting and excessive sweating, particularly in infants and young children.

Sometimes the child shows more severe neurological and psychological signs such as tics; or he may have severe personality disturbances or may even show psychotic behavior.

In some cases, of course, there really may be a behavior problem, and many associated psychic factors must be considered. But allergic illness should always be considered in an overall evaluation of an ill child.

Dr. Frederic Speer, allergist at the University of Kansas Medical Center, has described a number of children with allergic tension-fatigue syndrome. He tells of one seven-year-old boy brought in by his grandmother because of nausea, pains about the heart, poor appetite, listlessness, difficulty getting his breath and general nervousness. At times he would complain of feeling "hot all over," and at other times he would feel "shaky inside." Both his mother and grandmother had migraine headaches due to food allergy. The boy was pale and listless and appeared petulant and unhappy, but nothing physical could be found wrong. Dr. Speer thought there might be some psychogenic factors operative in causing the symptoms in this patient, since the boy's mother had been away from home for six months. But because of the history of multiple food allergies in the family, he decided temporarily to eliminate some of the foods well known as sensitizers. He omitted milk first. Within forty-eight hours "there was a dramatic improvement," Dr. Speer said. "The boy became relaxed, alert and cheerful. He was well aware of his improvement himself, and spoke of how much more energy he had and stated that he was without headache and general achiness for the first time in his memory." At the end of a week, as a test, milk was returned to his diet, and the boy developed a migraine headache and for the following two days was again pale, restless and irritable.

Other studies were done by Dr. William G. Crook and his colleagues in Jackson, Tennessee. They found that in a group of fifty children with this syndrome, all but one showed the five basic symptoms of fatigue, irritability and other emotional symptoms, paleness, circles under the eyes, and nasal congestion. In several children the need for sleep was so great that they would be found sleeping on their desks in school despite a full night's rest. One child slept thirteen hours a night and still could not be easily awakened in the morning. The doctors said that irritability, unhappiness, unruliness, emotional instability, rebellious behavior and even more serious emotional symptoms were present in all but one of the children.

"The pallor and circles under the eyes in combination with the stuffy nose are so characteristic of this condition," said Dr. Crook, "that the diagnosis in many of these children was suspected at a glance, even before the history was taken and diagnostic studies were performed."

One of his patients was an eleven-year-old girl with a history of recurrent generalized muscle and joint soreness, especially in the neck and shoulders. She also had frequent episodes of spasmodic wry neck. She had been seen by many physicians who had diagnosed everything from arthritis and psychoneurosis to rheumatic fever. Her symptoms were relieved completely by eliminating corn from her diet.

Some of these children had had other allergic symptoms, but not all of them.

There was one child who, influenced by the ads for a chocolate syrup on her family's new television set, soon was drinking a quart of chocolate milk a day. She became inattentive in class, her schoolwork became poor, she began to show obsessive-compulsive behavior. Her mother said she sometimes would sit in her room, would pay no attention to anyone, then would count things until she became hysterical. Two days after chocolate was eliminated from her diet, she began to improve. Within seven days the mother said she was "perfectly normal" and showed a complete personality change.

Another child was found to be allergic to milk, eggs and chocolate. Seven days after the troublemakers were removed from her diet, her mother said she did not seem like the same child; a teacher suspected she had been given pep pills, and even a problem of stammering disappeared.

The foods that are the most common offenders in causing allergic tension-fatigue syndrome are milk, chocolate, eggs and corn, in approximately that order.

It is treated as other allergies are, by finding out what the child is allergic to, avoiding the substance or substances as much as possible and, when this is not possible, having "desensitization shots."

The same principles of eliminating suspected foods from the diet should be followed as will be outlined in Chapter 9 on food.

We wonder how many children in this country with behavior problems really are reacting to some food in their diet or other allergenic substance.

■ ALLERGY AND EMOTIONS

There is much controversy over the role of emotional factors in allergy. Some psychiatrists and psychologists and a very few allergists still maintain that allergy is primarily a psychosomatic illness, that it is caused by emotional problems. However, nearly all other physicians now believe that allergy is based on physical causes, even when skin tests are negative. However, they do believe that in some, certainly not all, but in some patients, emotional factors play a role secondarily to the basic physical cause.

Ever since the time of Hippocrates, some relationship has been noted between allergy and human emotions. In fact, Hippocrates was familiar with asthma and warned that "the asthmatic must guard against anger." This does not necessarily mean that emotions *cause* allergies, but they can have a great deal of influence.

In fact, just as emotions and personality can have an effect on allergies, allergies in turn can have an effect on emotions and personality. The amount of influence differs in different people. In some patients there is no emotional component at all; in others there is a great deal of emotional impact.

Despite the fact that emotions don't often cause the basic allergic disease, they can sometimes trigger a specific individual attack of allergy. As we discussed earlier, any number of stimuli can set the mechanism off—infection, overexertion, change of climate, etc. An emotional occurrence can also set it off.

Conditioning seems to have some effect. This can be shown in animal experiments when animals are put in a special aerosol chamber to produce an asthma attack. Their attack stops when they are taken out. But when they are returned to the same chamber without being exposed to any special substances, they still have further asthma attacks.

Psychological pathways can be readily conditioned in real life, too. There is a classic example of a patient in 1886 who developed allergy symptoms after being exposed to an artificial rose. Another patient had a violent attack when he came into a physician's office where some artificial goldenrod was displayed. This mechanism is really the Pavlovian conditioned reflex by which the allergic attack is brought on through the association of ideas established by earlier attacks.

A second theory of how emotions can trigger attacks is that the emotional influences so prepare the nervous system that allergens that initially could not provoke a reaction become able to do so because the threshold is lowered significantly.

Another possibility is that emotional impulses emanate from higher brain centers and act on the blood vessels. Anger, laughter or embarrassment lead to dilatation of the capillaries, increased blood flow and increased mucus secretion. Since these are associated with the basic mechanisms of the allergic reaction, it is logical that anything that induces them will aggravate or trigger an allergic episode.

Because of all these influences, the whole patient must be considered with all his physical surroundings and with all his psychological influences and problems. A person is a product of his total environment; and his total environment, all his physical and psychological aspects, must be considered to completely understand his allergy.

The allergic reactions set up by physical factors are important, the physiology of the body is important, and the environment a person lives in is important. The emotions, in turn, act upon all these and are in turn acted upon by them. There *is* a relationship between mind and body, but it can work in both directions. Let's look at both ways that allergy and emotions are intertwined in the allergic child.

HOW YOUR CHILD'S ALLERGY CAN AFFECT HIS EMOTIONS

Both temporary emotional changes and permanent emotional scarring can result from the recurring impact of chronic allergic disease. Many allergic attacks are frightening, especially to children.

Upsets of normal routine, the constant medications and precautions, the maternal overprotection, the disruption of normal play and school experiences may all affect the child's psychological attitudes. All too frequently a vicious circle is established in which the consequences or accompaniments of the disease create tensions and difficulties which in turn tend to provoke the disease process. Fortunately the cycle can be broken by relieving the attacks medically and by relieving the emotional tensions psychologically.

Depression is almost universal in asthma patients during attacks, and many hayfever patients become very depressed when their pollen season starts. And well they might be, realizing as they start off again that they have another six to eight weeks of misery ahead to rob them of their normal life.

Organic changes also occur from allergy that may affect the emotions. The stress from allergies causes changes in several organs and glands, including the pituitary gland, the adrenal glands and the hypothalamus, all of which influence hormone secretion, and thus the emotions. So these hormonal changes can cause further personality changes on top of those caused by pure emotional factors.

Some of the repeated observations that we have made in patients who have recurrent allergic diseases are these:

Many children live in constant fear and anxiety. They feel that something they may do may initiate an attack, particularly an attack of asthma, which is a frightening experience. Many fear the suffocation accompanying the attacks of asthma and also either consciously or unconsciously fear death.

They may look for secondary gain. Children with allergies soon find, whether consciously or subconsciously, that the attacks can elicit emotional responses from persons close to them. They subsequently find that problems can be solved or gains achieved because of their allergic illness.

Allergic children often develop attitudes of overdependence as a result of their allergies. But it is difficult to determine whether the allergy is causing the overdependence or whether the overdependence is causing the allergy. Overdependence can be on a member of the immediate family or some strong figure, such as a friend or a physician symbolizing a parent figure.

Some children with allergy relate their allergy to feelings of aggression. A child might use his allergy to punish his parents, usually the mother. This might also be for his secondary gain so as to focus attention on himself or to control the family. Many children display aggressive hostility, probably because of the constant overprotection and restrictions imposed by parental figures.

Feelings of invalidism and of being different understandably develop also from repeated attacks of asthma. If a child has nasal allergy, he is constantly rubbing his nose. He breathes through his mouth, he sneezes at inopportune times, and he may manifest some facial disfiguration. These are bound to have psychic consequences. It becomes progressively more difficult for the child to be one of the group and to identify with his peers. Young people of dating age are increasingly concerned about nasal blockage, skin rashes and the anticipatory fear of sneezing or wheezing in public places. Also many patients with nasal allergies have accompanying bad breath, which frequently causes embarrassment.

Some allergic children seem nervous to adults and other children, but often this is because of their constant scratching, breathing through the mouth, or gasping efforts to get air, which gives an effect of nervousness.

Food allergies become intertwined with eating problems and child-mother relationships. Even with healthy children, maternal anxiety about the welfare of the family frequently becomes related to the problem of feedings, as is well known. A child with chronic allergy often desires air much more than food or fluid. Such children often lose weight, become pale and listless and have no energy. Thus, obvious reasons exist for the parental insistence on proper diet.

EFFECT ON THE PARENT

The allergy can affect the parent's personality, too.

Some parents, especially mothers, develop guilt feelings because their fruit—their offspring—is not completely normal. There is no logical reason for them to feel guilty; there is no reason for them to feel it is their fault, but somehow in our society today these feelings do sometimes occur. Sometimes the husbands or the grandparents feel that it is the mother's fault. Sometimes the woman simply imagines that they feel this way and develops the false guilt feelings.

There is no valid reason whatsoever for any parents to feel a child's allergy is their fault. If you find these guilt feelings arising in you, identify them for what they are, recognize them as being false, and then take positive steps to ignore them and be the best parent to your child that you can. If you don't get rid of these guilt feelings, they may cause you to reject your child or to overprotect him.

A typical reaction is that having envisioned a lovely, warm, healthy, happy child, the mother begins to get hostile and resentful, and rejects the child because of his illness. Then she can't face these feelings after being conditioned to believe mothers are all-loving, and so she feels guilty and anxious.

The parent also becomes resentful of the burden of caring for a physically ill child. With such a child, the mother has to modify household routine and family life. With his illness the child may try to manipulate his mother's life and irritate his father. He may also exhaust and monopolize his mother so that she has little or no time or patience for her husband or other children. He may also prove to be a drain economically on the family income, using money from what could be family luxuries and pleasures.

In contrast, parents sometimes become very overprotective. The mother may even sleep with the child or watch over him hour after hour. The parents may become so overprotective they retard the child's natural emotional growth and development. The mother may keep a "sickly" child at an infant level for too long a time, continually babying him. A child's allergy may indicate to one kind of mother that she is indispensable to his life, and she sometimes welcomes the chance to retain and control the situation.

Sometimes parents will alternate between overprotection and rejection, and this, of course, upsets the child even more.

Try to realize that it is natural for a sensible, sensitive, intelligent man or woman to feel hostile in a situation with a chronically ill child, and try not to feel guilty about it.

If you realize that some rejection of a child and some hostility are natural, your child's inevitable inability to function well in some respect will become less frustrating and less productive of anger. On the other hand, you will be able to offer love and affection without overprotecting and smothering the child. Simply understanding the situation and having some insight into the problem is helpful.

HOW THE EMOTIONS CAN AFFECT THE ALLERGY

Now let's look at the other side: how your child's emotions can influence his symptoms.

In *any* person the emotions have an influence on the body in both health and illness. And sometimes in allergy there can be a purely psychosomatic cause, but not very often. In one such case where there was an unhealthy relationship between a father and son, the son's symptoms of allergy—both asthma and eczema—became worse as he became older and increasingly eager to be independent. Even when he was twenty-three years old, he was still afraid of punishment by his father. When he joined the Navy, his symptoms disappeared. On his return home he became ill again. A year of psychotherapy with a competent therapist enabled him to separate himself from his father. He married, moved, went to work and had only occasional mild recurrences of his asthma. He remained free of serious attacks until he returned home after four years; then they recurred.

But basically in the larger number of patients allergic illness is physical. It is caused physically by substances that the person is sensitive to. There are emotional overtones, too, and these must always be investigated thoroughly and taken into account in treatment. However, we do not agree with the physicians who claim that allergies are initially caused by psychological reasons.

Some investigators say a specific personality pattern with specific psychological mechanisms can be found in allergic patients. Other investigators say that a study among any large group of people who have no allergy is going to reveal many who have psychological variations similar to those noted in allergic individuals. Actually, we have found that personality patterns and emotional factors are largely as normal and predictable in allergic children as in other children. There is no typical personality pattern for allergic patients.

Numerous theories have been proposed for supposed psychogenic causes of allergy. Causes cited have ranged from fear of separation from the mother and maternal rejection to fear of strong odors. Some psychiatrists interpret the gasping of asthma as a suppressed cry for the mother; the redness of the eyes and dripping nose as symbolic of weeping. Some theorize that asthma is a response to an unconscious fear of attack upon the respiratory apparatus. Some say hayfever results from latent, inadequately expressed sexual impulses based on smell. Some say the allergic child is rejected by his mother, and because he is anxious about expressing his hostility toward her, he turns it inward upon himself. Some say that the swelling of the air passages as occurs in bronchial asthma is a means of shutting out the world, and that the dripping and the mucus are an attempt to wash the world away. Some say the child is trying to engulf his parents. We do not believe in these theories.

One example of what happens with emotional instability in the family is the phenomenon we call "scapegoating." Just as several thousand years ago the Jewish people during the Yom Kippur days of atonement would put their sins on a goat and whip it and send it into the wilderness, now in disturbed homes the parents often heap their problems onto their children and psychologically whip them little by little. If the parents frequently quarrel, if they fail to achieve satisfaction or cannot cope with situations caused by the other parent, they tend to make their offspring a "scapegoat" of abuse, whether it is verbal or physical trauma. They generally will take the abuse out mostly on the ill child. If there are brothers or sisters, they often follow the same pattern and tend to abuse the weaker sick child.

In a psychologically poisoned home like this, the boy or girl who is sickly can develop a marked increase in physical symptoms or have considerable psychological disturbance from the abuse he receives.

The second outside stress frequently incriminated in allergic illness is parental rejection. It may be caused by many factors. A mother who was herself an unwelcome, unloved or neglected child may well reject her own offspring, almost without realizing it. Or a mother may, in her relations with her own child, be living through attitudes that were similarly expressed by her own mother.

The rejection might take the form of overt hostility and neglect or of expecting perfectionism in the child. In the first instance the mother might say bluntly that she disliked the child. In perfectionism, the mother would say the child cannot be loved as he is, but if he improved the situation might be different.

Rejection can take the form of minor nagging or threats, or there may be severe neglect or cruelty in punishment. Mothers sometimes deprive their infants or young children of fondling and handling or may not feed them properly.

The third factor, overprotection, can develop because of two diametrically opposed reasons: either because the child is very important to the parent, or because he was actually unwanted. Pampering is sometimes done because the parent feels guilty for not loving the child. The parent, martyrlike, tries to prove love by denying all his or her own pleasures for the welfare of the child. But in another instance, a woman who has lost one or more children, or who cannot have more, or who has waited a long time for her child, may feel she must always be on guard to prevent disaster, thus not permitting the child to develop independently.

Symptoms of overprotection are excessive contact, treating the child like an infant and preventing social maturity. Lack of love or overdemonstration, either one, disturbs and warps a developing personality.

Parents' attitudes are important, and you should consider what effect your attitudes have on your child's personality and in turn on his allergy. But on the other hand, many parents become *too* concerned about the relationship between emotional factors and their child's allergy. In some instances the concern and feeling of guilt *about* emotional factors have actually *caused* emotional problems in the child or in the family.

■ HOMES AND HOSPITALS FOR ALLERGIC CHILDREN

Usually a child's allergic illness can be quite adequately controlled by your own allergist; or you may obtain special treatment for him in an allergy clinic at a nearby hospital. Nine out of ten children will do very well under these circumstances; however, there is a small percentage of children (approximately 10 percent) whose allergies are so severe and crippling that they cannot be controlled this way. These cases that do not respond to customary treatment are termed "intractable." In such children, your allergist may recommend that you consider sending your child to a special home or hospital.

Many asthma homes were founded because increasing evidence of the emotional factors in some of these persistent intractable cases became apparent. The theory was to treat the children who did not respond to medical therapy by separating them temporarily from their parents and substituting psychologically oriented men or women in their place.

About forty years ago a doctor named M. Murray Peshkin, aware of this number of children who would not respond to adequate treatment, tried to establish the reason. Some of these severe asthmatics who lived only a few blocks away were hospitalized at Mount Sinai Hospital in New York City. In many of them the asthma cleared up within twenty-four hours without medication. Initially Dr. Peshkin believed that the children got better because they were removed from some allergy-causing substance in their home. However, subsequently he realized that it might also be the fact that they were removed from a home setting that was psychologically upsetting, that there might be a poor relationship with parents or other family members in a disturbed, unhappy or tense home environment. He arranged with a home in Denver to accept some of these children. The long-term separation from their parents he called "parentectomy." The children were now away from the emotional stresses that might have been caused by their own environment and at the same time were provided a physical environment free of the physical allergens that might have initiated their problem. Many of the children, after spending 18 months to two years at the home, returned to their parents vastly improved.

Now this home has become the Children's Asthma Research Institute and Hospital (CARIH). Children live at CARIH year-round, attending public school in a nearby community during the school year. In the summer there are swimming, sports, hobbies, hikes and picnics.

At CARIH, the skinny kids who had never done much of anything have climbed to the top of a mountain, bowled, hiked, skied and played baseball. Last summer the "Asthmatic Nine" won the public school league baseball championship.

Another one of the first homes that was founded was the National Jewish Hospital, also established in Denver. This hospital treats not only patients with asthma but also those with tuberculosis, emphysema and other chest diseases. Its staff includes allergists, chemists, geneticists, social workers, counselors, immunologists and rehabilitation counselors. One present excellent service is a rehabilitation program for patients who have made significant physical progress and so are able to work once more. Through contracts with some of the local industries, the adult patients when improved in health can gain work experience and once more begin to live full lives.

In these and other asthmatic homes the child is under close clinical observation. The center is devoid of many of the common environmental allergens such as pets, rugs, feathers and overstuffed furniture. Dietary control is given careful attention.

With close supervision the lowest possible doses of medicines are given, and in a few instances the medication needed to control the severe asthma can even be eliminated.

The children attend regular school classes. Many asthmatic children are below grade level because they are poorly motivated or have felt too ill to keep up with their work. Often because of their illness, teachers and parents have not required them to make up material missed during absences or have not held them up to the same work demands as other children. In the homes, teachers attempt to instill an attitude of attainment despite illness.

There is physical reconditioning. Because of the usually impaired physical growth and lack of physical activity, the asthmatic children not only have less strength and stamina, but often are actually small in size. Muscular strength and coordination are poor, especially in the arms and legs. The homes introduce the child to physical reconditioning as well as to group sports.

One of the best things about the asthma homes is that attacks are treated in a matter-of-fact way. If a child has an attack in the middle of a baseball game, he simply runs to a hospital in the center of the grounds, is given some medication, rests a few minutes and then dashes back to the game. Or if he has an attack of asthma in the middle of the night, he calmly climbs out of bed, pushes a button which flashes a light to call a nurse, and together they walk the short distance to the hospital for treatment.

The results of residential treatment vary, but are mostly very good when you consider that prior to the separation of the child from his home *nothing* helped him.

The medical director at CARIH, says that 30 percent of the arriving children are rapid remitters—they begin to improve the moment they arrive and remain well with virtually no medication for their entire stay. It has been said that much of this may be due to the change in climate, although recently Denver has become smoggier.

About one third of the children have sporadic bouts of asthma, varying in intensity and controllable with drugs.

The remainder do not show much improvement, and they have to remain on doses of medication throughout their stay. Occasionally, but not often, a child gets worse than before admission.

Other homes reflect somewhat different statistics, but the same overall good results are noted.

The major problem with these homes is that there are only a dozen or so in the United States and Canada, and they can take care of only about 625 intractable asthmatic children a year. There are about

300,000 of these children who desperately need this special treatment, so that nearly every home has a long waiting list. More homes are seriously needed.

If you feel an asthmatic home is necessary for your child, consult your allergist. If he agrees, you can pick one together, making sure that it incorporates all of the phases of a rehabilitation program and a warm accepting atmosphere.

And we stress again that these residential treatment centers are indicated only when your child's asthma is extremely severe and disabling, and cannot readily be managed in your local community.

The following is a list of the homes and hospitals. Application to them must be made in writing, and a full medical report must be sent by your physician:

Asthmatic Children's Foundation Residential Treatment Center 1800 N.E. 168th St. North Miami Beach, Florida 33160	Children with severe asthma. Ages 6 to 13.
Caverly Child Health Center Pittsford, Vermont 05763	
Children's Asthma Research Institute & Hospital 3447 W. 19th Avenue Denver, Colorado 80204	Will accept only the *intractable* asthmatic child.
Children's Convalescent Hospital Asthma Unit 1731 Bunker Hill Road N.E. Washington, D.C. 20017	Birth to 9 years.
Children's Heart Hospital Asthma Unit Conshohocken Avenue Philadelphia, Pennsylvania 19131	4 months to 14 years.
Convalescent Hospital for Crippled Children of the Cincinnati Orphan Asylum Auburn Avenue & Wellington Place Cincinnati, Ohio 45219	2 to 16 years.
Health Hill Hospital for Convalescent Children 2801 E. Blvd. Cleveland, Ohio 44104	

The National Foundation for Asthmatic Children (which maintains the Sahuaro School) 6015 East Broadway P.O. Box 1551 Tucson, Arizona 85711	Takes asthmatic children ages 6 through 12. Scholarships available in cases with financial need.
National Jewish Hospital at Denver 3800–4100 East Colfax Ave. Denver, Colorado 80206 or 49 West 45th St. New York, New York 10036	No age limit. Provides elementary and advanced schooling. Provides complete free medical care, rehabilitation education. Admits adults and children for asthma, emphysema, tuberculosis and other respiratory diseases.
Sahuaro School P.O. Box 12096 Tucson, Arizona 85711	6 to 12 years.
Saint Mary's Hospital for Children 29–01 216th Street Bayside, New York 11360	Infancy to 12 years.
Queen Alexandra Solarium for Crippled Children 2400 Arbutus Road Victoria, British Columbia, Canada	Infancy to teen-age.
Sunair Home & Hospital for Asthmatic Children Tujunga, California 91042	6 to 12 years. Regarding admissions write to: 920 S. Robertson Blvd., Suite 6 Los Angeles, California 90035
Stanford Convalescent Home 520 Willow Road Palo Alto, California 94304	Infancy to 16 years.
Sunny Hill Hospital for Children 2755 East 21st Avenue Vancouver, 12, B.C., Canada	
Villa Santa Cruz Box 398 Toltec, Arizona 85231	A boarding school.

■ SPECIAL CLASSES FOR ASTHMATIC CHILDREN

In many cities there are also special classes for children with instruction given in breathing exercises and physical conditioning. For example, in Oak Park, a suburb of Chicago, boys and girls between the ages of six and fourteen can attend classes at the local YMCA on Saturdays throughout the school year. Asthmatic children are taught how to use their abdominal muscles to improve breathing. By learning to slow down their breathing rate, they get better air flow during expiration. They often are less apprehensive during an acute attack because of the control, and they can usually decrease the severity and length of the attack.

In a children's asthmatic rehabilitation program in Kansas City, sessions are held weekly with instruction in breathing exercises, games, general athletic activities and swimming. The program teaches proper breathing methods and exercises to improve body tone and coordination. It also encourages the child to partake in all activities of other children of his age and size and helps rid him of psychological inhibition about his asthma.

Dr. Stanley L. Goldman, director of the program, says a four-year study has shown in most instances "good to excellent" results.

If you believe your child would be helped with such sessions, check with your allergist if any facilities like this are available in your city.

■ CAMP AND THE ALLERGIC CHILD

To send a child to camp or not when he has an allergy is a question that bothers many parents. If you choose your camp carefully and take a few special precautions, we think it good to send your child to camp. It's important to treat your child's allergy, but it's also important that he gets to do the things that other children do, and does not develop a sense of being an invalid or cripple.

Dr. Harold Lecks, a Philadelphia allergist, studied a group of children who were sent to camp despite their severe stubborn asthma. They were permitted a program of unrestricted camp activity for one to two weeks in an area of the country where there is a moderately severe concentration of pollens and molds. Physical examinations and laboratory tests were done every day before, during and after camp for evaluation. The children had very few problems, and actually improved physically and needed less medicine.

"Early in the session the counselors were oversolicitous," according to Dr. Lecks. "But when they were persuaded to adopt a more casual attitude, the number of attacks and infirmary visits declined markedly. Constant reassurance by the nurses and counselors and avoidance of treating these children as handicapped patients was fundamental to their improvement."

Here are some guidelines to sending your allergic child to camp:

If he goes to a regular summer camp, select one where a full-time physician is available at the camp at all times, not merely a nurse plus a standby doctor in a nearby town. Then your child can get his injections or other medication and be under proper medical supervision if he has an allergy attack.

Have him take his hayfever pills or other customary medicines with him. These should be plainly labeled, and the directions for use should be written out, preferably by your physician, with instructions to the camp's physician.

If your child has hayfever, find a camp located in an area that is low in the pollen he is sensitive to. Check our list of cities in the appendix for areas of low pollen count.

Swimming in fresh or salt water is permissible, although your child should not dive or swim underwater if he has a nasal allergy, because water may be forced into the sinuses and eustachian tubes, where the hypersensitive membranes in allergic people are highly susceptible to irritation and infection. The only thing that could keep your child from regular swimming is if he has the very unusual condition of allergic reaction to cold water.

If your child is allergic to sunlight, also a rare condition, he should not be exposed to excessive sunlight. In fact, rapid suntanning is generally harmful to any child who tends to get eczema reactions, so exposure to sunlight should be gradual. The child with eczema should also try to avoid overheating and excessive sweating to avoid itching and unfavorable skin conditions.

If your child is sensitive to animal dander, he should avoid horseback riding and other contact with animals. He should not take hay rides nor take overnight hikes that might include sleeping in barns.

If your child is allergic to insect bites or stings, especially stinging insects such as bee, wasp, hornet or yellow jacket, send this information along to the camp physician and counselors in writing so that he may avoid hazardous situations. He should be receiving treatment for this sensitivity. Also be sure to send along medications for emergencies.

There is no reason why the allergic child should not get tetanus toxoid. There are different types of tetanus toxoid—one form gives fewer reactions to allergic children than the others. So check with your doctor to see that his tetanus immunization is up-to-date before he goes to camp.

Most important of all is not to burden him with nagging, unnecessary admonitions and overconcern. Give him the necessary instructions, then let him have fun.

SPECIAL CAMPS FOR ASTHMATIC CHILDREN

If your child has a really severe case of asthma, we suggest you consider sending him to one of the camps that are specially set up to care for asthmatic children.

A typical one is Broncho Junction, an eight-week summer camp for children age eight through fifteen. Under the direction of allergist Dr. Merle Scherr, the camp not only gives the boys typical camping experience, but actively strives to make the often very sick asthmatic child feel like a normal child and one of the group. The camp is situated on 176 acres of rolling meadows and woods near Charleston, West Virginia. Its motif is trains, with the lodge set up like an old-time train station and campers living in railroad cabooses donated by railroad companies from across the country. The pun and fun of Broncho Junction is carried even further with a narrow-gauge express train running throughout the camp grounds. Dr. Scherr says, "It enables any camper having trouble with his asthma to get to and from the infirmary at any time. All he need do is call the counselor-engineer by walkie-talkie, sit down and relax. In a few minutes, he will be on his way without having drawn undue attention to himself in the process. Nor will any camper feel apprehensive about being left out of the fun because of a temporary inability to walk to an activity area."

On a typical camp day, there is breakfast and cleanup, a medication program, then calisthenics or judo, followed by a choice of archery, riflery, nature or railroad lore, camp craft, horseback riding, work projects or swimming. After lunch and a rest hour, there is further instruction, arts and crafts, or photography or free time for reading, chess or whatever. Evening brings musical performances, stunts, singing, council fires.

Belonging is stressed. Counselors work to fill the needs of these kids to share in a joint adventure, to enjoy the approval of the group and to experience the satisfaction of serving others. Campers often come up with new ideas themselves or pitch in with painting rooms or building outpost shelters. No matter what the job, the counselors say, it can accomplish miracles for the child's sense of self-respect, which up to this time has been sadly neglected.

The eight-week fee is $1,000. This includes all medication and medical treatment. In case of financial difficulty, fee reductions can sometimes be made through application for scholarship.

The following summer camps have been established especially for asthmatic children.

BRONCHO JUNCTION	Merle S. Scherr, M.D. 803 Atlas Bldg. Charleston, West Virginia 25301
THE NATIONAL ASTHMA CAMP	A division of the Silver Camps Durango, Colorado 81301
THE NATIONAL HAYFEVER RELIEF CAMP	National Hayfever Relief Association 401 Broadway New York, New York 10013 (Maintains a resort for adults and a camp for children in the White Mountains)
REDWOOD GLEN CAMP	The Allergy Foundation of Northern California, Inc. c/o E. James Young, M.D. 100 S. Ellsworth Avenue San Mateo, California 94401

■ SURGERY AND THE ALLERGIC CHILD

What special problems are there when the allergic child requires surgery?

In comparison with the nonallergic patient, the allergic child does run an increased risk. So when the family doctor or the surgeon or the anesthesiologist asks you questions when he takes your child's history, be sure that you give them full information on any current or previous drug treatment and be sure to tell them specifically what drugs work best on your child's allergies so that they may be on hand. Also tell them what drugs have failed in treating your child. And, of course, be sure to tell them of any of the drugs your child has had a reaction to.

The child should be kept as calm as possible before surgery so that he does not cry or become upset enough to bring on an allergic attack.

A doctor will usually give your child sedative drugs before surgery and might also find some that have an antihistamine effect that may counteract spasms of the airways. Morphine should never be given to allergic children.

Some anesthetics are contraindicated for allergic children, such as cyclopropane, barbiturates, narcotics or other agents that would tend to depress the nervous or respiratory system.

Children who have hayfever should never have their tonsils or adenoids removed during the hayfever season.

The important thing to remember in all childhood allergies is that early vigorous and correct treatment is important, not only to relieve today's discomfort but also to prevent occurrence of complications and development of more serious disease in the future. Most allergic diseases begin in childhood. See that your child gets proper treatment *early*.

Chapter 5

HAYFEVER

Allergy is perhaps the most variable of all diseases. It can appear and disappear like a magician's silk. It can change form like a chameleon, appearing in any organ system in any number of ways. It can masquerade as a cold, as bronchitis, as a stomachache, as a headache, as a skin rash or a dozen other things. It may yield to one treatment and not to another. It may even disappear suddenly without treatment, only to reappear inexplicably months or years later under a different guise.

But the most common form of all in adults—the one that causes the most discomfort, the most miserable days in the most people—is hayfever. Physicians call it seasonal allergic rhinitis or pollinosis. Patients may call it hayfever, rose fever, sinus trouble, catarrh, or they may just call it "hell."

An estimated one out of ten Americans has it; some say one out of five. Hayfever can be seasonal (the kind usually caused by pollens) or it can be perennial (the year-around off-and-on kind that can be caused by many things in the environment).

Sometimes both seasonal hayfever and year-around hayfever can exist in the same person. They have symptoms throughout the year, but the symptoms get much worse during certain seasons.

There are about 9 million days spent at home from work each year because of hayfever. In addition, chronic sinus trouble—which is often allergic in origin—is responsible for another 7 million lost workdays, and chronic bronchitis accounts for 4 million more days lost. It is estimated that some 97 million other days a year people have to restrict their activities because of hayfever, and 87 million more restricted days are caused by sinus trouble or chronic bronchitis.

This means that on any one day—like today—some 5,500,000 people had to cut down on production because of hayfever, asthma, sinus trouble and bronchitis. At least another 82,000 had to stay home from work because of the disorders.

Actually it is impossible to determine just how much damage and suffering and work loss are caused by hayfever because one cannot measure the loss of efficiency by people who are miserable and under par, who show up for work but are inefficient because of their symptoms. Nor can one really determine the cost of medicine or doctors' bills due to hayfever. Many hayfever victims do not even know they have it, merely complain of suffering from repeated or persistent colds, and their work records are spotted with days or weeks of absence year after year.

■ SYMPTOMS OF HAYFEVER

Sydney Smith, the English clergyman and writer, once wrote to his physician son-in-law in 1835:

"I am suffering from my old complaint, the hayfever (as it is called). My fear is of perishing by deliquescence—I melt away in nasal and lachrymal profluvia. . . . The membrane is so irritable, that light, dust, contradiction, an absurd remark, the sight of a dissenter—anything, sets me sneezing, and if I begin sneezing at twelve,

I don't leave off till two o'clock—and am heard distinctly in Taunton when the wind sets that way, at a distance of six miles. Turn your mind to this little curse. If consumption is too powerful for physicians, at least they should not suffer themselves to be outwitted by such a little upstart as the hayfever. . . ."

The symptoms are still about the same.

You may think you have a cold. Your eyes get red and itchy, swollen and puffy. Sometimes your eyes swell so much and the secretions are so bad that your eyelids are stuck together when you wake up in the morning.

You itch inside your ears, throat and mouth. Your ears feel full and there is often loss of hearing. You may cough or wheeze. You have the same general worn-out, tired feeling that you have with a cold. Breathing becomes difficult; and the trouble may extend into the bronchial tubes, causing suffocating attacks of asthma. The loss of sleep and the continual irritation and struggle for air wear the victim down so that it is not uncommon to have a significant loss of weight before the hayfever season ends.

The major symptoms of hayfever are in the nose. You sneeze, and sneeze. Your nose is stuffy or runny, or sometimes both.

Sensitivity to pollen usually begins in childhood, but sometimes people will suddenly develop hayfever in middle age. They breathe pollen for years before harmful side effects appear, and then suddenly it explodes into chainlike sneezing, coughing and weeping eyes. No one really knows the reason.

The noses of all of us are susceptible to infection, but the nose of a hayfever victim displays an extreme hyperirritable nasal reaction that nonhayfever sufferers do not have. His nose becomes an allergic "shock" organ.

Some people lose their sense of smell as a result of protracted and severe nasal allergy, especially if nasal obstruction is particularly persistent from swelling of the mucous membrane or obstruction. Many patients say that they have a greater loss of smell when the weather is damp. Others have more marked loss of smell during the height of the pollen season.

Hayfever can also cause symptoms of sinus trouble. It has been frequently established that the basis of a chronic sinus involvement is nothing but allergic illness in disguise.

Hayfever can also produce other serious complications: the

growths of nasal polyps or infections of the ear, nose or throat, for example.

And at least one out of every three hayfever sufferers goes on to develop asthma.

One strange pattern sometimes occurs that is very mystifying. A person will be allergic to ragweed pollen and yet will have no symptoms during the ragweed season but will become ill immediately *after* the season, with sore throat, sinus trouble, long-lasting colds, bronchitis or asthma. No one knows why this happens, but these people usually improve when treated with ragweed injections.

■ HOW TO TELL IF YOUR SUMMER COLDS ARE REALLY HAYFEVER

Usually a physician can tell if you have a pollen allergy by the times when your symptoms occur. For example, in the Midwest at least 95 percent of the pollen in the air during August and September is ragweed. In the southern states the ragweed season begins from one to four weeks earlier and lasts longer, usually through October. In Florida ragweed pollen may be found in the air from May until late October, and in southern California and Arizona there is an early spring ragweed season from March to May that is more troublesome.

But even if you decide that your bouts of summer colds are due to hayfever, it is still a problem to figure out specifically what you are allergic to. Different pollens are in the air in different seasons, and indeed may overlap and occur at the same time, especially in the South.

The chart by state in Appendix E will show you just what times the tree pollens, grass pollens, ragweed pollens and other troublemakers are most prevalent in your area. If your summer colds generally correlate with one of these time periods, it is a strong clue that this particular pollen is your personal troublemaker. To be absolutely sure of what you are allergic to, your doctor also will want to do skin tests. If the skin tests confirm it, your doctor will probably suggest that you begin desensitization injections to whatever you are allergic to.

There are several other ways to tell whether your condition is an allergy or an infection. The following are some of the guidelines that physicians use:

	ALLERGY	*INFECTION*
Onset	Sudden	Gradual
Sneezing	+++	–
Itching of nose	+++	–
Nasal discharge	Watery, mucoid, profuse	Thick, mucopurulent
Nasal congestion	Present	Marked
Constitutional symptoms	No	Yes
Attacks	Multiple, recurrent or constant	Occasional, free between attacks
Improvement with adrenaline or antihistamines	Yes	No
Associated allergies and allergic family history	Yes	Not necessarily
Allergic skin reactions	Yes	No

For example, in a true sinus infection the nasal discharge is thick and puslike. In hayfever, it is often colorless and runny. Also if you have a sinus infection instead of allergy, you will usually have headache or localized facial pain and tenderness, perhaps some fever. Your doctor can also check on your sinus areas by x-ray and by transillumination, in which he shines a light against your head in a darkened room to see if your sinus cavities are congested.

And there are other differences between infections and allergies. In an allergy, the mucous membrane of your nose is pale and swollen. In an infection, it is red. Also your doctor may examine your nasal secretions under a microscope to see if there are cells called eosinophils, which mark an allergy, or whether there are other white blood cells, which suggest infection.

OTHER DISORDERS THAT RESEMBLE HAYFEVER

Usually when you have a problem with nasal stuffiness that goes on and on, it is hayfever. However, there are other disorders that can cause the same nasal symptoms.

There may be some anatomical abnormality, such as a deviated septum—that is, the nasal cartilage is bent to one side or the other, narrowing the openings. Polyps or other growths may be protruding into the airway similarly reducing the nasal channel.

An underactive thyroid gland can sometimes cause nasal stuffiness and discharge, too. Usually if this is the cause, you will have other signs of too little thyroid hormone such as dry, cold, puffy skin or thin brittle nails or coarse dry hair. If your doctor suspects this, he will order some laboratory tests to see how effectively your thyroid is functioning.

There may be some simple irritant causing the nasal symptoms. Often a patient may not really be allergic to a substance, but is simply irritated by it. He may be in contact with chemical fumes, gasoline vapors or other strong pungent odors. Tobacco smoke can cause nasal stuffiness in some people by simple irritation, while other people have an actual allergy to the smoke. Some drugs, particularly drugs used to treat high blood pressure, may also induce nasal stuffiness.

Emotional upsets are sometimes involved. Many people react to stressful situations by developing nasal symptoms. Depressed patients especially are prone to excessive nasal and eye discharge.

■ RAGWEED HAYFEVER

Hayfever is rarely caused by hay and it hardly ever results in fever. A rise in temperature usually means some other illness has been added to the basic allergy. However, sufferers from hayfever often have low-grade fever of approximately 100°F during the height of the season.

Nearly anything in the air can cause an allergy: pollens from grasses, weeds and trees, as well as dust, feathers, hair, animal danders, mold, algae and the dust from insect wings.

The symptoms of hayfever were first described scientifically by an Italian, Botallus de Pavie, in 1565, but not till 1819 did Dr. John Bostock of London use the term "hayfever." He noted that he began to sneeze in June when farmers started haying and finally found relief in mid-July when British hay is all stacked. He thought his hayfever was caused either by hay or by sunlight and stayed indoors as much as possible. Later Dr. Charles H. Blakely, also English and also a hayfever victim, put in fourteen years of research and in 1866 published a book on his theory that pollen was the cause of hayfever. He also sneezed when he walked through a hay field, but he then discovered that pollen from grass put in a test tube caused hayfever if inhaled at any season of the year, and that a bit of pollen rubbed into a scratch in his skin caused a swelling similar to a hive. But Dr. Blackley's work was largely ignored, and the cause of hayfever remained a subject of controversy. In fact, it was about 1910 before the pollen theory as a basis for nasal allergy began to receive some degree of acceptance.

Today we know that ragweed pollen is the major cause of hayfever in the United States. The ragweeds—there are hundreds of varieties—are found from Canada through South America. In the United States alone, allergists estimate that more than 250,000 tons of ragweed pollen each year are blown across the nation for sometimes hundreds of miles. A single plant produces about a billion grains per season.

Victims who are sensitive to the ragweed pollen grains may be affected when there are only two or three pollen grains in a cubic foot of air! A ragweed pollen under the microscope looks like a battered up little golfball. The diameter of one is about 1/25,000 of an inch—that is, 25,000 of them would have to crowd up side-to-side to stretch to one inch.

Most pollen grains are transferred from the male flower parts to the female flower parts by insects. However, a few species which have very light pollen depend solely on wind to transport the pollen to the waiting ovary. These are the ones that cause hayfever. Insect-pollinated plants usually have colorful flowers, sticky and heavy pollen, sweet odors and nectar that attract flying insects. The plants that are pollinated by wind action are generally drab, inconspicuous, and have no perfume or nectar. Their pollen grains are not sticky and are produced in huge quantities.

So the goldenrods and roses are usually perfectly innocent bystanders. However, *close* contact with zinnias, cosmos, golden glow and goldenrod may sometimes cause symptoms in patients who are sensitive to ragweed because the pollen of these flowers, while mostly heavy and insect-borne, is closely related to ragweed.

At the University of Michigan in Ann Arbor a team of scientists have studied the mechanism of pollen grain discharge. They find that early in the morning, between 4:00 and 6:00 A.M., a tiny floret which is ready to release its pollen swells slightly and projects out of the other florets. The petals that have been tightly closed over the pollen sacs slowly open; then the pollen sacs themselves deepen and open, and the pollen is released in sticky clusters. As the fluid dries, the grains separate and are picked up by the wind. This all takes ten to thirty minutes. In the next hour or so another primitive sex organ extends out from the inside of the floret and pushes out any remaining pollen. The pollen continues to be discharged until 8:30 A.M., so that about 60 percent of the pollen is given off in just four hours in the morning. By noon the level has decreased, and the discharge remains low all through the night. The organs withdraw back into the petals, the floret closes tightly, and never opens again.

The University of Michigan researchers also found a scientific basis for the statement made by many hayfever sufferers that on damp or rainy days their hayfever symptoms are not as bad. They found that the florets do not release the pollen if the humidity is more than 80 percent.

Much of the ragweed pollen that falls around the plant stays there and is never refloated by the wind. Some travels a short distance. And some may be carried upward by air currents, soaring 4,000, 5,000, sometimes 10,000 feet in the air, sometimes floating hundreds of miles on the crest of the wind.

At night as the air cools and the wind turbulence dies down, the pollen descends at about 3 feet per minute. A particular pollen following this route to, say, 2,000 feet starting downward that evening would reach the ground about 12 hours later some 100 or so miles from the source of the original ragweed plant.

Much of the blame for the prevalence of ragweed should be placed on subdivision builders and farmers, according to the Michigan scientists. They say many construction crews and farmers leave the ground bare, providing the perfect bed for ragweed to take root. The researchers found 172,000 ragweed plants per acre in southern Michigan fields where grains had been harvested, more than 300 times the plant density in fields covered with pasturage. In urban areas they found almost all of the ragweed was in new building areas where the disturbed soil was left untouched during spring and summer.

They recommend that construction companies be required to clean up building sites and plant some fast-growing ground cover as early as possible, since ragweed is easily crowded out by other plants. Similarly, farmers should not leave harvested, plowed fields uncared for.

The best way to destroy ragweed over large areas is by use several times yearly of a weed spray such as 2-4-D. In small areas you can cut the plant low near the roots.

To help ease the pollen problem in your own neighborhood, make certain that your property is free of ragweed and check vacant lots. Report the presence of ragweed to local health authorities since there is a law that weeds must be cut.

Ragweed is relatively inconspicuous and can be just a few inches tall or as high as fifteen feet. But you can recognize it by its hairy green stems, feathery parted leaves and long spikes of flowers that produce the pollen.

■ OTHER POLLENS

Ragweed hayfever is the most common type of pollinosis, but there are many other pollens that can cause hayfever—pollens from other weeds, trees and grasses.

The types of plants and the seasons in which they produce pollen vary in different parts of the country. In the Midwest and East there are three distinct hayfever seasons.

The fall season is caused mainly by ragweed, and lasts from mid-August to the end of September. In the South and Southwest the grass season is considerably longer, and may in some areas last all year long. About half of all ragweed hayfever sufferers are sensitive to grasses as well.

The relatively mild spring season, from about the first of April to the end of May, is caused by the pollen of trees, such as elm, maple, birch, poplar, ash and oak.

The midsummer season, resulting in a condition commonly known by the misnomer "rose fever," is more frequent and more common, and lasts from about the middle of May to the end of July and is the result of the release of pollen grains of grasses, such as orchard grass, June grass, red top, timothy and rye.

In other areas of the country other types of pollen are important as a cause of symptoms: Russian thistle, Mexican firebrush, mesquite, English plantain, cedar, sage, walnut, pecan and many others.

If a patient has a history of symptoms during May, June and early July in the northern half of the United States, and gives positive reactions to grass pollens on skin tests, then grass pollen treatment is indicated. If the symptoms occur during the spring, begin earlier than mid-May or last beyond mid-July, the patient should be tested with pollens other than those of the grasses, and treatment should include these factors.

If your hayfever is from grasses or trees, your chances of escape by moving are limited. These pollens are very widespread, and grow diffusely in all states. Changes of climate must be undertaken with great caution and with full knowledge about the particular allergy and the territory considered for the move. The very arid regions and very high altitudes may be helpful in that there are fewer pollen factors to cope with; but costly mistakes are often made.

In the appendix at the back of the book is a chart of all the common weeds and grasses that cause hayfever and the states they occur in.

■ MOLD ALLERGY

More and more molds are being discovered to play an important role in allergic diseases. They are now known to be major causes of bronchial asthma, seasonal and perennial hayfever, and eczema. They often complicate and confuse the picture of pollen sensitivity.

Allergy to molds was once believed to be rather rare, affecting only people whose occupations exposed them to large numbers of mold spores, as, for example, farmers and mill workers. It also was thought that mold spores occurred in large quantities only in the Midwest, and were not present in the East in sufficient quantities to cause allergic symptoms. Recent studies, however, show that mold spore allergy is important everywhere.

In the northern part of the United States and in the grain belts of the Midwest the most common molds are *Alternaria* and *Hormodendrum*. Their spores begin to appear in May. As plant debris begins to increase in the late spring, with dying flowers of early blooming trees and plants, and as warmth and humidity increase, molds begin to propagate. In the North and Midwest, the growth is at a peak from July to October, depending on local crops and foliage and the weather.

In the South, molds can be found the year round and are prime causes of respiratory allergy for at least ten months of the year.

Mold grows nearly everywhere. It spoils bread, rots fruit, mildews clothes and grows in abundance on wheat, corn, oats, grasses, leaves, straw, hay and even on soil. Cases have been reported of hayfever or asthma in sawmill workers who were exposed to mold spores in bark or mill dust and in greenhouse workers exposed to mold on tomato leaves. One man who worked for a coffin manufacturer was found to be allergic to the mold that grew in the excelsior padding and lining of the coffins. A farmer was allergic to molds that grew in his chicken-house. Allergies to mold are frequently encountered among furniture repairers who work with old bedding and overstuffed furniture, among gardeners, fruit and vegetable workers, farmers or botanists, and among others who work in damp or musty places.

In the house, molds are especially found in furniture and mattress dust and stuffed animal toys. Molds also attack paper products, wallpaper paste, paint, wood, natural and synthetic fibers, and leather. They have been found on rubber gaskets around refrigerator doors and air conditioners, on the underside of leaves of house plants, in foods, in damp cellars, in summer cottages that have been closed for long periods, and in resort hotels and motels where they may lie dormant throughout the winter, but flourish with the first rise in temperature.

Mildew of textiles is generally due to mold that is introduced in the raw material during manufacture or acquired in exposure to air and damp environment. In damp areas be particularly careful of awnings, tents, draperies, window shades, wallpaper, canvas and upholstered furniture and mattresses with cotton or kapok.

People who are allergic to molds may even react to foods naturally containing molds, such as cheeses, beers and wines, bread and certain cakes, and soy sauce.

Molds are not killed by frost. So a warm spell after a frost may result in a new crop of molds and new symptoms. Persons who are around hay, straw or grain may have attacks even in the winter.

Molds are part of the fungus family. One that causes much hayfever is *Aspergillus*. Many patients in Great Britain have had severe hayfever and asthma at the unusual time of late fall and early winter. A few of them also developed a low-grade fever with lung complications, and were thought to have tuberculosis or pneumonia. It was discovered that the cause was the large amount of *Aspergillus* in the air at that time. The patients with hayfever and asthma did well when treated with injections of extracts of *Aspergillus* because they were allergic to the mold. The patients thought to have tuberculosis or pneumonia were not allergic to the mold but were actually infected with it. So it can cause problems by causing either an allergy or an infection.

Some of the other common forms of mold that produce allergy are *Penicillium, Fusarium, Alternaria, Helminthosporium, Hormodendrum* and *Mucorales*. Many others have simply not been investigated.

Mold allergy is more or less of a problem in every part of the country, but there are fewer molds at high altitudes and in dry regions of the Northwest or in southwest California.

The severity of mold hayfever, as with other hayfevers, varies from season to season and day to day. The severity depends largely on the weather conditions during the growth of the plant and the temperature, humidity, sunshine and wind velocity during ripening time. The most sensitive mold allergy patients have symptoms for most of the year and are well only when the ground is frozen or covered with snow. Even during winter, when the wind blows the soil dust, there are enough mold spores to produce symptoms in some sufferers.

People who react to mold usually have bronchial asthma or hayfever, with the same symptoms as those of people allergic to ragweed or other pollens. Eczema of the skin can also be caused.

If you have summer asthma or hayfever, but your symptoms do not occur at the time of pollination shown on the chart on page 396 and you do not show positive reactions to skin tests to pollen, you may have mold sensitivity. Also mold allergy is suspected if your attacks occur in musty rooms, in damp basements, in barns or similar places.

Many people are sensitive to both pollens and molds. All patients who have hayfever should be routinely tested with mold extracts.

Failure of a physician to consider mold sensitivity is often responsible for poor clinical results achieved with injection therapy.

The treatment of mold allergy begins with avoidance. As far as possible, all suspicious material such as old books, old furniture and bedding should be removed from the environment. Damp cellars should be dried with dehumidifiers. Synthetic materials, where possible, should be used for furniture and bedding. Mold-proof paint should be used in place of wallpaper. Mold-inhibiting products can be sprayed or painted on walls and in cellars, but must be repeated at regular intervals.

In areas of high humidity take special care to see that shoes, gloves, suitcases and clothing are not allowed to become mold-infested. Keep an electric light burning in a clothes closet to keep it warm and dry. If you live in an apartment, live in an upstairs apartment where it is often much drier and less conducive to mold growth than are ground floor or basement rooms.

Desensitization treatment of mold-sensitive patients and administration of palliative medication are similar to the methods employed for the treatment of pollen allergy.

■ DUST ALLERGY

If you often feel like you're catching a cold on cleaning day, or if you sneeze and sniffle when you go through old things in the attic, change the draperies, or take up rugs for cleaning, you probably are allergic to dust.

Dust is made up of tiny particles resulting from the deterioration of carpets, carpet padding, upholstered furniture, pillows and mattresses. Many people think they sneeze only from the tickle of the dust balls in the nose, but usually the sneezing is an allergic reaction of the entire body.

Various studies to determine the incidence of allergy to dust shows that anywhere from 45 to 80 percent of hayfever and asthma patients are sensitive to it. Strangely enough the older dust becomes, the more potent it is in causing allergic symptoms.

Be suspicious of allergy to house dust whenever the following things occur:

If your symptoms get worse when you are confined indoors.

If your symptoms are worse at night and relieved during the day.

If your symptoms increase when you dust, clean or carry out other household duties.

If your symptoms increase while washing or ironing.

If your symptoms increase when you turn on the heating units and close the windows as the weather turns cold.

Physicians give victims of house-dust allergy the same type of hyposensitization treatment that they use for other allergies, patients actually being injected with extracts of house dust.

Keeping your house dust-free is of utmost importance. We give you details on this later in this chapter.

■ HAYFEVER FROM INSECT DUST

Many substances are being discovered as major causes of hayfever that were never before even suspected. Bits of dust from insect wings and other bug parts are one of these newly discovered causes.

Just as ragweed, grass and other pollens get into the air, so do the tiny disintegrated bits of dust that are given off by the millions of insects in the world.

Insects have only been investigated for a few years as sources of allergy, but already it has been learned that allergy can be produced by mayflies, silk cocoons, grasshoppers, ant eggs, houseflies, mosquitoes, bees, water fleas, mites and fruit flies. With hundreds of millions of insects and other small life present in the air and in the ground nearly all dust contains insect substances. You don't even have to be in direct contact with insects, just with ordinary dust.

The fact that insect dust can cause allergy may be the reason so many of the people who have hayfever have not reacted to the commonly known allergens and have not been helped by usual immunizing injections.

For example, at Northwestern University Medical School where much of the early work on insect dust was done, one woman came in who had had a stuffed-up nose and watery eyes for nearly all of her adult life. She had some symptoms the entire year and was severely disabled from May through October. All efforts to find the cause of her allergy failed. The most scientific and extensive testing revealed nothing that she was allergic to. She was given drugs, but they weren't much relief.

Three allergists at Northwestern—Alan Feinberg, Samuel Feinberg and Carlos Benaim-Pinto from Venezuela—were working on the possibility of insects as allergy-causers. They knew there had to be some explanation for patients who had flare-ups of symptoms during the warm months, but showed no reaction to pollens or molds. There had to be some seasonal cause. Then they noticed several patients whose skin tests showed sensitivity to silk. When given desensitizing shots of silk extract, they were relieved of hayfever symptoms. But they were almost never exposed to silk fabrics! What caused the allergy?

They began collecting different insects by the hundreds to make extracts. Then they tested some of their patients and found that many were sensitive to the insect extracts.

They gave injections of insect extracts to the woman who had been helped by nothing. All of her symptoms disappeared in a few months.

Others were tested. Nearly 30 percent of all the hayfever and asthma patients tested were found to be sensitive to one or more insects. Of the patients who showed sensitivity, three out of every four when given the injection were helped.

Now more and more different insects are being discovered as allergy-causers.

In Africa an unexplained outbreak of hayfever occurred every summer in people working or living near a sewage works. It was found the hayfever was caused by dust from the disintegration of dead sewage flies which appear in large numbers at the sewage plants in the summer.

A study at George Washington School of Medicine has implicated the cockroach as a factor in allergic reactions. In a survey there, 44 percent of hayfever and asthma patients living in insect-infested surroundings had positive reactions to tests with the common cockroach.

Just recently some Dutch scientists have reported evidence that house-dust allergy may really be caused by a tiny insect called the house-dust mite. Until the mite was discovered, the actual allergen in house dust had never been isolated. Now it may be that the tiny—1/50 of an inch—dried-up bodies of the thousands of these mites present in dust are responsible for dust allergy.

■ OTHER HAYFEVER CAUSES

Other nonseasonal airborne substances also commonly cause allergy. If you have a dog or bird, there is a fair chance that it may be the cause of any allergy in the family. If you have a cat, the chance is even greater. Rats, mice, guinea pigs, gerbils and rabbits frequently cause allergies in laboratory workers. In fact, one patient who is a laboratory worker and who is severely allergic to rat dander must wear a gas mask in the lab to keep from having severe asthma attacks.

Almost any organic dust can produce allergy. Among the numerous items—the starch of face powders, the vegetable gums of hair-setting fluids, the cottonseed meal dust used as animal food, castor bean dust used as fertilizer or contaminating the air during castor oil production. Penicillin sprays and dust may cause allergy among pharmaceutical workers.

Three new substances—algae, a fungus called actinomycetes, and a slime mold called myxomycetes—have been incriminated as major causes by researchers at the University of Texas. Drs. Thomas R. McElhenney, John P. McGovern and Donald Larson say these three air contaminants are much more prevalent than had ever been believed and may explain why some patients are not relieved by standard therapy for ragweed and other well-known allergens.

These substances had not been recognized previously as possible major factors in inducing allergic symptoms because they were so small or so lightweight that the usual air sampling instruments were not able to record them. Most pollen counts, the Texas researchers believe, are misleading because they ignore the wide variety of organisms that may cause hayfever and usually record only the major offender, ragweed. The three newly discovered allergy-causers could well explain the lack of correlation between reported pollen counts and the frequency and severity of patients' hayfever symptoms.

In a study at ground level, at nose level, on rooftops, and from airplanes, algae were found to be fantastically common. On the ground they ranged anywhere from 1,000 to 800,000 algae per gram of soil, and a dust cloud blowing off from a fertile field usually contained over 5,000 algae per cubic yard of air, more than enough to send any sensitive person into paroxysms of sneezing. Airplane samples showed the algae present at levels as high as 20,000 feet.

In correlating the contaminants to actual clinical cases of allergies, the doctors found that 45 percent of hayfever patients had positive skin test reactions to it.

Patients may be treated successfully with extracts of these algae.

The implications are vast. There are hundreds and hundreds of species of the algae, the fungi and the slime molds. All of them are found nearly everywhere in the world; for example, the green algae commonly found throughout the United States in ponds and lakes appear to cause hayfever and asthma and eczema. The algae have been reported to be able to cause a reaction within a few minutes, whether you breathe the dried particles or swim in them in the water.

■ OUTSIDE INFLUENCES

As we mentioned in Chapter 2, there are many outside influences that can singly or collectively lower your allergic threshold and increase your symptoms. Infection, emotional upsets, exertion, fatigue, hormone imbalance, poor nutritional status, lack of sleep and other factors can all aggravate your allergy. These outside influences can make your hayfever sometimes more severe even on a day when the pollen count is low.

Atmospheric conditions can be a major modifying influence also. For example, if you have an asthmatic condition with your hayfever, you may get a heaviness or tightening of your chest or wheezing when you step into cold air. High humidity or an approaching electrical storm can have the same effect.

It sometimes takes a combination of meteorological factors to set off an allergic attack. A recent experiment showed that when both the temperature and barometric pressure were lowered rapidly in a laboratory setting, asthmatics began to cough and choke up; but if only the temperature or the pressure alone were dropped, it had no effect.

During hayfever season, doctors often note that patients phone to complain about their hayfever and asthma before and during a storm. Rain decreases the pollen count tremendously by washing the pollen out of the air, but this is the very time when people get worse symptoms because of the other factors. Sometimes, of course, this can also occur because they are allergic to something else besides pollen, such as mold.

Eating foods you are allergic to can aggravate and contribute to a hayfever condition.

Hormone changes can also affect allergy symptoms. Sometimes the symptoms will suddenly appear or disappear during puberty or pregnancy or at menopause. Some women find that their hayfever becomes worse during their premenstrual period, while others find it becomes aggravated during menstruation. There doesn't seem to be any logic to it, but there is certainly some significant relationship between hayfever and hormones that awaits clarification.

■ POLLEN COUNTS

Daily pollen counts as reported in newspapers and on radio and television are counts taken of the pollen grains that land on a glass slide or other apparatus, usually on the rooftop of a laboratory, medical center or weather station. Pollen counts are valuable, but they have limitations and inaccuracies.

Usually the pollen count represents the average level in the *previous* twenty-four hours rather than the current level, and there is considerable shift in count from hour to hour, with the count only giving the average of the day's pollen level. The pollen count also differs markedly from one part of town to another, so that the count reported may be different from where you live or work. The count at any sampling station on a roof is going to reflect the pollen in the air from the weeds immediately surrounding the building, and it will also be influenced by the wind speed, wind direction and humidity in that particular area and may very well be different from that on the street five stories down.

Further, the pollen count presently reported to the public usually measures only the ragweed. If your hayfever is caused by any other substance, such as mold, then the count has no meaning for you at all.

What pollen counts do give us is a *qualitative* comparison of times, seasons and places and an approximate gauge of the effects of treatment from one season to the next.

There are two major ways to avoid whatever in the air is causing your particular hayfever. One is to keep the troublemakers out of your environment. The other is to get yourself out of the environment—by moving to another area of the country, either permanently or temporarily. Let's look at both of these possibilities.

■ HOW TO ALLERGY-PROOF YOUR HOME

If we could eliminate from the air all the allergens to which a patient is sensitive he would have no symptoms. Complete elimination isn't possible, of course, but even partial removal of allergens in the air will be helpful to any patient with hayfever.

The instructions in this section may seem unnecessarily severe, but experience has shown that an allergen-free environment for even part of a day will give substantial benefits.

Carry out as many of these instructions as possible even though it is difficult, and you will find hayfever symptoms substantially improved.

The infiltration of dust and other microscopic allergens in the air into every crevice of the room and furniture is insidious and cannot be controlled by ordinary housecleaning methods. Dust slips in through the windows and through the spaces around the doors; it comes in on people's clothes; it is circulated around through the heating system.

Most housewives feel that they are constantly cleaning house, but most of them don't realize just how big the job is. A study by an international home furnishings organization showed that the average six-room house in a metropolitan area collects some 40 pounds of dust in a year. In Chicago an average of more than 37,000 tons of dust per square mile comes sifting down. You can see how much dust there is on days when a beam of sunlight shines in the room, lighting up the tiny dots drifting about.

FURNISHINGS AND HOUSEKEEPING

The chief source of house dust and other allergens is upholstered furniture, mattresses, box springs, mattress pads, pillows, rugs, rug pads, stuffed toys, blankets, bedspreads, comforters, quilts and drapes. Old upholstered furniture is especially troublesome. Usually the older the furniture, the more allergy it causes.

The hayfever sufferer's bedroom should contain as little overstuffed furniture as possible. Keep furnishings simple. Avoid anything that might collect dust such as rugs and drapes, knickknacks, pictures, books. Use wooden chairs, lintless rag rugs or cotton rugs that can be washed every week or so. Rug pads should not be used unless made of rubber. Use no curtains or drapes or use simple ones that can be washed once a week, or try plastic curtains that can be wiped with a damp cloth every day or so.

Shag and chenille type fabrics are unsatisfactory. Mattresses and box springs and pillows should be of foam rubber, Dacron or other synthetic fiber. Do not use kapok, cotton linters, animal hairs, feathers or down for mattresses or pillows. Mattresses and pillows must be covered and air-tight. Try using two pillow cases on each pillow, with the second pillow case put on in reverse, thereby sealing both ends. Wool blankets are acceptable, but avoid the fuzzy type. Quilts and comforters are not recommended. All bedding should be easily washable. Blankets should be washed every four to six weeks. Pillows should be vacuumed frequently.

Do not keep toys or other items which will accumulate dust in the room. Avoid stuffed animals. Use only washable toys.

Frequent heavy cleaning of the hayfever patient's bedroom is essential. More time is spent in the bedroom than any other room in the house. A child will spend even more time in his bedroom than an adult, often spending close to twelve out of every twenty-four hours—half his childhood—in his bedroom. Preparatory to cleaning, as much as possible of the furniture, carpets, curtains and drapes should be taken from the room or moved to the center, and all the closets should be emptied. The closet should contain only necessary things in current use and should be as dust-free as the room. Seal off the registers and furnace pipes if the room is warm enough without them; or if the heat is necessary, put several layers of cheesecloth across and under the register to help filter out the dust coming through with the hot air. Wash down the walls and ceilings, the woodwork, the floors, the radiators or registers, the closets, the furniture. Be sure to wash off things like the backs and corners of furniture, the tops of doors, window frames, sills, moldings, lights and closet shelves. An excellent way to obtain this kind of thorough cleaning is through professional cleaning services available now in many cities.

Brooms or dusters should never be used; instead use oil mops, vacuum cleaners, or frequently changed damp cloths.

If the walls are papered, use wallpaper cleaner every four to six months and in-between times brush walls down with a dampened brush.

The patient should always be out of the room or out of the house when it is being cleaned.

Many allergists recommend that all overstuffed furniture and rugs in the house be vacuumed daily. This is sometimes impossible, and we feel that except in very severe hayfever cases, twice a week is sufficient. The vacuuming should include not only the furniture and rugs, but also the drapes, the pillows, mattresses and box springs. Again this vacuuming should be done while the patient is out of the house.

Try the several products available that inhibit dust formation on furniture, rugs, drapes and blankets. They tend to immobilize old dust and retard the formation of new dust. You can rinse fabrics in them, spray them on furniture, rugs or car upholstery. Some hayfever victims even sponge them on their pet animals.

If possible keep the bedroom primarily for sleeping. Do your dressing in another room, and if possible keep your clothes in a closet in another room. Keep the doors and windows of the bedroom closed as much as possible, and prevent drafts from going through it. During the height of the hayfever season, it pays to keep the entire house closed and sealed.

If your home is being remodeled or built new, there are a number of ways to help avoid allergens.

If a heating choice is possible, electric heat or hot water is preferable to forced air heat. The type of heating is not as important as the location of the furnace. (The fumes from natural and manufactured gas, coal, oil and even lubricating grease from the blower might irritate the allergic person.) Therefore, it's best to place the furnace in a separate room with an outside entrance; outside combustion is important.

Some people are also allergic to the gases and dusts in their heating systems—either furnaces or electric heaters. Thousands of tiny lint particles in the air are burned into carbon cinders which irritate the membranes of the nose, throat and lungs. Of even more serious impact are the plastic and synthetic materials in the air which, when they hit the high temperature surfaces of furnaces and electric heaters, vaporize into toxic gases that cause allergy. Hot water heat will correct the problem.

In homes heated by a forced air system, insert a good two-stage electronic air cleaner within the ducts which will filter out most of the household air contaminants, particularly dust and mold.

When choosing building materials, sheet vinyls are the easiest to keep dust-free, since they can be damp mopped and have fewer cracks to collect dust and mold spores (a 12- by 18-foot room covered with 9-inch tiles has more than 600 feet of dust-collecting seams).

In the bathroom, laminated plastic panels are superior to small ceramic or plastic tiles which allow more moisture to seep through the seal and cause mold growth. The new flexible silicone rubber mastics offer the most impregnable seal between wall and tub. The clothes dryer should be vented to the outdoors.

PROTECTING AGAINST MOLD ALLERGY

Mold is one of the more potent allergens and is impossible to avoid completely, since like dust it is present all year round in the air. If your furniture or clothes tend to smell musty or moldy, then this is a problem that you must be especially careful of.

Molds are mostly a problem in humid areas, and if a house is kept dry, it will help decrease the amount of mold spores within the house. However, very low humidity has a drying and damaging effect on the mucous membrane of the respiratory tract and skin. It is best for allergic people to keep a humidity of approximately 40 percent within the house.

The measures carried out to help reduce house dust and other allergens will also reduce mold spores. There are also several commercial preparations available as paints or sprays that may be applied to the walls and other areas to decrease the amount of mold and keep it from growing.

ANIMAL PETS

There should be no animal pets with fur or feathers in the house of any person with hayfever. Not only dogs and cats but pet birds can be a significant cause of respiratory allergies. Animal hair and dander and even animal saliva are potent allergens and should be avoided by allergic persons. Patients sensitive to animal hair and dander should also avoid zoos, circuses, rodeos, horse and dog shows, other pet shows, barns and stables. If anyone in your family has hayfever and you do not have pets, do not get any, no matter how much you love animals or how much your children beg you for them. And if you have a pet now and it dies, do not replace it.

If the allergic person in your family has only a mild case of hayfever and you can keep the pet outside the house, then he may be kept if he is never allowed in the house.

In a distressing number of instances we have worked for years with patients trying to overcome their hayfever, then find they have lied to us about getting rid of their pet. If you already have a pet and are not sure whether it is causing your allergy and skin tests do not give a specific answer, then have the dog boarded away for several months, clean your house from top to bottom, vacuuming twice a week for those several months to get rid of all lingering hairs and danders, and see if your hayfever is improved.

Feathers and animal hair and dander are present in many common household items also, and you must be alert to the danger from these. For example, avoid feather pillows. Use Dacron, Orlon, acrilan, nylon or foam rubber instead. Avoid rug pads with cow hair or hog hair. Rabbit hair mattresses used to be one of the major causes of allergic illness, but are less commonly so now, since rabbit hair stuffing has been forbidden. If you or your doctor think wool might be a problem, then use cotton or synthetic fabrics. Be on the lookout for horsehair. It is often found in brushes, mattresses, shoe linings, gloves, pressing cloths, some sacks and bags, and even as a binder in plaster.

Allergic patients with a sensitivity to horsehair and dander, by the way, may also have a severe allergic reaction to tetanus antitoxin, which is obtained from horses. Therefore it is imperative for such a person to keep his tetanus toxoid level up-to-date by receiving regular booster injections. If you are allergic to horsehair or dander or have ever had a reaction to tetanus antitoxin, see your doctor about getting proper amounts of protection to tetanus. There is now available a tetanus antitoxin made from human origin.

AIR CONDITIONING

Efficient well-maintained air conditioning can be a big benefit to hayfever sufferers. Central air conditioning units that function for the entire house are the most efficient, but individual units in several rooms or the most frequently used rooms are also effective.

Air conditioners decrease the amount of dust, pollens and other allergens by filtering the air within the house. Temporary filters should be replaced frequently, the time interval being determined by the amount of dust that accumulates on the filter, usually varying from two weeks to a month. Some patients don't have to examine the the filters. They know the morning they wake up sneezing that it's time to change the filter.

It also pays to have an air conditioner in the car, not only to filter out the pollens, but also to make it possible to keep the car windows closed and thus prevent pollen-laden air from rushing into your face as you drive.

Filtering the air is always of value to the hayfever patient, but it is not good for him to be overly chilled or to have sudden temperature changes. Keep the temperature of the house or car at a comfortable level and avoid sudden changes. The temperature should not be lowered drastically because the sudden chill can irritate the nose and bronchial tubes. Moderate cooling with temperatures not more than twelve degrees lower than outdoors is best. Some of the new, large electrostatic systems for taking the dust and other foreign elements out of the air are effective, too. But some of the smaller units sold at retail stores have been labeled ineffective by the Food and Drug Administration for respiratory and allergic conditions.

The most effective presently available air conditioning unit is the microstatic precipitator which has been demonstrated to have considerable value in minimizing the amount of pollens and dusts which may come into the room.

When you use an air conditioner turn it on a few hours before using the room if possible, keeping it closed up to get rid of the pollen. Do not use exhaust or fresh air vents, but use only the "re-circulated" adjustment. Keep the doors and windows shut to that room all day.

OTHER ADVICE

There are several other things that can be done to minimize the amount of pollution and irritants in the home environment. See that your house has no tobacco smoke, kerosene or oil burners or chalk dust, and try to keep the hayfever sufferer away from cooking odors and paint or varnish fumes. Use only hypoallergenic insect sprays or powders. Avoid any sprays that have odors of camphor or tar.

Don't drive in the country with the car windows open. Avoid fields and farms where ragweed grows. Avoid garden work where pollen gets stirred up from the weeds and dirt. Avoid handling objects covered with dust, such as books, boxes or clothing that has been stored in closets or chests.

If you are allergic to any foods, even mildly, avoid them during the hayfever season, because their ingestion will add to your symptoms, even though they may not give you much trouble the rest of the year.

■ GETTING AWAY FROM IT ALL

Many ragweed sufferers find that the simplest thing to do is to take their vacation during the ragweed season, going to some part of the world where there is no ragweed pollen. The American Academy of Allergy has compiled statistics about various cities in the country and the degree of their pollen pollution. They find that ragweed pollen is largely absent in deserts and forest regions and in the wooded areas of the northern tips of Michigan, Minnesota, New Hampshire and Maine, as well as the central Adirondacks and the extreme southern tip of Florida.

Unfortunately as many of these relief areas become populated and developed, the ragweed begins to grow there, so that many places that were pollen-free for hayfever holidays ten or twenty years ago are no longer satisfactory.

If you are considering moving to any of these places permanently, you should also realize that some people, after they move to a new area, develop new allergies to substances growing in that particular area. However, this is not true of everyone.

If you think that moving to a new climate is the answer for you, we suggest that you don't sell your house and belongings and make a permanent move right away. Try the new location out for at least a year to see how much benefit you have before you make the move permanent. If you're troubled by ragweed pollen, you have a fair chance of getting away from it by moving to another part of the United States that is free of ragweed or to another country. However, if your hayfever is caused by grasses or trees, escape is less likely, since these are generally more widespread.

We believe the lists of cities and areas and the charts and maps in Appendix E will help you make decisions about locations for moves or vacations. You might also want to consider an ocean voyage for a vacation, which will remove you from all pollens during the hayfever season.

Because other pollens such as brush and thistle and amaranths and molds may complicate the problem of your finding a suitable haven you should always consult your physician about your particular allergy.

■ AIR POLLUTION

There is still some controversy about how much effect air pollution has on allergy. It certainly aggravates the condition, and in heavy smog episodes many people with asthma and other respiratory problems have great distress. It has been recorded that the death rate from asthma climbs during periods and places of high pollution.

To check your city as to its air pollution see the following page for the ranking that has been done by the U.S. Public Health Service's National Center for Air Pollution Control of 65 of the largest metropolitan areas in the nation. The worst cities are listed first, with the numbers shown referring to the relative amount of suspended particles, gasoline, and sulfur dioxide in the air.

■ TREATING THE SYMPTOMS

When Dr. Oliver Wendell Holmes was asked to prescribe a treatment for hayfever, he said, "Gravel is an effective remedy. It should be taken about eight feet deep."

Matters aren't quite that bad nowadays. When you go to your doctor, you will find that he has many medications that are of help in alleviating symptoms. In fact, there are at least forty drug preparations on today's market that offer temporary relief. They include pills, capsules, nose drops and nasal sprays. Most of them are designed to dry up nasal secretions or counteract sneezing, itching, eye irritation, nasal stuffiness and other symptoms.

RELATIVE SEVERITY OF AIR POLLUTION IN THE 65 STANDARD METROPOLITAN STATISTICAL AREAS WITH INDUSTRIAL POPULATION OF 40,000 OR MORE

New York	457	Youngstown–Warren	294	Worcester	234
Chicago	422	Toledo	287	Houston	233
Philadelphia	404	Kansas City	285	Chattanooga	232
Los Angeles–Long Beach	393	Dayton	280	Memphis	232
Cleveland	390	Denver	280	Columbus, Ohio	231
Pittsburgh	390	Bridgeport	261	Richmond	230
Boston	389	Providence–Pawtucket	261	San Jose	217
Newark	376	Buffalo	260	Portland, Ore.	210
Detroit	370	Birmingham	259	Syracuse	209
St. Louis	369	Minneapolis–St. Paul	257	Atlanta	208
Gary–Hammond–East Chicago	368	Hartford	254	Grand Rapids	204
Akron	367	Nashville	253	Rochester	200
Baltimore	355	San Francisco–Oakland	253	Reading	196
Indianapolis	351	Seattle	252	Albany–Schenectady–Troy	187
Wilmington	342	New Haven	246	Lancaster	181
Louisville	338	York	246	Dallas	178
Jersey City	333	Springfield–Chicopee–Holyoke	241	Flint	171
Washington	327	Allentown–Bethlehem–Easton	239	New Orleans	160
Cincinnati	325			Fort Worth	156
Milwaukee	301			San Diego	151
Passaic	304			Utica–Rome	130
Canton	302			Miami	117
				Wichita	102

Some of these drugs work better than others in different people, and what is most effective for one person is not necessarily what is best for another person. Only trial and error and cooperation with your doctor will tell you which are the best ones for you and in what dosage.

Antihistamine drugs will lessen your nasal and sinus congestion and relieve itching. Most of them are effective for only three or four hours and so must be taken several times a day, but some of them are combination or delayed-action pills that last eight to twelve hours. This allows you to sleep without waking up in the middle of the night to take another pill. Many people find it works well to take regular four-hour pills during the day only when they really need the relief and then, when they go to bed, to take an eight-hour pill to last throughout the night.

Many antihistamines make you drowsy or sleepy. This can be a decided disadvantage if you have a lethargic-type job like reading editorial proofs, and it can be extremely dangerous if you pilot an airplane, work around machinery, or drive a bus or the family car when you are taking the medicine. In fact, a lawsuit was instigated recently in Washington state because a passenger on a bus was injured after the driver, who had taken an antihistamine, fell asleep at the wheel. Don't take an antihistamine when you have to be alert.

Some brands of hayfever pills combine antihistamine with amphetamine or caffeine to overcome this sedative effect, but this sometimes increases your pulse rate and must be carefully watched.

Surprisingly enough, some persons are allergic to the antihistamine drugs themselves, so all antihistamines must be used under the direction of a physician.

Hayfever pills sold in drugstores and grocery stores over-the-counter—that is, without a doctor's prescription—will help mild hayfever symptoms. But if your symptoms are at all severe, you need the stronger medicine you can obtain only by prescription from a doctor.

Sometimes after you have carefully tried several antihistamines and have found that one that works best and has the fewest side effects for you, you discover that you have built up tolerance to it. Use another one for several weeks. Then you may be able to return to the first one.

Sometimes the antihistamine tablets also contain other drugs to help asthma symptoms or may contain stimulants, aspirin or cough medicine. A mild tranquilizer or relaxant is often helpful when given in addition to regular hayfever medicines.

Your physician may suggest that if you have an allergic cough or asthma, an aerosol spray form of antihistamine or other drugs may be effective. For mild wheezing, ephedrine is helpful, and the ubiquitous, not-understood but usually helpful aspirin sometimes has value, too.

Nose drops or sprays often help, but you must be careful not to use them excessively. You must also be careful to find one for you that does not cause a "rebound phenomenon"; that is, after the drops or spray open up your nose, it then reacts and becomes worse than it was before.

If the membranes in your nose are dry, insert Vaseline in the morning when you wake up and before you go to bed.

Eyedrops are helpful for itching and burning eyes. Drops containing a local anesthetic and epinephrine or hydrocortisone are helpful, as is one made up of epinephrine, cocaine and distilled water. Some eyedrops also use solutions of antihistamines. One product made up of extract of rose petals gives many people help. Ask your doctor if he will prescribe some medication that might help you.

Simple things can help, too. During hayfever season, stay out of the wind and away from drafts. The wind blowing pollen and dust at you can quickly set severe symptoms off. Drink warm sugared tea or coffee to toast up your insides and boost your energy level. Many patients find eating frequently helps them. Their symptoms are worst just before a meal when they are hungriest, and the symptoms clear up as soon as food is eaten.

Complications of hayfever must be recognized and treated as well.

If there are nasal polyps and if they cause nasal blockage or lead to repeated secondary infections, they must be removed.

If there are repeated sinus infections, they will usually be reduced as the allergy itself is brought under control, but sometimes antibiotics will also be needed for acute attacks.

If there is enlargement of the tonsils and adenoids, they may have to be removed. However, with the help of a knowledgeable physician, one should always get the allergic problem under good control before considering surgery, because often the tonsil and adenoid problem is solved as the allergy problem is resolved.

If ear infections occur frequently, they too will be helped as the allergy is moderated. For acute attacks, antibiotics may be indicated.

There are also a number of surgical procedures that are sometimes of value.

When infection of the respiratory tract is associated with hayfever, treatment is the same as that used for similar infections in nonallergic patients, except that sometimes treatment must be a little stronger or used for longer periods.

There are also some things that *don't* work for hayfever. Gamma globulin has not proved effective, unless the person has a low level. Local treatment to the nose consisting of x-ray or cauterization of the nasal mucous membrane is not helpful and indeed can be harmful.

Some hayfever sufferers claim that smoking marijuana during hayfever season helps in clearing symptoms. However, we know of no scientific studies that have been done on this.

Hormones (cortisone, hydrocortisone, prednisone, prednisolone, and ACTH) are sometimes used for hayfever and for asthma. They are needed in only the occasional patient—the very severe case—and they should be used only when all other treatment has failed. The use of these hormones requires a number of precautions and close medical supervision, and in certain disease conditions they cannot be used safely. They, as well as the other treatments, are powerful drugs and are never to be used without a physician's advice and direction.

Also, since hayfever varies in kind and intensity from area to area and from person to person, you should not regard your case as identical with that of your friends, and you should not consider the advice given by his or her physician as applying to you. Different patients need different treatment. See your family physician or an allergist to find out what is best for you.

■ GETTING TO THE CAUSE —HYPOSENSITIZATION

Treating your symptoms of hayfever with drugs as the symptoms occur can work quite effectively if you have only mild or moderate symptoms. But if you have severe and constantly recurring symptoms, you need to consider the more basic and permanent treatment of your illness—desensitization, also called hyposensitization.

This technique of immunizing you to whatever is causing your hayfever involves three general steps:

First, the doctor does skin tests to determine what substances are causing your hayfever.

Second, he prepares specific extracts of the substance causing your allergy.

Third, he begins a series of injections, starting out with very small doses and gradually, over a period of visits, increasing the amount injected.

Sometimes injections are given only before the season, sometimes both before and during the season, and sometimes all year round. Usually they are given once or twice a week.

If you have a respiratory allergy that is due to pollens and molds, injections are generally quite effective. If you are allergic to foods or drugs, injection treatment is usually unnecessary. Avoiding the food or drug is easier. If you have a contact allergy—that is, you are allergic to substances that you come in contact with by touching—injections are not necessary either.

The medicines used for desensitization injections are made of the substance you are allergic to. If you are allergic to ragweed pollen, you are given injections of extracts of ground-up sterilized pollen diluted with physiological saline solution. If you are allergic to dust, you are given extracts of dust diluted the same way.

Sometimes if you do not seem to be allergic to the ordinary dust that your doctor has available for testing and injecting, he may ask you to collect dust in your home or place of business by using a vacuum cleaner. You vacuum bookcases, overstuffed furniture, carpets, drapes, rugs, rafters, shelves, closets and the attic, including the fluff as well as the more solid particles. You collect about a pint of the sample, and your doctor sends it to a laboratory for extraction. Then you have a custom-made solution for your injections.

Within the last few years the repository or so-called one-shot hay-fever treatment has been used in many people. With the one-shot injection the extract of the substance you are allergic to is suspended in a long-lasting oil preparation so that it will release slowly in your body, eliminating the need for frequent injections. Sometimes if you are very sensitive, several of the regular injections are given first to build your immunity up gradually, and then the one-shot injection is given to replace the rest of the series.

There is still considerable controversy about this form of treatment, mostly because if an extract of a substance is given to a person who is not allergic to that particular substance, he may actually be caused in the future to develop an allergy to it. Because of this danger, also because of the rare but possible chance that an abscess might develop at the site of the injection, and because there was some fear that the oil base of the injection might cause cancer, the U.S. Food and Drug Administration took the one-shot treatment medicine off the market except for experimental use. At present the one-shot treatment use is restricted, and it is administered on an experimental basis only.

When infection recurs as an important factor in a person's allergic illness, vaccines and filtrates prepared from bacteria are often of great benefit. Sometimes the vaccine is prepared from the cultures of bacteria from the patient himself, or it may be a stock vaccine containing a mixture of the strains of bacteria most frequently encountered in the respiratory passages. Injections are usually given at weekly intervals starting in the fall of the year and continuing until late the following spring.

As to the effectiveness of hyposensitization treatments, most allergists report that satisfactory immunity is achieved in about 80 to 90 percent of patients who receive injections of specific pollen extract. About half of these receiving treatment become completely free of symptoms and require no medication whatsoever, and another one out of three are markedly improved, needing only minimal medication during the hayfever season. About one of five receive only minimal benefit or no help at all.

Even when relief is incomplete, the severity of symptoms is often reduced by the treatment, making the patient more comfortable. The remaining milder symptoms can then be treated with medication.

Hyposensitization treatment should be continued until the patient is relatively free of symptoms for at least twelve months, maintaining it through all four seasons of the year without symptoms. In fact, many allergists feel that a patient should remain under treatment until he has been without symptoms for two years. Then treatment may be discontinued, but with visits being made back to the doctor once a year for the subsequent two years. Any recurrence of symptoms should be promptly reported to the doctor.

The treatment of even a simple case of hayfever is a long-term project, requiring careful and constant attention over many years. You must understand this at the beginning of your treatment so that you do not become discouraged when you are not cured overnight.

Chapter 6

ASTHMA

At first your chest feels a little tight. Then it gets tighter and tighter, and soon feels like a giant hand squeezing you in the throat and chest.

It's hard to breathe. Your mouth opens trying to get as much air as possible. You try lying down, but that makes it worse. You feel like you're choking. You sit up on the side of the bed and lean forward. The labored breathing knots the muscles of your neck and shoulders, chest and abdomen, and they strain with every breath. The wheezing in your chest is so loud it can be heard across the room. As the attack goes on, the mucus begins to accumulate in your bronchial tubes and you try to cough it up, the spasms of coughing growing more and more uncontrollable and body-wracking. You sweat, and you may even turn slightly blue.

You are tired, you are discouraged and you are afraid.

This is how it feels to have an attack of asthma.

Asthma has been known through the ages.

Hippocrates and his followers spoke of "asthma," which in Greek means panting. Greek physician Aretaeus gave an excellent description of it in the second century. "Wheezers" are referred to in the Bible in Deuteronomy; and in the Ebers Papyrus from ancient Egypt there are a series of prescriptions for asthma.

But it was 1698 before Sir John Floyer noted for the first time that asthma was due to a "contracture of the muscular fibers of the bronchi."

The problem is not only still with us, it is growing worse.

Today millions of people suffer attack after attack through the year—the estimates vary from four to ten million people in the United States, many times more than persons with cancer. And many are killed by it each year—the latest estimate is ten thousand.

And the problem is still growing. In just one recent four-year period there was a net increase of more than 20 percent in the number of patient visits to physicians in the United States for asthma.

In many medical centers the number of patients having acute asthmatic episodes has increased *100 percent* in the past few years.

The death rate from asthma has gone up at alarming rates around the world, but the worst reports, the grimmest statistics, have been from England and Wales. In less than ten years there the death rate for asthmatics aged five to thirty-four has increased to three times what it was before! Between the ages of ten to fourteen, the death rate from asthma has increased by nearly *eight times!*

The asthmatic person is often handicapped throughout his life, and may be invalided. His life is a combination of chronic disability and frequent rushed interruptions of racing to his physician or to the hospital for emergency treatment of acute attacks. His productivity in school and on the job is greatly impaired, and his happiness is destroyed.

He may function well for many years and then pant into old age. But usually the asthma patient's incapacities grow, often despite all that is done to help them, so that many must limit or stop working, spend much of their savings and wind up economically helpless.

Asthma results in an estimated 128 million days lost from work, school and other necessary activities in the United States.

■ WHAT ASTHMA REALLY IS

Bronchial asthma is recurring shortness of breath and difficulty in breathing, with coughing and wheezing. Let's look at how it works.

The respiratory system is composed of an upper and lower respiratory tract. In normal breathing, air is breathed in about sixteen times a minute through the mouth and nose and passes through the trachea (the windpipe) to the large bronchial tubes (bronchi). These large tubes divide into smaller and smaller ones (bronchioles) until they are the size of fine threads. At the end of each small tube there is a cluster of tiny air sacs (alveoli). In these sacs, the oxygen from the air is picked up by the blood, to be pumped through the entire body. At the same time, the waste product, carbon dioxide, is removed from the blood and breathed out.

There are also passageways to a number of other structures associated with the respiratory system such as the ear, the eye, the sinuses. Because of the many connections, complications can affect the related structures, such as the ears and the sinuses.

Almost all the respiratory tract is lined with moist mucous membrane, and most of the cells in the membrane have microscopic hair-like structures called cilia on their surfaces. These wave rhythmically toward the mouth. Some of the cells in the membrane are mucus-producing, secreting a fluid which coats the membranes. The cilia function like tiny conveyor belts, slowing pushing bacteria, dirt particles or other foreign substances out of the air passages and into the mouth where they are usually swallowed down to the stomach and eliminated.

In asthma there is a difficulty in breathing and choking caused by obstruction of the small bronchial tubes. Breathing is like trying to force air through a narrowed or clamped tube. The patient has the feeling of suffocating.

Bronchial obstruction can be caused by any one or a combination of three factors: (1) The membranes lining the bronchial tubes swell. (2) The tiny muscles around the tubes contract in a spasm, making the airways smaller. (3) The tubes become plugged by mucus. As a result, the linings become distended, breathing out becomes increasingly difficult and labored, the chest swells, there are wheezing noises.

One of the characteristics of asthma is that there is a cycle of progressive vulnerability. One attack leads to another attack. And each repeated attack leaves the person more vulnerable to the next attack and to many successive respiratory infections because of a lowered threshold of resistance. Asthma attacks and infections become more frequent and more protracted. Asthma that is only occasional may become recurrent, and asthma that is repetitive may become chronic. Attacks related to a particular pollen season may after several years be prolonged beyond the pollen season and then may become chronic, lasting throughout most of the year. Infective asthma is particularly apt to become chronic in elderly patients.

One of the reasons for this progressive vulnerability is that during each attack some of the tiny cilia that usually propel normal mucus up from the bronchi toward the throat are destroyed during an attack. Because some of these cilia are lost, there is less propelling of the mucus upward, and the patient is more likely to get a next attack because he has less protection against infections, allergens or pollution in the air. Also the mucous blanket that usually moves upward to carry bacteria out now becomes slowed up or stagnant and becomes just the right medium for bacteria to grow in.

Asthma may occur in occasional attacks or in frequent ones, or it may become almost continuous. The attacks may last for hours or, if untreated, last for days or weeks until the patient is exhausted. Occasionally they end in collapse and death.

Fortunately, most attacks of asthma are mild. They are more distressing than dangerous and can be relieved by modern medical treatment. However, with repeated attacks, the person may develop chronic bronchitis. Or his continual forced breathing may stretch the lung tissue and may damage it permanently. When this happens, the person no longer breathes out completely, and a good deal of residual air remains trapped, causing a condition known as emphysema. He then has less endurance and may be short of breath after only slight exertion. In addition, an extra load is placed on the heart, which must work harder to force blood through the damaged lungs.

The sooner the asthma attacks are controlled, the less permanent damage will be done to the lungs and heart.

Asthma may appear at any age. A two-month-old baby may develop a choking cough and wheeze, and an eighty-year-old man who never had allergy in his life may suddenly develop it. But it's generally more apt to appear before age ten, often following childhood eczema and hayfever. The frequency of onset of new cases diminishes greatly after age forty.

Although asthma has its roots in childhood, the asthmatic child rarely outgrows the condition without the contributory causes being treated. If it does clear up spontaneously, it is more likely to occur at about age eight. But there are more people who grow *into* asthma than there are those who grow *out* of it. There is no present method by which the physician can predict which cases will be self-adjusting. Therefore medical care gives an asthmatic person the best chance against illness. The earlier the treatment, the better the prospects.

■ CAUSES OF ASTHMA

Wheezing, shortness of breath, and coughing do not always mean asthma. They can also be caused by other illnesses such as heart trouble, nasal polyps, thyroid nodules, tuberculosis, emphysema, enlarged nymph nodes, kidney trouble or anemia; or they can be due to bronchial obstruction from cancer of the lung, benign tumors, cysts, scars in the bronchi or simply a choked-on foreign body. Only your doctor can determine the difference.

One specific kind of asthma, called "cardiac asthma," is really a serious form of heart failure in which the patient wheezes.

But when one talks of asthma, he usually means bronchial asthma, where the interference with respiration occurs in the bronchial tubes, where the bronchial muscles tighten up in spasm, the lining membranes become thick and swollen, and mucus pours out into the tubes. This asthma can be due to an allergy, an infection, air pollution or other factors. In some cases the underlying cause simply cannot be determined.

When the asthma is due to an allergy, as it most commonly is, then it may be a reaction response to pollens, molds, dust, animal danders, foods—any of the same allergens that can cause hayfever. The same sort of allergic reactions take place, only with the bronchial tubes in the chest being the target organs rather than the eyes and nose, as in hayfever.

Most asthma is caused by inhaled allergens from the air such as dust, pollen, molds and animal dander. Foods are a less common cause, but still an important one. Drugs can cause asthma also, especially aspirin, aminopyrine (Pyramidon), quinine and penicillin.

Also as in hayfever, asthma may occur only at certain seasons or may occur all year round, depending on what the person is sensitive to. And again as in hayfever, many contributory factors play a role, such as changes in the weather, smoke, smog, general health of the individual, fatigue and emotional upsets.

Many people have both hayfever and asthma, about one of three.

Infections of the sinuses sometimes precede asthma and may cause attacks, and in children infections of the tonsils and adenoids may also precipitate asthma.

Nonallergic irritants may cause an attack also, since the mucous membranes of the bronchial tubes are more easily irritated in asthmatic patients than in other people. For instance, ordinary street dust, chalk dust, chemical fumes, paint, strong odors, coal smoke and other irritants may bring on an attack.

Some of the most interesting recent research concerns evidence linking asthma with the presence of intestinal parasites. Dr. David C. H. Tullis, a Canadian physician, studied 201 bronchial asthma patients and found intestinal worms in 198 of them. A control group of patients without asthma had no worms. It is believed that the larvae of the worms migrate to the lungs to cause the symptoms. If future research proves the evidence valid, then physicians may be able to treat asthma by treating the parasitic infection.

ALLERGIC ASTHMA

Finding the cause of allergic asthma is not always simple.

One physician reported a puzzling case of a garage mechanic who had attacks of asthma that couldn't be explained. Skin tests showed that he was sensitive to a mold found in red clay, but there was no such clay for at least thirty miles from his work and from his home. Then the mechanic remembered that he had a customer, a farmer in the red clay area who brought his tractor in for repairs. The cause of the mechanic's asthma was the dust from the bottom of the tractor that he inhaled whenever he crawled under the tractor to work on it.

Another man was found to have asthma attacks because he was allergic to karaya gum contained in the material used to keep his upper denture in place.

A strange cause was also found in a great number of persons in the oyster-shucking and pearl-culture industry. One out of four workers was coming down with asthma and hayfever symptoms. From October through April they worked in cold, poorly ventilated rooms, striking oyster shells with hammers to open them, the working area saturated with water and shell fragments. After much investigation allergy specialists found that the workers were allergic to tiny animals called sea squirts that were attached to the oyster shells like barnacles. Most of them were relieved of their symptoms when they changed jobs or received injections specially prepared from the strange little sea squirts.

In California, an asthmatic condition was found to be caused by giant redwood trees. Researchers at Stanford University School of Medicine identified the condition when they studied a thirty-eight-year-old sawmill worker who had an unexplained lung disease for four years. He suffered shortness of breath and coughing and finally lost forty pounds. After intensive study the researchers determined that inhaled redwood sawdust had found its way into the air sacs of his lungs and had provoked an allergic reaction there. His condition improved when he was no longer in the sawmill.

A similar disease is farmer's lung disease, associated with moldy hay.

Sometimes the causes are not so readily established. For example, mysterious outbreaks of asthma have occurred in New Orleans many times in the past two decades. Known as "New Orleans epidemic asthma," at the height of a typical outbreak it is often responsible for two hundred admissions daily in just one city hospital. The various New Orleans outbreaks seem to be due to different substances in the air at different times. One study showed that some outbreaks were due to huge amounts of ragweed in the air, and other outbreaks were due to spores of certain fungi. But another study indicates that the asthma attacks were related to emissions from the city dumps polluting the air.

A recent statistical analysis of visits for asthma to the emergency clinics in four New York City hospitals revealed that abrupt increases in the number of asthma clinic visits occurred on the same days at all four hospitals in the fall. These days were not distinguished by an increase in pollens or molds, but coincided with the onset of early cold spells and the beginning of the heating season.

When you visit your doctor for treatment of your asthma, he will search for the factors causing your asthma just as he does for hayfever, checking into your daily life to see what might bear on the problem.

Just as with hayfever allergy he will take a detailed history of when the attacks take place. And as in hayfever, if you have symptoms only at certain times of the year when pollens and molds are present, these are suspected. If you cough and gasp when you have been with a cat or dog, the dander of these animals is suspected. The doctor will also want to do a physical examination, and will study the nose and sinuses for evidence of chronic infection and will examine your heart and lungs to determine if any damage has been done to them. He may also take x-rays and do laboratory tests.

He will probably do skin tests, too. They will provide the clues to the cause in about three fourths of the people with asthma. They are very reliable in detecting airborne substances that are causes, but are less reliable, although still somewhat useful, in detecting foods that may be contributing to the allergic symptoms.

You and your doctor will have to play the Sherlock Holmes–Doctor Watson bit again, looking for telltale clues. And it isn't always easy because asthma often has many 007 tricks up its wheezy sleeve. For example, you might be sensitive to feathers. But you say smugly, "I have no feather pillows. I have no parrots or parakeets." But! Feathers aren't always in your pillows or in your parakeet's cage. One farmer developed asthma whenever he went into his chicken coop. One little girl developed it whenever she fed pigeons in the park. And one woman's asthma was traced to sparrows nesting in vines under her bedroom window.

You must investigate your environment and activities with the same diligent detective search that we outlined for investigating food allergies and hayfever. Look over these chapters again for some clues to what might be causing the asthma.

Dr. Bernard Berman and Dr. James J. A. Cavanaugh, two allergists from Boston, Massachusetts, outlined one way to visualize the many problems and causes that may be factors in bronchial asthma. Here is what they suggested at an exhibit at an American Medical Association meeting for investigating asthma in children. You can adapt it to your own circumstances.

Try to visualize the many problems that may arise as a consequence of an unsatisfactory allergic environment.

BEDROOM—The rug in the child's room may have a hair pad.

PLAYROOM—A favorite old chair may have down cushions.

PARENTS' BEDROOM—The youngsters may watch TV from the parents' bed which has feather pillows.

PETS, AT HOME OR IN GRANDPARENTS' HOME—"Pets" mean cats and dogs to some parents—we mean any fur- or feather-bearing animal.

CELLAR OR ATTIC USED FOR PLAY—A damp cellar means mold, and an unused attic means dust.

FRIEND'S HOME—Perhaps there is a dog or a parakeet in a house where your child frequently visits.

SCHOOL—A kindergarten teacher may have animals in the room.

WEEKEND COTTAGE IN COUNTRY—There may be old feather pillows

and dust, or the previous owner may have housed chickens and horses in the barn.

PLAYGROUND—Ragweed or other pollen-producing plants may be in abundance around the periphery of a play area.

FATHER'S ACTIVITIES AT HOME—Father performs his own improvements, with paint and varnish fumes in abundance.

Look over the following list and check off those that seem to bring on your asthma:

Head colds
Chest colds
Overexertion
Rainy weather
Cold weather
Excitement
Worry
Anger
Sadness
Laughing
Damp weather
Arguing
Crying
Coughing
Pollens
Dust
Animals
Foods
Drugs

Of those you checked off, decide which ones are most important and give you the worst symptoms. Also before you see your doctor, try to determine what the time interval is between when you are exposed to the cause and when you have the asthma attack, and how often the attacks occur.

All of these bits of information will be greatly useful to him in tracking down your problem.

ASTHMA AND INFECTIONS

Asthma is usually caused by an allergy, but it can also be caused by an infection. Even more confusing, it can be caused by an allergy to an infecting bacteria or virus. Or it may be a combination. There are many complex tie-ins between allergy and infections.

Patients with respiratory allergy are more prone to infections. This is due partially to the fact that the mucous membranes of the respiratory tract are modified by the allergic state so that there is lowered tissue resistance, allowing infection of these tissues to occur more easily. Also, swelling of the allergic membranes may cause blockage of the nose, the openings to the eustachian tubes from the inner ear, the sinuses, and the bronchial tubes. Thus, bacteria are able to multiply in the trapped and more abundant secretions, which may lead to repeated middle ear infections, sinusitis, bronchitis and pneumonia. The secondary infection can also cause labyrinthitis (poor balance), tonsillitis, adenoiditis, sore throat, laryngitis, croup and tracheitis ("-itis," in case you haven't guessed by now, means "inflammation of").

So patients with hayfever or asthma, for example, are usually more vulnerable to bacterial sinus infections. And in sensitive patients, exposure to allergens will often trigger recurrent upper respiratory infections, as well as regular hayfever and asthma symptoms. Staphylococcal bacteria are often found in asthmatic patients and their families, causing colds, pimples, boils and abscesses.

And in just the reverse, infections can affect allergies. Infection can raise subclinical allergy to clinical allergy. It can temporarily induce a sensitivity to foods, inhalants from the air, or bacteria. A rabbit, for example, normally insensitive to ragweed, becomes sensitive to it in the presence of staphylococcal toxin given off by staphylococcus germs. Asthma has been known to follow virtually all types of respiratory infections—bacterial, viral and fungal. In fact, many times asthma follows an acute contagious disease of childhood such as whooping cough or measles.

As an example of the complex interactions, the common cold, usually caused by a virus, may be then followed by a bacterial infection which continues to produce the cold symptoms, and then may set up an allergic reaction because the person is sensitive to the bacteria involved.

If you think you're confused, imagine your doctor trying to figure out a differential diagnosis so he can give you the best advice for treating your particular case of asthma.

AIR POLLUTION

There is growing evidence that air pollution plays an important role in causing asthma. Many patients suffer attacks after exposure to smog.

In fact, recent experiments show that air pollutants cause direct release of histamine in lung tissue. Histamine release—the same H substance that is the basis of all allergic reactions—was shown to be caused by ozone, sulfur dioxide, cigarette smoke and nitrogen dioxide.

In cities across the nation our skies are polluted by the burning of wood, coal and petroleum products, the smelting of steel, aluminum, magnesium, beryllium and other metals, and the manufacture of fertilizer and plastics. Chimney smoke, open dumps, cement plants, brick and enamel works, petroleum and oil refineries, soap, paint and other chemical manufacturing processes pollute the air, while exhaust fumes pour out from railroad locomotives, ships, automobiles, trucks, buses and planes. Cigarette smoking, burning leaves, cooking, sewage disposal, insecticides, herbicides and fertilizers all add to the problem.

Pollution is getting worse, and some firm legal means of controlling it must be brought to bear on the problem.

Air pollution laws are not completely new, by the way. The first smoke-abatement law appears to have been enacted in the reign of Edward I, in the year 1273. The law was aimed particularly at silversmiths who used soft coal or peat in their shops. Control was somewhat stricter than occurs today. In 1307 one violator of the law was prosecuted, condemned and executed for creating too much smoke.

Recent evidence has shown a clear correlation between the level of air pollution and the number of days missed from work because of respiratory disorders and the number of hospital admissions due to them. The number of asthma attacks increases during smog and pollution days, and the death rate from asthma escalates as well. This has been seen in the choking, killing fog of October 1948 in Donora, Pennsylvania, in the almost epidemic outbreaks in New Orleans over the past decade and more, and during the "flu epidemics" in January and February of 1963 in New York and in recent incidents in many cities across the nation.

An outstanding example of air pollution as a cause of asthma was the so-called Tokyo-Yokohama asthma that occurred in military personnel stationed in Japan. These patients could be relieved of their asthma only by permanent transfer away from these urban areas of high air pollution.

Many chronic ailments are brought on by persistent intake of minute quantities of pollutants. Ultimately, these may involve the respiratory tract, causing bronchitis, asthma, nasal, sinus or eye problems, or they may also cause problems in the liver, kidneys and central nervous system.

The following list of air pollutants and what they can cause was prepared by Dr. George L. Waldbott, allergist of Detroit, for physicians. It indicates just how widespread the effects of air pollution are.

SOME COMMON AIR POLLUTANTS AND THE SYMPTOMS THEY CAUSE

Agent	*Source*	*Symptoms*
Sulfur dioxide	Paper pulp industry, refineries, chemical plants, coal	Pulmonary, conjunctival
Hydrofluoric acid	Fertilizer, aluminum, steel	Pulmonary, gastro-intestinal, neuro-logical, nephropathy
Carbon monoxide	Automobiles, cigarettes	Headaches, dizziness
Nitrogen dioxide	Automobile exhaust	Pulmonary
Ozone (peroxyacetyl nitrate)	Automobile exhaust	Pulmonary fibrosis, conjunctivitis
Hydrocarbons	Gasoline, oil	Carcinogenic
Chlorinated hydrocarbons (i.e., DDT, etc.)	Pesticides, rodenticides	Gastrointestinal, hepatitis, carcinogenic
Lead	Paint, coal, automobiles, cigarettes	Anemia, neuropathy
Manganese	Metallurgy	Lenticular, degenera-tive (Parkinson's disease)
Nickel	Metallurgy	Loeffler's syndrome, dermatitis
Beryllium	Fluorescent lamps	Pulmonary granuloma, fibrosis, dermatitis
Radioactive fallout	Cosmic rays, nuclear detonations	Pulmonary fibrosis, leukemia

If you have asthma and you live in an area where air pollution is high, you might consider moving, if not to a new city at least to an area of your city that has the least pollution. Many doctors have advised their asthma patients to move from the smog-polluted environs of Los Angeles. In fact, some sixty members of the UCLA medical faculty wrote to the *Los Angeles Times* that "air pollution has now become a major health hazard to most of this community during most of the year." They advised "anyone who does not have compelling reasons to remain to move out of smoggy portions of Los Angeles, San Bernardino and Riverside County to avoid chronic respiratory diseases like bronchitis and emphysema."

It may be of some help now that meteorologists are able to forecast the arrival of a period of high air pollution. When the criteria for possible stagnation of air pollutants in any one area exist, air pollution officials can transmit an alert to that area. Then the city affected can begin to use emergency measures necessary to reduce all contaminants arising from daily living and manufacturing activities. Factories and grain mills can be shut down, furnaces turned off and automobiles kept off the streets. By doing this, the rate of discharge of pollutants from industrial smokestacks, power plants, heating units and motor vehicles can be vastly reduced. However, not many cities are fully utilizing the possibilities of such a system.

If your area has such alerts, any members of your family with asthma should stay in as much as possible during one.

You can help decrease air pollution in your area by not doing any backyard burning of leaves or trash and by reporting to your local air pollution control committee any examples of pollution from smokestacks, factories, electric plants or auto-wrecking plants.

PSYCHOLOGICAL FACTORS

Asthma presents special problems psychologically over other allergic illnesses.

Fear is an inevitable consequence of severe asthma—fear of death during attacks and the fear of attacks while you're waiting for them during the intervals between. The fear affects not only the patient but also his family. There is a constant atmosphere of apprehension and tension because of the ever-present possibility of an attack—from a food, from some unknown substance in the air, from emotional excitement, laughter, exertion, or any seemingly ordinary everyday activity.

Further, time lost from work and school and limitations on activity tend to make the asthmatic person feel different or make him feel he is losing out on both learning and good grades in school and promotions on the job. He may become overdependent and preoccupied with his illness or perhaps hostile and aggressive or more easily distressed.

Asthma and other allergies can also have a direct effect on behavior by producing irritation of the nervous system, headache, fatigue and other problems.

However, as we pointed out in the chapter on childhood allergy, asthma, as other allergic diseases, is not *caused* by "nerves" or other psychological factors. Asthma is caused by physical factors. The emotions can have an effect on the asthma, however, and the asthma can have an effect on the emotions. Periods of gloom, despair, grief, loneliness, anger, misfortune or other emotional stress can aggravate asthma as they can any illness, just as feelings of confidence, tranquility and peace of mind tend to contribute to good health.

And although a person has his original asthma because of physical reasons, specific attacks can subsequently be triggered psychosomatically. For example, Dr. Harold A. Lyons and his colleagues at Downstate Medical Center in Brooklyn report that they were able to induce asthmatic reactions in nineteen of forty persons by deliberately tricking them into believing that they had been breathing dust, pollen and animal dander, when they really were breathing only air with a saltwater mist. In the same way, when given a fake treatment, actually more of the same saltwater mist, many (but not all) improved.

Every allergy clinic has many records of patients whose asthma attacks are precipitated by excitement or by anticipation of an exciting experience, even when these are happy or festive occasions that the patient is looking forward to. Sometimes patients report having a feeling of tension before they have such an asthma attack. Sometimes these predictive sensations are angry and anxious; sometimes they are erotic, with a feeling of great well-being.

Here is what one psychiatrist, Dr. Aaron Paley, chief of the department of psychiatry at the National Jewish Hospital in Denver, has to say about psychological factors:

"Asthma is never a purely psychological disease; it always has an allergic cause, although stress can bring on an attack.

"While it is true that, like all of us, the patient with asthma does have psychological attributes that can be described, there is no underlying conflict, no personality type, no special trait or family pattern that is common to and unique for all asthmatic patients. The disease is not a purely psychological entity. It has an immunological, biochemical, or histopathological foundation.

"One can do a vast amount of good for the patient by simply remembering that he is a complex, but still understandable, individual trying to get along with a difficult burden in a difficult world."

He stresses the importance of attitudes, not only of the patient but of his family, friends and doctor, all of whom may show too much apprehension, anxiety and oversolicitude, making the patient react with either self-pity or anger.

■ TREATMENT OF YOUR ASTHMA

It used to be considered pretty hopeless when you had asthma, that little could be done. You simply lived with the disease and put up with it. But now with the progress that has been made in medicine, asthma no longer need mean lifelong invalidism. Much can be done for asthma, first, to protect the asthmatic person against attacks and, second, when attacks cannot be avoided, to minimize the symptoms.

New knowledge about the disease, improved diagnostic techniques, new discoveries about causes plus the use of hyposensitization injections and modern drugs have meant new hope and a new life for most asthmatics.

The major problem now is that there are so many asthmatics who are suffering with their disease needlessly—who could be helped if they would see their doctors early and take advantage of these new advances, and who could also be helped more if there was not such a lag in facts on the new advances reaching many doctors.

Unfortunately, but true, many doctors simply are not treating asthma in the proper way. They are not learning about or taking advantage of the newest methods of diagnosis and treatment.

In fact, a former president of the American College of Allergists says, "In spite of its obvious importance, few physicians treat asthma with the same skill and confidence with which they treat diabetes, peptic ulcer, and a host of other disorders less common than asthma. . . . There are nearly three million asthmatics who are not being treated by methods best calculated to give them lasting relief."

A similar story was told by a pediatric allergist of New York to his colleagues at a recent meeting of the American Medical Association—that too many physicians are settling for the temporary alleviation of symptoms without attempting to discover the reasons for the symptoms and treating the disease itself for more permanent results.

Most asthmatics can be successfully treated by avoidance of the allergens they are sensitive to, plus hyposensitization and rehabilitation. But too many doctors are simply prescribing medication without taking the time to search for the troublemaking allergens causing the patient's asthma.

In many asthmatic children sent to allergists for referral by other doctors, we find that often no environmental changes have been prescribed to eliminate pollen, molds or dust, and that many children have animals at home or are on completely unrestricted diets. Some already have emphysema, chest deformities, the "moon" facial appearance typical of asthmatic children, and marked growth retardation.

Every attempt should be made to find the cause of your asthma so that the *right* treatment can be given to you.

There are no quick cures for asthma. It is still a chronic disease that usually requires treatment over a long period. But if you cooperate with your doctor, it can generally be treated successfully. Don't try to diagnose or treat yourself. You will be running a great risk of unnecessary illness and permanent damage to your lungs.

AVOIDING THE CAUSE

The first step in the treatment of asthma is to determine the allergen causing your symptoms. If you are fortunate, the troublemaker will be something easily avoided, and your problem will be solved quickly.

If your asthma is caused by a food, you must exclude this food from your diet. If your diet has to be restricted greatly because of your allergy, then you should work out a well-balanced diet with your doctor that will give you all the proper vitamins and nutriments while at the same time keeping you free from your trouble-food. Keep in mind that thorough cooking often makes food less allergenic. For example, boiled and evaporated milk are less likely to cause trouble than fresh milk.

If you believe your asthma is due to cosmetics, then be particularly careful of orris root in face powder, karaya gum used in hair setting and hand lotions. You may buy preparations now available that are less likely to cause allergy.

If your asthma is due to infection, then any measure that helps remove the infection will help you. This may be accomplished in some cases by antibiotics, in others by local treatment of the sinuses. Try to avoid respiratory infections by avoiding others who have such infections. Many times infections may be minimized by a series of injections with a bacterial vaccine. When influenza vaccines are available, take them to help prevent viral infections of the respiratory tract.

If your asthma is due to dust, read the directions again on how to allergy-proof your house in Chapter 5.

HYPOSENSITIZATION

If your particular troublemaker is not easy to avoid, then, as in hayfever, you will need to consider injections to build up your immunity. These are usually quite effective in reducing symptoms, but there are sometimes failures. One reason—the patient may actually be allergic to two or three allergens. If he receives injections for just one troublemaker, the others can still cause symptoms to continue.

Sometimes, too, once desensitized against one allergen, a patient may become sensitive to a *new* allergen. Hospitals report cases in which the offending allergen was quickly found, desensitization brought relief, and then six months or a year later the patient was back with an allergy to a substance not even suspected earlier.

Also there are factors involved that often make evaluation difficult. Not only may the pollen season be of different intensity from one year to the next, but the patient may be living a different kind of life, exposing himself to a different amount of pollen. During one year's pollen season he may take a deep breath and run from his air-conditioned home to his air-conditioned car and then take another deep breath and run from his air-conditioned car to his air-conditioned office. The year after he has taken his injections he may play golf three times a week and drive in the country with his car-top down and wonder why his symptoms are unchanged or even worse.

A CHANGE IN LOCATION

Many asthma patients claim that a change in climate helps them, but many others disagree. The U.S. Public Health Service receives thousands of letters every year asking about the best climate for those with asthma.

Many find that they feel better in places like southern Arizona, Colorado, New Mexico, in the desert areas of southern California, in southwestern Texas or the southernmost tip of Florida. It depends on whether your asthma is caused by a particular pollen or by an infection or some other factor. Actually some people feel better in the climate of the Southwest, while others feel worse because of the very dry air. Deserts can become extremely hot in summer, and too much heat can be dangerous to people who have heart trouble.

Before you consider a move because of climate, find out what is causing your asthma; then working with your doctor, find an area that is free of that particular substance. Try it for a temporary period before you make any drastic permanent moves. There are many examples of people who moved from New York to Arizona to avoid asthma when all they had to do was get rid of their old hair-filled sofa, which they, of course, took with them.

One kind of asthmatic patient who does often benefit from a change in climate is the one who suffers from chronic sinus or pulmonary infections and who has frequent attacks of asthma associated with cold and damp weather in the winter. For these patients, moving to a dry warm climate often helps if smoggy areas are avoided. Even in such cases there should be consultation with your physician before making a decision, and a trial period of not less than six months.

Another factor in whether a new area would improve your asthma is whether the weather conditions are relatively stable or whether changes are sudden and frequent. Asthma is made worse when there is a sudden increase in the general turbulence of the atmosphere, an influx of cold air, or a sudden sharp drop in temperature.

Sometimes a short move within the area you now live is enough. For example, if you live in a smog area, you may want to move to a part of town with less pollution. If you live on a farm and your child is allergic to pollen, you may want to move in closer to the city. If you live near a zoo and you are allergic to animals, move away from it.

Or sometimes you can stay where you are and change your pattern of living. Farmers who have trouble should try to stay away from areas in which the thresher or combine is operating and should avoid enclosed dusty areas such as the barn, henhouse, hoghouse and corncrib, especially when the dust is being stirred up. They should also see whether contact with animals is causing their problem. Many horse-sensitive individuals can ride a horse but cannot curry one or stay in the same room with clothes carrying horse dander.

TREATMENT FOR THE ACUTE ATTACK

It is rare indeed that anyone dies of asthma—far more rare than the odds of dying in an automobile accident. If you have an attack of asthma, keep calm. It can usually be relieved at home by taking medicine which your doctor can prescribe and which can be taken by mouth or by rectum. If you cannot get relief by these means, then an injection of epinephrine (Adrenalin) or aminophylline will almost always relieve you.

The essence of treatment of acute attacks of asthma is early use of bronchodilation, hydration and sedation. Patients can often sense an impending attack of asthma. And there are often certain objective factors that tend to precipitate asthma and can be looked out for, such as sudden changes in climate or temperature, overexertion, colds and emotional stimuli. Knowing these things, it is possible to begin therapy very early in an attack—in fact, almost before it begins. This is the time when an attack of asthma is easiest to block, for asthma tends to progress and become fixed once it gets fully started.

THE FIRST STEPS

At the first sign, or prodrome, of asthma, allergists usually advise patients to take a mild medication to effect bronchodilation and sedation. A mixture of ephedrine and a sedative taken by mouth is effective. Sedation, however, should not be used in asthmatic children, since it can decrease respiration even more.

While bronchodilation and sedation are being carried out, you also must think in terms of keeping the mucus loose and liquefied should an attack progress. The best expectorant treatment is to drink lots of fluid. It is extremely important to keep the mucus thin and watery. Take small amounts of liquids frequently in the form of juices, water, coffee, tea or soft drinks. Whatever fluid is used, it should be neither very hot nor very cold.

Dr. Irvin Caplin, allergist of Indianapolis, calls water *the* most important aid to asthma. "Keep your tongue wet and your urine running and you are not apt to get into severe difficulty with your asthma," he says.

Coffee is particularly good to drink because the caffeine in it dilates the bronchial tubes and makes breathing easier.

Iodide salts in tablet form or in solution also are good expectorants, dislodging the plugs of mucus in the bronchial tubes. Many tablets contain ephedrine, sedatives, potassium iodide and other substances combined.

Aspirin is a good home remedy.

Sometimes the easiest relief of all is simply to sit and rest for a few minutes until the attack subsides.

BRONCHODILATORS

If the ephedrine and sedative don't stop the attack, then a bronchodilator drug such as epinephrine (Adrenalin) should be administered by injection. In proper dose it usually gives prompt and dramatic relief by relaxing the contracted muscle bands and opening the bronchi.

Bronchodilators can be given orally in liquid or tablet form or by breathing them directly into the respiratory system in the form of a fine mist or powder that will penetrate deeply into the lungs. It can be done by a hand-operated squeeze bulb or a stream of air or oxygen, or with a pocket-sized pressurized aerosol device.

The whether, when and how often of inhalation therapy should be determined and periodically reevaluated only by an experienced allergist. Many patients abuse and overuse aerosol bronchodilators.

In fact, reports have come in recently that excessive use of aerosol sprays that are designed to relieve asthmatic attacks can actually trigger attacks in some patients. Dr. John F. Keighley of Syracuse, New York, tells of several patients in whom attacks were caused when they used the sprays. When eleven frequent aerosol users were given aerosols while their asthma was in remission, six had either severe asthma attacks or decreased pulmonary function. When the patients stopped using the spray, they had fewer asthma attacks and needed less medication of other kinds.

The aerosol hazard was discovered purely by chance. Several years ago an unresponsive asthma patient, who had spent the previous few years in and out of hospitals, suddenly improved after stopping all medication. But the man's physicians could not pinpoint the drug that had been doing him more harm than good. Then, while studying different ways of administering aerosol sprays, they inadvertently put a patient into an acute asthma attack. They repeated the procedure several times, causing a new attack each time. The doctors then brought back the first patient and had him use the inhaler. The result was his first attack of asthma in two years.

The side reactions from the use of bronchodilators have become so prevalent lately that some allergists urge that they not be used in asthma at all, nor in emphysema or bronchitis. Others feel that they can still be used, but in great moderation.

Nearly all allergists believe that the laws should be changed so that the devices are available only by prescription instead of over the counter as they are now dispensed in most areas.

Dr. Irvin Caplin warns that the bronchodilators can even cause death. He tells of a growing number of reports of high school and college students attending a football game on a cold wintry day, sniffing repeatedly at their bronchodilators to open up their lung passages, then going into a hot smoky congested discotheque and dropping dead.

He also warns that trouble can occur with the bronchodilators if people think they have asthma when actually their symptoms are from heart trouble (the symptoms are sometimes very similar). The medication can readily cause death by its effect on an already weakened heart.

Caplin tells of more than two hundred patients using bronchodilators whose asthma became more severe. Some of them were even placed on maintenance levels of cortisone, but despite this they continued having severe symptoms. When they were taken off bronchodilators, they improved very shortly and were able to give up cortisone and many of their other medications.

Dr. Sawyer Eisenstadt, of Minneapolis, Minnesota, did a similar study with forty-five patients who had chronic asthma severe enough to require regular maintenance with corticosteroids. There was often dramatic improvement after discontinuing their nebulizers, he reported, and a significant decrease in the amount of corticosteroids they needed, many being able to give up the corticosteroids completely. He found over 70 percent of the entire group were clinically improved.

"One wonders how many corticosteroid-dependent patients today would not require corticosteroids if not for the use of their nebulizers," Dr. Eisenstadt commented in reporting his results to other allergists.

Many asthma sufferers are "nebulizer clutchers," taking a squirt or sniff simply from habit, whether it is necessary or not. If you use a device more than three times a day, you are using it too much, allergists say, and you had better consult with your doctor immediately for an adjustment in your management.

One woman had hayfever and asthma for years. She was helped with hyposensitization injections, but still had wheezing when she was exposed to tobacco, smoke or house dust. When she was living with two heavy smokers she developed chronic asthma to the point where she was using an inhaler every few minutes. Her physician put her on steroids to try to control the asthma, but despite this she still became worse. She refused to give up her inhaler and was soon in the hospital with a severe attack of status asthmaticus. During hospitalization the inhaler was taken away from her forcibly to save her life. Within three days, she became asthma-free and has remained so ever since.

OTHER DRUGS

In addition to injections of epinephrine in difficult cases, aminophylline (theophylline) given orally or rectally also is effective. It is a diuretic, antispasmodic and cardiovascular agent as well as a powerful bronchodilator.

Daily doses of potassium iodide have also been of help to about two thirds of asthmatics using it.

Several new drugs are being developed and tested now that are reported as having value. One called fenspiride has been developed in France. Another called cromolyn sodium has been developed in Great Britain. More studies are being done on both of them.

If significant bacterial infection is present in either early or advanced stages of an asthmatic episode, a broad-spectrum antibiotic (not penicillin) is usually given.

Corticosteroids can dramatically relieve asthmatic symptoms, but they should not be used unless absolutely necessary because of their possible side effects. Unexplained deaths during surgery have been reported in patients who have been taking corticosteroids before surgery. And in a number of automobile accidents, victims who have been taking prolonged corticosteroids have died even though they apparently had *not* suffered lethal injury. Autopsy showed many with atrophy of the adrenal glands.

There apparently is a relationship between the long-term use of steroids and the malfunction of the adrenal glands, so that the person is unable to survive massive effects of sudden stress. Nevertheless, these hormone medications still constitute a very valuable adjunct in the therapy of severe asthma when the indications for their use outweigh the contraindications. Short-term use of steroids is not harmful. If other measures have failed to block an attack that has continued during a period of twenty-four hours, and the attack becomes more severe, then corticotropin (ACTH) or corticosteroid should be considered to minimize the attack. An initial dose is given by mouth and repeated every six hours, then is reduced so that the treatment will last only five to ten days. If, in the process of reduction of dose, relapses are noted, then a much slower schedule of reduction is employed.

The long-term use of corticosteroids is sometimes necessary, but should be used only when the patient's response to other medication has been poor.

Ways have been developed for cutting down some of the side reactions of cortisone and its derivatives in recent years so that they are less likely to cause side effects and are less likely to depress the action of the patient's own adrenal glands. By keeping the dosages low and by taking the drug at particular times of the day or even every other day instead of daily, many of the complications can be avoided. It has also been shown recently that certain other drugs can heighten the effect of steroids so smaller doses can be taken.

HOME THERAPY UNITS

When a great production of mist is required and one that can be continued constantly for several minutes, home therapy units have proven successful. Several aerosol drugs or water can be used to produce a fine aerosol mist which is introduced into the respiratory system through a mask by an air compressor or pump. The unit is small enough to be portable for visiting, traveling or vacationing. However, many physicians prefer a hand-operated atomizer so that excess pressure cannot be built up.

INTERMITTENT POSITIVE PRESSURE BREATHING

Sometimes a machine is needed to deliver air, oxygen and medicines under increased pressure. This pressure is controlled for amount and frequency—hence the name intermittent positive pressure breathing. The positive pressure helps to open and inflate collapsed areas of the lungs. It increases the flow of fresh air into and stale air out of the lungs, and it improves bronchial drainage by the increased force of the expired air. Slow, deep breathing is desirable. The mask is held firmly over the nose and the chin so there are no air leaks. The person should be allowed to stop and cough up secretions. A sitting position in a straight-backed chair enhances full ventilation without restriction of chest muscles or diaphragm movements. Treatments can be given at home, in the office or in the hospital as many times a day as indicated, but must be controlled and supervised, of course, by a knowledgeable person.

VAPORIZERS

Steam works excellently as an expectorant, liquefying mucus and giving considerable relief. Recently it has been shown that cool mist is best in the treatment of most respiratory problems. Cool mist generators can be bought for home use just as the old type of heated vaporizers were.

Aerosols of heated mist are still useful, however, when the loosening of thick secretions is desired, as in severe asthmatic cases or in cystic fibrosis. Heated nebulizers can be utilized alone or together with positive pressure breathing therapy units. Ultrasonic nebulizers run by high-frequency sound waves can also be used, and are becoming increasingly more appreciated, some physicians considering them the most effective of all.

TRANQUILIZERS

It is understandable that persons who have difficulty in breathing or other distressing symptoms of asthma will be nervous, tense and irritable from the wear and tear. Members of the family, naturally concerned with the patient's discomfort, frequently feel the tension and become tense themselves. Therefore, many physicians recommend medication to relax tension both for the patient and for members of the immediate family. Diversions of a relaxing nature, such as walks and car rides, often are helpful too.

But oversedation for an asthmatic is a serious and sometimes fatal situation, particularly if opiates or their counterparts are used. Opiates suppress cough, retain secretions and increase bronchial plugging and anoxia. They are a common cause of death in asthma. Mild sedation with barbiturates or chloral hydrate is usually sufficient to produce comfort.

All of these drugs and techniques should be used under the direction of a physician, of course. For most of them a prescription is necessary. But even if it weren't, the drugs are powerful and when misused can be dangerous. So always work with your physician. Self-medication can be dangerous in any condition as serious as asthma.

A further word of advice: Beware of patent medicines. They may be insufficiently effective or may produce serious side effects.

WHAT TO DO WHEN ASTHMA RESISTS TREATMENT OR WORSENS

The patient with chronic asthma that recurs and recurs is the most difficult to treat. It taxes the ingenuity of both the patient and the physician. An attack may last for a short time or it may persist for days or weeks, disappearing, then coming back again; or the patient may just remain in a chronic state of mild asthma all the time, hardly noticing his symptoms when he is resting, but with shortness of breath and wheezing becoming apparent whenever he exerts himself or eats a big meal, laughs, sings or becomes excited. For these people continuous use of bronchodilator drugs and antibiotics is often recommended.

Sometimes a patient will cough up yellow-green mucus, and the problem does not respond to antibiotics, expectorants or bronchodilating agents. He just cannot seem to get rid of excess mucus. Sometimes a lung lavage with salt water will successfully wash out excess mucus and will temporarily solve the problem. Such patients often get relief for months or years from a lung washout, after which the procedure can be repeated if necessary.

Many people with asthma work too hard at coughing up mucus. They cough and spit up most of the day and night, piling their wastebaskets high with tissues. The more they cough up, the more mucus is formed. Sometimes stopping the coughing habit will do more than anything else to clear up symptoms. Avoid anything that makes you cough.

Sometimes drainage of the bronchi or lungs is helpful. This requires positioning of the patient so that the head is considerably lower than the chest. The more elevation that can be obtained, the more satisfactory the drainage will be. Place the patient over four to six pillows, clap gently but rapidly with cupped hands, or with the fingertips, over the back, encouraging the patient at the same time to exhale slowly and thoroughly and to cough up as much sputum as possible. Drainage should continue as long as the cough is productive. Postural drainage should be carried out several times a day, for ten to fifteen minutes, following any type of inhalation therapy. Your physician will give you more details concerning the various positions that give the most effective drainage.

If you have been working closely with your physician and have carried out his recommendations, but your asthma still does not become better, here are several things that you and your physician should consider.

Allergy. It is possible that your particular troublemaker has not been identified properly; or perhaps in addition to the allergens that have been discovered, you may be allergic to one or two additional things. Or are you really conscientiously avoiding the offending allergens? Check with your doctor and check where your particular allergens are found. If you are allergic to horses, for example, there may be horsehair in your antique sofa that you were not aware of. Have you been taking aspirin? Perhaps you are sensitive to it. Check labels of medicines. If a label says acetylsalicylic acid, this is aspirin. Try another salicylate such as sodium salicylate which does not have aspirin's aggravating effect on asthma. Are you taking any other drugs?

Respiratory Infection. Do you have respiratory infections that are frequently triggering asthmatic symptoms? Do you have yellow or green nasal discharge or sputum that you spit up? Perhaps you should be taking antibiotics. Have your doctor check whether you are one of the very few people who suffer from a deficiency of gamma globulin. If so, injections of this might help.

Bronchospasm. Are you taking full advantage of bronchodilators, expectorants and inhalants? If you have not been using them because of gastric irritation, try taking your pills after each meal and at bedtime to reduce this problem. If you have been waking up in the middle of the night with respiratory problems, take a long-action form of your medicine which will last throughout the night and ensure more sleep and help keep your resistance from running down.

Hormone Factors. Sometimes asthma attacks are tied in with hormone levels. For women who get asthma at menopause, estrogen is often helpful. For those who have asthma with menstrual periods, relief is sometimes obtained with ammonium chloride and with restriction of salt and water before menses.

Emotional Reactions. Are you overly anxious and afraid of your asthma attacks? Are you under some particular emotional stress? Try to relax more and ease up on the worrying and tension if possible. Solve the problems that can be solved and try to float over the ones that cannot. Have your doctor check into the drugs that you might be taking for bronchodilation. Sometimes they can cause excessive nervous stimulation.

A relaxed mental state will help in both preventing and shortening attacks. Worrying about asthma won't help, but relaxing and *not* worrying about it *will* help. For those who have emotional problems that have resulted from their long-standing illness, help from a psychologist or psychiatrist can be of aid.

Acidosis. Sometimes your blood and body fluids become acid during an attack because the exchange of gases through your lungs is not complete. This may reduce responsiveness to epinephrine and other drugs. Blood studies will clarify the problem.

Dehydration. In a severe attack guard against dehydration that reduces the effectiveness of expectorants. See that you get plenty of fluids.

WHAT YOU SHOULD DO WHEN YOU GET A COLD

One of the major problems in the management of asthma is upper respiratory infections because they usually act as a precipitating factor, triggering the patient into an asthma attack. Many allergists feel that it is very important to try to abort a cold the minute you realize it's coming on. The first thing to do when you feel the beginnings of a stuffy, runny nose or itchy watery eyes is to determine whether you are having an allergic reaction or are actually catching a cold. If you think it is an allergy attack, then you should take your medication and prepare to keep the oncoming asthma under control.

However, if you feel achy, with a sore throat and a fever, and you look sick, or if you have been exposed to the flu or a cold among family or friends, then you probably have a viral or bacterial infection working. Ordinarily physicians do not believe in giving antibiotics for simple respiratory infections. However, in asthma patients, since the infections do set off more serious complications, they sometimes recommend taking antibiotics. Antibiotics are not effective against viruses, but some physicians believe in giving antibiotics anyway, even with flu, to prevent the further secondary infection that often occurs with bacteria. If the infection is bacterial, the antibiotic will be able to begin its work right away. Sometimes a physician will give you a prescription for an antibiotic to have filled and have on hand so that no matter what time of day or night you feel a cold coming on, you have an antibiotic ready to use without waiting.

Different antibiotics should be alternated for different episodes of colds to decrease chances of your becoming sensitive to one of the antibiotic drugs and so your bacteria do not acquire a resistance to one drug. You should not use penicillin. You should never suck lozenges or troches containing any antibiotics. And you should not use any ointments or salves containing sulfa, penicillin, mycins or other antibiotics. They are all notorious for inducing drug sensitivity.

Also when you feel a cold coming on, many physicians recommend that you do deep breathing exercises as often as you can. If you usually do them twice a day, do them four times a day.

One controversial treatment for colds caused by virus is the administration of high doses of vitamin C. Although there is a great deal of controversy over the value of vitamin C for colds, some doctors attest to its value.

Dr. H. Curtis Wood, Jr., of Philadelphia, for example, says that he has prescribed high doses of vitamin C to hundreds of patients with very effective results. Other physicians deprecate its value completely.

Dr. Wood recommends taking 500 mg of vitamin C as soon as cold symptoms start, continuing every two hours until the symptoms improve, usually on the second day, then reducing treatment to every four hours. The third day, the symptoms should be gone, but take 500 mg two or three times during the day. For children, use half the dosage.

A great number of people are deficient in vitamin C, and the problem is especially bad in smokers, since nicotine destroys vitamin C. Some physicians recommend that smokers take 250 mg of vitamin C for each 10 cigarettes they smoke to keep their body levels up and help prevent colds.

Regular vitamins taken every day can also help in preventing colds. A survey in Philadelphia of 500 known users of vitamin and food supplements showed that most people who had four to five colds a year before taking vitamins became free of them or had less severe colds after they began daily vitamin and mineral supplements.

If a person usually develops asthma after a cold, some physicians recommend that he have an immediate intramuscular injection of epinephrine at the beginning of a cold. It will usually prevent the asthma, although it won't affect the cold.

If you are in the habit of taking aspirins for colds, take great care. Many people are sensitive to aspirin, and so by its own allergenic properties it can cause asthma. Secondly, it inhibits certain enzymes and so may contribute to increased spasm of the bronchial tubes in the chest, making the asthma worse. It can also increase symptoms by causing vasodilation and secretion of mucus. Frequent ingestion of aspirins has also been shown to contribute to the development of ulcers.

For the asthmatic person who often gets colds, bacterial vaccines can be very valuable. They don't prevent every cold, but they do an excellent job of minimizing most of them and avoiding the complications of respiratory infections such as sinusitis, bronchitis and bronchial pneumonia.

The bacterial vaccine, usually made of a number of common bacteria, is also very effective against infectious asthma itself. Dr. Harry Mueller, chief of allergy at Children's Hospital Medical Center, Boston, reports 80 percent effectiveness. Treatment with this bacterial vaccine takes about three years of injections. In 75 percent of the patients marked improvement appeared within four months. At the end of three years, two thirds of the patients were completely free of asthma, and others averaged less than one mild attack a year. Most had continued good results even a year after the vaccination was stopped. The beneficial effects were also corroborated in animal studies. At the Second International Symposium on Pediatric Allergy held in Mexico City, Dr. A. Eisen, chief of children's allergy at Montreal Children's Hospital, reported that the bacterial vaccines were effective in rabbits.

It also benefits asthma patients to take advantage of flu vaccines when they are made available, usually in the fall or early winter.

HYPNOSIS TREATMENT

Hypnosis has been successful for a few allergists in treating asthma patients. One Boston allergist claims to have regressed patients under hypnosis to infantile breathing patterns, and he was able to terminate asthma attacks in just a few minutes without the use of drugs. When the asthma is caused by pollen or infection, however, there is little response to hypnosis or any tranquilizing agents.

Dr. Raymond L. LaScola, a pediatrician of Santa Monica, California, says he treats twenty-five to thirty patients with severe refractory asthma each year with hypnosis. He includes instruction in autohypnosis. Following therapy, he reports, they usually need no medication at all, and rarely have another attack. During the first one-hour session and two or three half-hour sessions after that, he explains the physiology of an asthma attack to the patient and the role of emotional factors. Then he teaches the patient how to make himself relax by autohypnosis to control the wheezing. Other physicians who have watched his demonstrations report that patients hypnotized during an attack usually have complete relief within fifteen minutes.

However, both allergists and psychiatrists warn against the indiscriminate use of hypnosis, and of course it should not be used to treat asthma unless under the direction of a physician.

ELECTROSLEEP THERAPY

Electrically induced sleep therapy, much publicized in Russia, has now been tried in several other countries. Electrodes from a simple battery-operated apparatus are attached to the head and neck, sometimes throughout the night. Studies at Tel Hashomer Hospital, Tel Aviv, and at Hadassah-Hebrew University Medical School, Jerusalem, show promising results in asthma. Many patients, especially children, with severe or intractable bronchial asthma get a "long-term and beneficial effect," reports Dr. Israel Glazer there.

The studies are still experimental.

GLOMECTOMY

There is still controversy over surgery to remove the carotid body, (glomus caroticum), a small structure in the neck, to treat asthma.

Most studies indicate glomectomy to be of little or no value, but some surgeons still remove the carotid body, and the American Academy of Allergy still receives inquiries about the procedure from patients and physicians.

In an attempt to settle the matter once and for all, the Research Council of the Academy organized a special glomectomy study group a few years ago. The fourteen-man team of investigators from the

United States and Canada concluded in their official report that glomectomy *is not* an effective therapeutic measure in the treatment of asthma.

An estimated 5,000 to 10,000 glomectomies have been performed in the United States since the technique was introduced in Japan during the late 1940s. A few surgeons are still performing a number each year, but most surgeons feel it is without value. It has been abandoned by the Japanese surgeon who initially introduced it.

One proponent of the procedure, Dr. Richard H. Overholt, who pioneered the technique in this country, says, however, in a series of more than 1,600 glomectomies for asthma he observed long-term improvement in about one third of his patients. Another one third showed "some improvement." No improvement occurred in the remaining one third.

Asked to comment on the controversial procedure, Dr. Overholt said, "We are continuing to employ this method," although "we are up in the air as to why it helps some people."

■ ASTHMA AND EXERCISE

Many people used to believe that victims of asthma must be lifelong invalids. They were often routinely put to bed, kept away from school and work, forced to live restricted lives. Fortunately this is no longer the case. Work, normal activity and exercise are all part of the regular day of asthmatic people receiving modern treatment.

In fact, body-building exercises and activities are one of the do-it-yourself things that seem to help asthma.

At National Jewish Hospital in Denver the value of exercise was assessed in asthma patients aged fifteen to thirty-five who had failed to respond to other treatment. Every day they did calisthenics for one hour: push-ups, sit-ups, weight-lifting, pedaling a bicycle. For the second hour they played competitive sports such as basketball. A second control group of patients participated only in routine hospital activities without additional physical exercise. At the end of three months the groups exchanged places.

Result: Three out of every four patients were better able to use oxygen after the exercising. None of the patients showed harmful effects.

However, there is still controversy over the real value of planned exercising. Many doctors say it helps. Others say if you do it for fun, fine; but it doesn't really improve the asthma. The answer is still not known.

There is less controversy over the value of breathing exercises. Most allergists feel they are of value. Asthmatics frequently lose the mobility of the chest. Elasticity of the lung tissue is lost, muscles of the chest and diaphragm are affected, and the rib cage becomes rigid. Breathing exercises help counteract this and improve breathing.

Breathing exercises are especially good in early cases of asthma before the chest muscles have been altered by the overdistention of the lungs, so best results are often found with children, although adults can be helped also. Only patients with far-advanced obstructive lung disease cannot be helped with the exercises. In fact, these conditions could be aggravated by the exercises.

Dr. Bernard T. Fein, chief of the allergy clinic of the Veterans Administration office in San Antonio, has used breathing exercises extensively in his patients. He says, "Without exercises, the breathing of the asthmatic tends to become shallow and rapid, with difficulty on expansion. The breathing is entirely in the upper chest. We believe that reeducation of the asthmatic patient in breathing is possible, with the lower chest expanding almost to its maximum after good training." The exercises often make it possible to reduce medications, he says.

Exercises don't help during an attack, but are useful when done routinely over a long time to prevent attacks.

The exercises should be done for about ten minutes, three or four times a day, changed later to twenty minutes twice a day. When the exercises have been mastered, which usually requires two or three months, the exercise periods may be reduced to five minutes daily. They should be continued for at least a year.

The following exercises have been found beneficial to asthma patients.

DIAPHRAGMATIC BREATHING

Before beginning the exercise, blow your nose to ensure a clear airway. Lie on your back with your knees drawn up and one hand resting over your chest. Complete relaxation is essential. As the object of the exercise is to empty the lungs, each exercise begins with a short sniff through the nose followed by a long expiration through the mouth, making an F or S sound with the lips and teeth.

Exhale slowly while gently "sinking" the chest as much as possible and then the upper part of the abdomen. Following expiration, the fingers rest lightly on the upper abdomen or lower front margins of the ribs.

Relax the upper part of the abdomen so that it and the lower chest are felt to expand slightly while air is inhaled through the nose quickly but silently. The chest is not raised. The exercise is repeated eight to sixteen times with rest as needed and should be practiced frequently—as often as you think of it—throughout the day.

BREATHING AGAINST RESISTANCE

To learn synchronization of abdominal and diaphragmatic breathing, place a medium-sized book or weight on the abdomen just below the first ribs. The book gently rises and falls with inhalation and exhalation. Under the book is where the diaphragm is.

Elevate the foot of the bed or use a tilt board to encourage diaphragmatic breathing without conscious effort. Then lying flat in bed, place a weighted object on the abdomen. Start with a 15-pound shot or sandbag, or books, and gradually increase the weight to 20, 25, 30 pounds. Make the stomach push the weight upward when breathing in, let it fall back when breathing out. The increase in weight over a period of time strengthens the inspiratory diaphragmatic contraction.

MOBILITY EXERCISES

These exercises are to assist the return of a "barrel chest" to its normal size and shape.

Stand with your arms swinging loosely and rotate the trunk to each side, twisting your body rhythmically as far as you can.

Then still standing, alternately bend to each side.

Also standing, swing the arms rhythmically in a circle in front of and close to the trunk in a windmill fashion.

STRAIGHT-LEG RAISING

Lie on your back, a small pillow under your head. Keep the knee straight and raise one leg from the floor or bed until it reaches about a 45-degree angle. Repeat with the other leg.

EXERCISES FOR ASTHMA PATIENTS

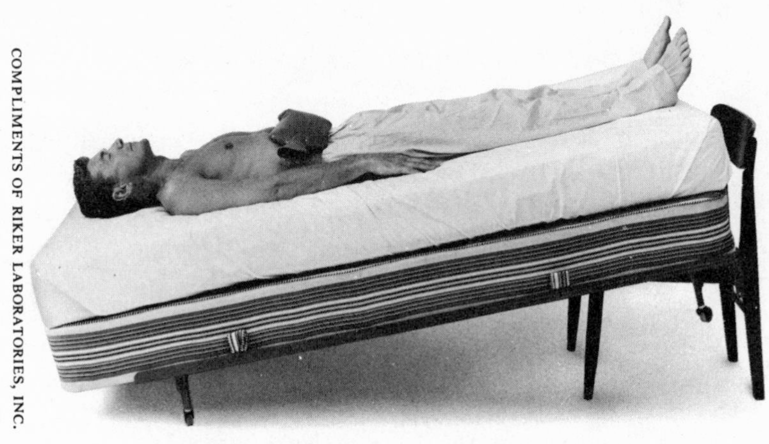

COMPLIMENTS OF RIKER LABORATORIES, INC.

BREATHING AGAINST RESISTANCE

Then continue slowly to raise first one leg and then the other, but exhale as you raise the leg and inhale as you lower the leg.

HEAD AND SHOULDER RAISING

Still lying on your back, raise head and shoulders off the floor or bed and exhale while raising them and inhale while lowering them to the starting position.

SIDE EXPANSION BREATHING

This exercise may be done sitting with the back against a support or while lying on your back. Place your hands with the little fingers resting on the lowest ribs. Keep the shoulders down during the exercises. Begin with a short sniff through the nose.

Breathe out slowly through the mouth, first sinking the chest as much as possible, then the lower ribs, and, finally, squeezing the ribs to help expel the air from the lungs. Repeat eight to sixteen times, with rest when necessary. This exercise may be modified by the use of a belt instead of the hands for pressure over the lower ribs. The loose ends of the belt are grasped with the hands and pulled together, exerting an even compression of the lower ribs.

ELBOW CIRCLING EXERCISE

This exercise is done between breathing exercises in the sitting position. The fingers are placed on the shoulders with the elbows kept parallel to the floor. Move the elbows in circles, forward, up and back and down. Movement must take place in the shoulder joints and not in the back.

FORWARD BENDING

This encourages relaxation and counteracts tenseness.

Sit with the arms relaxed at the sides. Breathe out slowly while dropping the head. Sink your chest and bend forward until your head is above or between your knees. Contract the abdominal muscles firmly during the last part of the bending.

Breathe in gradually while raising the body so that your hips come back first, followed by the back, shoulders, neck and finally the head.

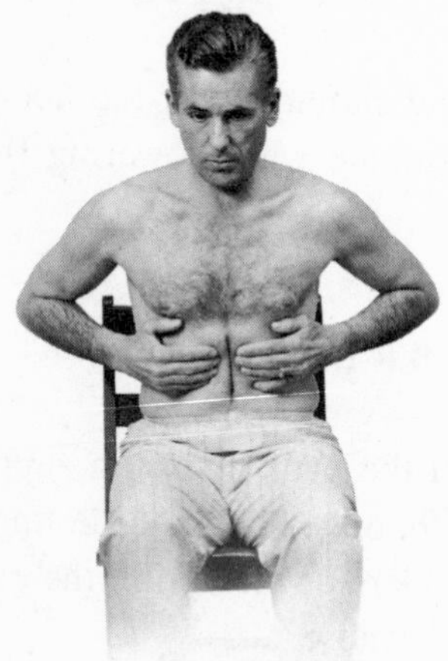

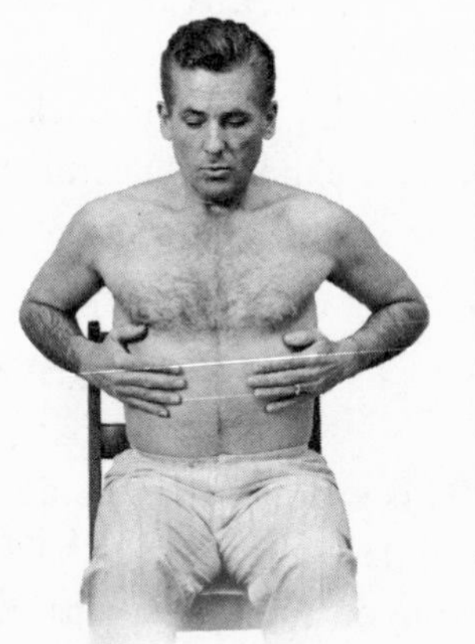

COMPLIMENTS OF RIKER LABORATORIES, INC.

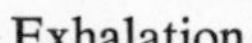

Exhalation Inhalation

SIDE EXPANSION BREATHING

POSTURE EXERCISES

Stand with your back against a door or similar support. In a relaxed manner, bend down and breathe out diaphragmatically. Then raise yourself slowly, uncurling your spine and trying to flatten your back, shoulders and neck against the door. The abdominal muscles remain contracted to press back the lower spine against the door and only relax when this area has been uncurled.

WALKING WITH OXYGEN

Exercise tolerance can be restored by performing a program of walking exercises while inhaling oxygen from a portable oxygen tank to develop breathing muscles. Walk 50 to 100 steps while inhaling oxygen; then walk half that number of steps without oxygen. Over a period of 10 days the number of steps is gradually increased to 1,000 steps with and 500 steps without oxygen twice daily. Thereafter, decrease the number of steps taken while breathing oxygen; increase breathing air. This program is first begun walking on a level, then on an incline, and, after two weeks, climbing stairs.

PURSED-LIP BREATHING

Slow exhalation with the lips partly closed, after a full deep breath, requires increased effort of the muscles between the lower ribs and of the upper abdomen, and helps empty the lungs of stale air.

A. Place a candle on a table and adjust the height of the wick to the level of your mouth; use books to raise it to the proper height. The flame should be about six inches from your lips. Place both hands on the upper abdomen. Inhale deeply, pressing your hands inward and upward and blow against the flame so as to bend it without extinguishing the candle. Do this exercise for five minutes once or twice daily. Increase the candle distance two to four inches each day until you are able to bend the flame at thirty-six inches.

B. Place a blanket on a table and roll the edges so as to form a small curb on either side. Place two or three ping-pong balls on the blanket near you. Sit or kneel so that your chin is slightly above the level of the table. Inhale deeply, and blow against the balls with long continuous exhalations to blow the balls to the far side of the table. Children may stand up for this exercise. Keep the shoulders down rather than hunched up.

C. Fill a drinking glass with water about one-third full. Place a straw in the water and blow bubbles, using abdominal breathing. Do this for three minutes, three or four times daily.

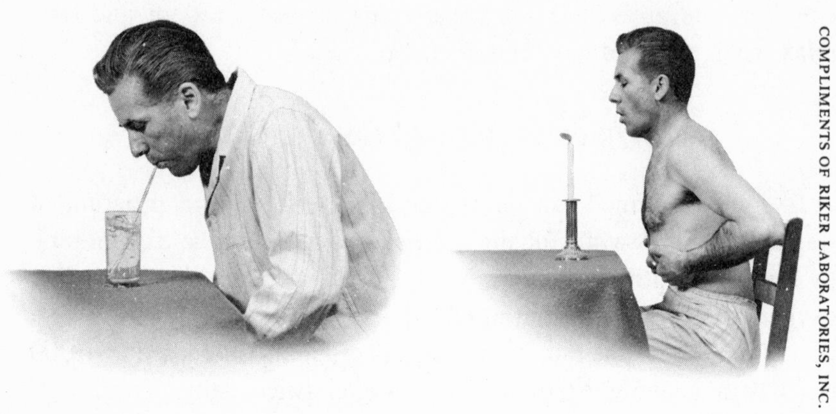

COMPLIMENTS OF RIKER LABORATORIES, INC.

PURSED LIP BREATHING

GENERAL INSTRUCTIONS

You should constantly remind yourself to maintain good posture.

Use pursed-lip breathing during activities such as shaving, washing, walking, driving the car. Squeeze the excess air from your chest while exhaling through pursed lips.

Leaning forward in the sitting position increases intra-abdominal pressure to push the diaphragm up during expiration to help breathing. The leaning-forward position may also be assumed when standing or walking. Breathe with the diaphragm at all times and assume the leaning-forward position as often as possible during the day's activities.

Some patients derive considerable benefit from wearing a special Gordon-Barach abdominal belt. The belt overcomes the depression of the diaphragm caused by the downward pull of your abdominal viscera when you sit upright. You can determine whether you will benefit from a surgical belt by walking briskly until short of breath. Then have someone stand behind you and lift your lower abdomen against the diaphragm, holding it there for twenty to thirty seconds. If relief of difficult breathing occurs with the manual support, the surgical belt is definitely indicated.

■ GENERAL ADVICE ON PREVENTION OF ATTACKS

A good deal can be done to prevent attacks.

Keep in generally good physical condition. Try to avoid colds and respiratory infections and take prompt and adequate treatment if a cold threatens. Avoid extremes of heat and cold and dampness, and if you must go out in inclement weather, dress warmly. The asthmatic person does not tolerate cold weather as well as the average person. You should wear a hat in cold weather, and when you jump out of bed in the morning, don't jump onto a cold floor. This will often precipitate an attack. Have a throw rug at the side of the bed or keep your slippers and robe ready. Keep the windows in the bedroom closed at night, and don't allow the room to get colder than 65 degrees.

On the other hand, air that is too dry, as in many homes in the winter, may be harmful. The linings of the upper and lower respiratory tract become parched. Try for a relative humidity of 45 to 50 percent.

Infected teeth, infected sinuses and adenoids should be cleared up. The diet should be as well balanced and nutritious as possible, with foods selected to compensate for any allergic food which is being eliminated. Keep away from paint fumes, dust and tobacco smoke that may irritate the bronchial tubes.

Get enough exercise. In persistent or severe asthma, exercise should be moderate. In mild asthma or between infrequent attacks, all sports are permissible. Check with your physician.

Get plenty of rest. Enteric-coated tablets containing theophylline, ephedrine and phenobarbital can be prescribed by your physician to give comfort at night.

If you have asthma, you should give up cigarette smoking absolutely, completely, permanently, irrevocably.

Also to cut down emotional factors try to arrange your life so as to be relatively free from emotional strain and anxiety; try to develop the capacity to take things easy, to worry less.

■ ASTHMA AND ALCOHOL

There is disagreement as to whether persons with asthma should give up alcohol or not. The type of alcohol is one factor. If, for example, a person is allergic to corn, then bourbon, which is made from corn, might trigger his attacks. If he were allergic to malt, then beer would give him trouble. Alcohol can also make allergy attacks worse if you drink at the same time that you eat some food that you're allergic to because alcohol hastens absorption from the stomach. So if any food that you're sensitive to is present in the stomach when you drink, the effects will be more pronounced. Alcohol also increases local circulation to the tissue in the lungs and so may result in more allergens being delivered to the lungs by the increased circulation.

In general, minimal alcoholic intake in the absence of specific allergy to the ingredients is acceptable. In fact, it may have a tonic effect.

■ ASTHMA IN PREGNANCY

All allergies, including asthma, are usually improved during pregnancy because of the increased production of hormones. However, sometimes the intra-abdominal pressure during the later months of pregnancy increases breathing difficulties in an asthmatic woman. Treatment is generally the same during pregnancy as any other time, with no contraindication to continuing regular asthma treatment during pregnancy unless the patient is prone to severe reactions from treatment. Then dosage must be carefully modified.

■ STATUS ASTHMATICUS

Status asthmaticus is a sudden intense and continuous asthmatic attack marked by shortness of breath that is so bad that the patient becomes exhausted and collapses.

It is serious, often leading to death.

It may occur at any age.

Respiratory tract infection would seem an important contributory factor to the development of status asthmaticus because there is a high rate of mild pneumonia found in patients hospitalized with the attacks.

As the attack continues, the patient's lungs and circulation become excessive in carbon dioxide and low in oxygen, and the body goes into acidosis. Headache and dizziness occur, and eventually the central nervous system is depressed. Heart rate goes up, blood pressure increases and then may suddenly plummet. Heart rhythms may be disturbed, and the heart may stop beating.

Because of the imbalance in blood gases, what are usually adequate doses of epinephrine (Adrenalin) do not help, and the severe wheezing and other symptoms persist. The person may become restless, agitated, incoherent, irrational and finally lapse into coma.

Whenever a patient with a severe asthma attack finds that epinephrine is not helping him, he should contact his physician, who will usually suggest that he should go to the hospital, where he can get any necessary special treatment.

■ ALLERGIC PNEUMONIA

If a person is ill with pneumonia and does not respond to antibacterial treatment, it may well be that he has pneumonia due to allergy rather than the usual type of pneumonia due to infection. Dr. Charles B. Carrington, of Yale University School of Medicine, described five such patients at a recent meeting of the American Thoracic Society. The patients, all middle-aged or older, appeared with high fever, weight loss and shortness of breath. All were severely ill, and some appeared close to death when hospitalized. When the doctors realized that the pneumonia was allergic, they began therapy with adrenocortical steroids, and improvement began within forty-eight hours. Within a week the x-rays were clear, and the patients were well.

■ OUTLOOK FOR THE ASTHMATIC PATIENT

What is the outlook for you if you have asthma, or for any member of your family who may develop asthma?

The Allergy Foundation of America says that if the onset of asthma is early in life and the disease has not been persistent for a long time, if attacks are infrequent and the management of the illness not too complicated, the outlook is good. If the asthma occurs in middle life with complications of bronchitis, emphysema, sinusitis, if it is of long duration and there is difficulty in establishing the source of sensitivity, the outlook is not as good. In either event, given a physician skilled and experienced in allergy, it is a rare asthmatic who cannot obtain relief and comfort so that he can lead a useful life.

The essential point is to recognize asthma early and take effective measures.

In the final analysis, the earlier the disease is recognized and the earlier that proper treatment is begun, the better are the prospects for controlling the asthma and permitting the return of the person to normal life.

The biggest danger is if asthma is untreated; then it may lead to chronic bronchitis and emphysema with progressive lung damage and possible death. We will look at these two conditions in the next chapter.

Chapter 7

EMPHYSEMA AND CHRONIC BRONCHITIS

"C.O.L.D." the doctors call it—chronic obstructive lung disease. It's a term that refers collectively to emphysema and chronic bronchitis, and sometimes asthma. Together these lung illnesses have become the fastest growing cause of death in this country, now killing an estimated 20,000 to 70,000 people every year.

The diseases have sprung from relative obscurity to grim prominence as their incidence has risen.

No one knows how much the occurrence of the disease has skyrocketed. Many studies are being done trying to determine the true incidence. But because these studies are done on different people in different areas, the results from the reports often vary and so the total truth is not really known.

However, here are some of the grim statistics that have been coming in. The U.S. Public Health Service reports that the number of deaths from emphysema have doubled every five years since 1945, that it is the most rapidly increasing cause of death in men over age forty. *New* cases are now *doubling* in number every three to four years.

The National Heart Institute calculates that deaths from emphysema were only around 3,000 in 1953, then climbed to 18,000 in the next ten years.

One doctor warns that it is likely that the deaths from emphysema and chronic bronchitis soon will exceed those from lung cancer, asthma and pulmonary tuberculosis combined. The deaths undoubtedly already exceed those from lung cancer.

Estimates of prevalence are alarming—some say more than 10 percent of middle-aged and elderly Americans probably are afflicted. Other investigators believe it may already be as prevalent as arthritis. Another said, "Each new report reveals an alarming situation."

The Social Security Administration now gives more disability allowances to persons in their fifties and early sixties because of emphysema than any other disease except heart trouble. They say the disease disables more than 15,000 workers a year, with the disability payments totaling more than $80,000,000 a year.

A spokesman for the American College of Chest Physicians said, "I am convinced that emphysema in some form affects about one in ten persons around the age of forty and the percentage increases with age."

A director of a pulmonary screening program in Massachusetts says, "Emphysema and chronic bronchitis have become a health problem of almost epidemic proportions."

In addition to the already alarming statistics, some physicians say that emphysema and chronic bronchitis cause even more deaths, but are often missed, that often deaths are attributed to heart disease or pneumonia when actually the cause is C.O.L.D. One group of Denver medical researchers report that the real death rate from emphysema may even be 40 to 50 percent greater than that reflected by death certificates. With autopsy studies they found that death was directly related to chronic airway obstruction in many people, but in only about three out of four of these had emphysema or chronic bronchitis been declared as the cause of death on the death certificates.

A speaker at a special conference on research on emphysema said that one large Eastern hospital had written off 30 percent of emphysema cases as heart failures and 25 percent as asthma.

So the condition may be even worse than the already frightening statistics indicate.

■ WHAT THEY ARE

These diseases are called chronic obstructive lung diseases because their main feature is interference with the movement of air in and out of the lungs.

All three conditions—asthma, emphysema and chronic bronchitis—have the same major symptoms: cough, wheezing, excess production of mucus, shortness of breath and difficulty in breathing. And all three act by slow suffocation that produces disability, debilitation, despair, discouragement and sometimes death.

Differentiating these three conditions is not easy, and the guidelines that have been published for physicians have been called a "wilderness" with confusing and conflicting sets of definitions and fuzzy areas in differential diagnosis.

For example, some physicians consider chronic bronchitis an integral part of asthma; others consider it a long-term complication, as they do emphysema. Further confusion—the British use the term chronic bronchitis to cover the same condition that Americans call emphysema.

These are the usual accepted characteristics of the conditions, at least in the United States:

Asthma is an illness in which variable degrees of airway obstruction are present. In many instances, the obstruction tends to respond to bronchodilators or clear spontaneously. The disease is common from infancy and through the teens, but can occur at any age. It is periodical and is reversible in its early stages. As it progresses, the asthmatic episodes may become longer and more severe, so as to produce more or less chronic continuous airway obstruction, cough and mucus production. This is especially so in the asthmatic over age forty-five. In this latter phase it is difficult to distinguish bronchial asthma from chronic bronchitis. By and large the pathological changes demonstrated in the lungs and bronchi are *not destructive*.

Bronchitis is defined differently by different authorities. Some use the term to refer to the early stages of asthma when the patient coughs and has extra secretions of mucus but does not have wheezing or shortness of breath. Others say that bronchitis is a result of long-standing asthma.

The pure definition of bronchitis is "inflammation of the bronchial tubes." There are so many variations to the definition that there are thirty-three separate entries for different kinds of bronchitis in one medical dictionary. It can last a short time, or be chronic, there can be coughing or spitting up or not, there can be lung damage or not. There may or may not be shortness of breath. There is excess production of mucus and an irritating cough, and the hazards of constant coughing are serious. Each repeated violent episode of coughing can break down the delicate architecture of the air sacs of the lungs and tear off the tiny cilia of the bronchi, making the person more likely to develop other illnesses and eventually shortening his life-span.

Emphysema in many ways is similar to chronic bronchitis, but the chief symptom is shortness of breath. Sometimes it is the only one. The trouble in emphysema takes place down in the smaller and finer air spaces or sacs, whereas in chronic bronchitis the blocking of the tubes and the excess mucus are higher up in the air passages. In emphysema there is overdilation and overextension of the lungs. The lungs lose their mobility. There is permanent stretching of the lung sacs and a loss of elasticity of fibers around the sacs, so that they become permanently distended, losing their balloonlike capacity to expand and contract in normal breathing. The blood doesn't get enough oxygen, and the victim becomes short of breath with the slightest exertion or sometimes even at rest.

Many patients have features suggesting a mixture of both bronchitis and emphysema, and the two may well be manifestations of the same or related problems. Because of this, many physicians feel that it is more accurate to refer to the condition as a whole, calling it C.O.L.D. or emphysema-bronchitis syndrome. Whatever you call them and however you define them, the chronic obstructive lung diseases are dangerous and of increasing concern to physicians around the world.

The result in both emphysema and chronic bronchitis, left untreated, is more and more progressive lung damage with airway obstruction that finally becomes irreversible, causing—suffocatingly—disability, then death.

The tragedy is that many of the nearly one million new cases discovered each year are discovered too late. If C.O.L.D. is discovered early, it can be treated, but in more than one third of cases diagnosed in doctors' offices, the diagnosis is late and the disability and death rates in these people are consequently high.

BRONCHIECTASIS

Another chronic lung disease that is not as common as bronchitis or emphysema, but can be a complication of asthma and other allergies, is bronchiectasis. In this condition the small bronchial tubes are damaged, and pockets of infection and pus are produced in the lungs. The person often has bouts of coughing, with or without sputum, and usually has a persistently bad breath. Occasionally blood may be spit up.

The only way to make a definite diagnosis of this condition is by physical examination, x-rays and sputum studies. Sometimes the doctor will instill an opaque oil into the respiratory system to help outline any diseased portions of the lung.

Sucking out of the secretions and pus with special equipment will often relieve bronchiectasis, but it will not cure the disease. Usually for a permanent cure, surgery is necessary to remove the portions of the lungs that contain the sacs of pus.

■ WHO GETS C.O.L.D.?

The typical patient with chronic obstructive lung disease is a man, usually white, and usually between forty and seventy years old. He is *frequently a heavy smoker,* and has been most of his life. He often complains of shortness of breath and sometimes believes falsely that he has heart trouble.

Women get emphysema too, but ten times more men get it than women. And when women get it, they tend to have a milder form. We don't know why. Very few children develop it, and when they do it is with much less severity.

It occurs twice as often in people in the city as in the country.

So far no major relationship has been found between emphysema and a person's occupation. There doesn't seem to be, for example, any excessive incidence of the disease in people exposed to industrial dust.

Evidence up to the present indicates that there are two general patterns in the development of the disease. The more common pattern involves a slowly developing airway obstruction which begins in early adult life and becomes recognizable on physiological testing by the age of 30 or 40. However, it takes twenty to forty years for these individuals to develop sufficient airway obstruction to produce chronic labored breathing. Patients with this pattern of the disease generally complain of weakness and labored breathing. A mild cough often begins before or with the onset of the breathing impairment.

The second pattern of the disease seems to begin earlier, sometimes in childhood. It is characterized by recurrent respiratory infections, recurrent airway obstruction, and early chronic irritation and coughing.

The disease never develops suddenly, but is insidious. It creeps up on people. A typical victim probably has several very bad colds for a few years, usually accompanied by a heavy cough that persists beyond the cold.

The problem that usually brings him to the doctor is that he begins to feel short of breath in the morning. He sometimes thinks he has asthma. His problem may begin with only a slight morning and evening inconvenience in breathing, then mild effort or exertion such as a short walk may be enough to bring on breathlessness. Unless promptly recognized and treated, a day-in, day-out struggle to keep the lungs functioning efficiently can develop, so that every breath requires a major effort.

The disease leaves the patients gasping for air and they are unable to fully empty their lungs so that the proper air exchange can take place. Breathing rates may almost double. The lungs may eventually be permanently damaged and the extra load put on the heart requires it to pump harder and often causes the chambers of the heart to weaken. Heart failure results.

The degree of emphysema found is usually closely associated with a person's age, the severity of the disease and the death rate from it increasing progressively after age forty until age seventy. After that, it does not change much.

The tendency for C.O.L.D. to be progressive is clearly brought out by a ten-year follow-up study of postal worker patients in London. Half of the men who were diagnosed as having C.O.L.D. were dead within the ten-year period of the study.

The outlook is worst for those who have severe breathlessness as an initial symptom.

It is important to diagnose chronic obstructive lung disease *before* breathlessness occurs and then treat it vigorously so that the physician who is planning a program of treatment may take full advantage of the reversible elements of the disease.

■ WHAT CAUSES C.O.L.D.?

There is an aura of mystery around chronic obstructive lung disease, a whole series of unanswered questions. We don't know why in the past ten years the incidence has skyrocketed so tremendously, making it the fastest-growing cause of death. We don't even know what the basic cause is or whether there are several causes.

All of us, in the course of our lives, have chest colds, pneumonia, bad coughs, heavy doses of polluted air. Yet not all of us develop the inflammation and swelling of the air tubes and overproduction of mucus that add up to chronic bronchitis; and not all of us develop the worn and stretched air sacs and shortness of breath of emphysema. Why is it that some do, some don't?

We don't know. But it seems clear that for certain people the repeated insults of years of infections and irritations in the lungs, especially by cigarette smoke, can have this effect. The person with C.O.L.D. can usually recall a long history of chest illnesses, bad air, heavy smoking and other such abuses to the delicate breathing machine within his chest. But some people who say that they rarely had bad chest colds, never experienced chronic cough lasting for years, and never smoked a cigarette in their lives may turn out to have it. Maybe their colds and other ailments were more severe than they remembered. Perhaps they lasted longer than they thought.

On the other hand, perhaps some people are particularly sensitive for some reason. Perhaps the colds and coughing spells that would do no damage to other people's lung tissues were enough to start damage to their bronchi and air sac walls. This may be a personal susceptibility, an inborn part of heredity. Some studies indicate that emphysema runs in families.

Emphysema may have some relation to the hormones and to the changes that the passage of time brings in the operation of the hormone-secreting glands of the body. The fact that the occurrence of the disease differs so sharply in men and women may indicate some such hormonal relationship.

We do know that a history of respiratory diseases is a factor, and that cigarette smoking and air pollution are major causes.

The risk of death from bronchitis and emphysema is currently estimated at six times greater for cigarette smokers than for nonsmokers.

And much of the higher disability rates of smokers and the greater number of days lost from work is due to C.O.L.D.

How smoking harms the lungs is far from clear. But one thing is known: cigarette smoke interferes with the lungs' cleaning system of hairlike cilia that line the air tubes. The cilia no longer are able to rid the lungs of germs and chemicals by the steady movement upward and outward. This interference with the natural cleaning process means that cigarette smoke stays longer against the tissues and may be the mechanism by which damage is done. In addition, dryness in the tubes and tissues is a part of the trouble for many patients with breathing problems. Smoking tends to increase such dryness.

There also appears to be a close relationship to air pollution, because the incidence of bronchitis and emphysema is higher in heavily industrialized cities. The National Center for Air Pollution Control says that dirty air is a major factor in emphysema and chronic bronchitis.

One study was done comparing emphysema in Winnipeg, an agricultural city, and St. Louis, a heavily industrialized urban community. Autopsy studies were done on 300 persons who died in each city. There was more emphysema in smokers than in nonsmokers in both cities. In fact, *all* cases of severe emphysema occurred in smokers, and only mild cases were found in nonsmokers. But environmental pollution was important too, because the incidence of severe emphysema in comparable groups of cigarette smokers was four times higher in St. Louis than it was in Winnipeg. The investigators in the study reported that "these findings suggested that the development of emphysema may be related to a synergistic effect of smoking and environment."

■ COUGH, COUGH, HACK, HACK, BUT IS IT SERIOUS?

Coughing and shortness of breath are not diseases themselves, but symptoms of disease that can be due to many things—something as simple and temporary as breathing in fumes of a household cleaning compound, or something very serious, such as emphysema, cancer, tuberculosis or heart trouble. Coughing can be caused by irritation of the respiratory tract by gas, dust or infection, by postnasal drip, by excessive singing or talking, or by cigarette smoking. It can even be caused by temperature extremes; hot dry air parches the throat of some people and causes them to cough, while others are sensitive to cold air and so cough during the winter. One type of heart disorder causes a cough every time it produces an extra beat. Or a cough can be caused psychologically. Some children use a cough to get attention. Other people use it as a nervous habit or as a defense against embarrassment and anxiety.

Or it can be that coughing has simply become a habit after an infection or other cause has been eliminated. Habitual unnecessary coughing often persists, for example, after a bout of whooping cough.

Sometimes when the physician cannot find a cause of a cough, an examination of the bronchi must be done by bronchoscopy. In some instances a foreign body may be found lodged along the respiratory tract. The hidden objects can often go unnoticed for long periods of time while all manner of cough medications are tried unsuccessfully.

Sometimes the cough can be caused by bronchial obstruction from enlarged lymph nodes or a cancer tumor that acts just the same way that a foreign body would in causing the cough.

Other coughs are due to reflexes from some irritant in another part of the body that is connected by nerves to the cough center. There are several such sensitive spots in the nose that can cause a person to cough. These can be stimulated by swelling, polyps or pus to trigger the reflex. In a similar manner there can be a cough due to small growths situated on the thyroid gland, at the base of the tongue or in the sinuses. One man who had a lasting cough had rounds of examinations until it was finally discovered that the cause was a hair in his ear that was tickling him and setting off a reflex.

All coughs are not alike. There are productive coughs, useful ones that succeed in getting mucus up and out of the tracheal tree or lungs. There are dry unproductive ones that are useless, get no mucus out and simply tire the cougher and irritate his throat and windpipe, and irritate the people who have to listen to him.

Sometimes patients have impaired consciousness after coughing. After a coughing attack, they feel giddy and dizzy and often temporarily lose consciousness. The condition commonly affects middle-aged, thick-set, overweight men who have chronic respiratory disease.

It doesn't matter if you cough only in the morning or only at night or only in the winter—if it has been hanging on for several months, your cough is chronic. Other signs of a chronic cough: buying a lot of cough medicine, routinely carrying a package of cough drops for a nagging hack, or considering a cough so usual that you just take a dose of medicine and forget it.

You may call it just a cigarette cough, but it can be serious. If a cough has gone on a month or more, see a doctor. If the doctor finds the cause of a chronic cough early, even if it's caused by bronchitis or emphysema, he can do something about it. He can start treatment before it becomes too persistent. If it's not serious, you will have saved several weeks and months of needless worrying.

■ SHORTNESS OF BREATH

Just as some people cough so constantly that they don't notice it, so some people are short of breath so often that they aren't aware of it. You can tell when you are short of breath when you are aware of labored, uncomfortable breathing or if you have to struggle and gasp to breathe.

Usually the breathing difficulty comes on gradually so that you do not notice it for some time. Only if you think back over weeks or months do you realize that there has been a change in your breathing. The flight of stairs seem higher now than it was a few months ago. Your breathlessness is not really new. You actually have been experiencing it for weeks, perhaps months, with it growing steadily worse for some time. Usually in the same period you have been troubled by "bad colds" or persistent coughing that often lasted long after the other symptoms. Or you may have awakened every morning with a coughing spell for months.

Sometimes shortness of breath is normal. For example, it is natural if you have done sitting-up exercises, mowed the lawn, shoveled snow or played tennis. It is natural when you start getting around again after an illness.

But normal shortness of breath disappears after a few minutes if you rest. If shortness of breath persists, it may a sign of something wrong.

Many people find themselves short of breath as they get older. Some of them simply get out of breath once in a while because they let themselves get out of condition or need to go on a diet and take off some of the excess weight they carry around. But years alone do not usually bring shortness of breath. A middle-aged or even older man or woman in good health should have no trouble with his or her breathing when walking—even rapidly. Shortness of breath on little or no exertion is never normal regardless of your age, your out-of-condition state or your general way of life. If you have unusual trouble with shortness of breath that is not due to being out of shape or being overweight or that comes at times and in activities that did not bother you before—you should see your doctor.

The symptoms are especially serious and foreboding if they are combined with other symptoms such as chest pain, cough, spitting up of blood or wheezing.

If you notice that you are becoming short of breath you should see your doctor so that the underlying condition can be diagnosed and treated. Other conditions besides C.O.L.D. most likely to cause shortness of breath are pneumonia and heart disease.

The only first aid measure for an immediate occurrence of shortness of breath is to rest. If rest does not bring immediate relief, if the shortness of breath continues, you should send for a doctor right away.

■ WHAT CAN BE DONE?

When chronic obstructive lung disease has developed, there is a distressing tendency to regard it as untreatable. But if the disease is diagnosed early enough, it can still be contained. And even in advanced cases, some things can be done to make the person feel better. Medical treatment should be started as soon as the condition is discovered, no matter what any other factors are.

This is often not done. Both the public and the medical profession have remained relatively ignorant of the advances in treatment that have been made against bronchitis and emphysema. The conditions *are* difficult to treat, but not always impossible, and the complete cloud of pessimism often found is not necessary. The new knowledge that has been obtained is often not being put to use. Communication about new facts concerning the causes and treatment of these conditions, as of all allergy conditions, is simply not effective, is not reaching the public.

Says one official report, "For more than twenty years, the U.S. Public Health Service has supported extensive research into the nature and causes of chronic respiratory diseases. However, because of defeatism and misinformation, private and public medical authorities have lagged in the systematic application of existing medical knowledge for their relief."

Other quotes from doctors in the field:

"There is great apathy among our colleagues in respect to chronic obstructive lung disease."

"The pessimism of the medical profession toward pulmonary emphysema, which has been termed 'our most neglected disease,' is unwarranted."

"The most common cause of inadequate therapy is failure of recognition; however, even when the proper diagnosis has been made, there has been a tendency to underestimate its significance and consequently to undertreat; furthermore, the therapeutic armamentarium available does not seem to be common knowledge."

"At the present time, dramatic results can be obtained in the advanced, disabled cases of pulmonary disease; however, these rehabilitation services are not yet widely available for the pulmonary cripples who need them."

"Respiratory failure constitutes one of the most desperate pictures in medicine. The need for adequate facilities to dispense intensive treatment of acute respiratory insufficiency is well known."

But progress is being made, as the growing importance of the problem begins to be recognized.

Many government and private organizations are spearheading programs to fight C.O.L.D. The U.S. Public Health Service and several national organizations, for example, are conducting a national campaign to make both physicians and laymen more aware of emphysema and other respiratory diseases and what can be done to detect and treat them. They have developed educational conferences and workshops for professional people and for the public.

Emphysema clubs are being formed so that persons with the disorder can help each other meet their special problems, and efforts are being organized to fight air pollution on both a national and local level.

SCREENING PROGRAMS

In the past few years there has been an increased interest in the use of screening programs to detect C.O.L.D., and in many communities screening for C.O.L.D. is combined with screenings for tuberculosis.

One of the first screening programs was set up in St. Luke's Hospital in New Bedford, Massachusetts. Educational and publicity programs were set up. Questionnaires were sent out that included questions on the history of cough, sputum production, dizziness, wheezing, effects of weather, nasal symptoms, chest illness, smoking and occupation. Mobile units traveled to various points in the city. Persons filled out their questionnaires ahead of time, and then went to the mobile stations for evaluation of lung function. A major test was a single forced exhalation, the volume of which was measured on a spirometer. Questionnaires and test results were recorded and evaluated by computer.

Say the directors of the study, Drs. Paul Chervinsky, Stanton Belinkoff, Franklyn Berry and Myron Stein, "Our preliminary experiences indicate that a simple and inexpensive survey program can be set up to screen patients for chronic obstructive lung disease. The cooperation of the public can be obtained."

A simple at-home test you can do is the match test. Light a match and permit the initial flare to subside; when the match is burning steadily, hold it six inches from your open mouth. Take as deep a breath as possible and then exhale rapidly in one strong blow in an attempt to put out the flame. Do not purse the lips. Repeat it several times to be sure you have made a maximal effort. Patients with advanced C.O.L.D. will not be able to blow out the match.

TREATMENT

Besides the tremendous need for community-wide screening programs to detect cases of C.O.L.D., there is a need for programs of treatment and rehabilitation of people found to have it.

Recognizing the seriousness of the problem, the U.S. Public Health Service is organizing and supporting model rehabilitation projects in communities to demonstrate the feasibility of restoring these people to normal rather than crippled lives. Physicians, nurses and technicians will be trained in modern rehabilitation techniques.

Model intensive respiratory care units are also being set up where well-trained teams can give rapid emergency treatment to save the patient who has gone into acute respiratory failure.

In Minneapolis, a successful pilot project has been set up combining home treatment programs with periodic checkups in hospital clinics. Patients receive complete physical examinations, x-rays, laboratory studies, lung function studies and exercise tolerance tests using stair-climbing and treadmill walking to determine the presence

QUESTIONNAIRE FOR C.O.L.D. SCREENING

NAME____________ AGE____ MALE____ FEMALE____ DATE____.
ADDRESS____________ PHONE______ HEIGHT______ WEIGHT______

Please Circle Below:

A—Cough

1. Do you usually cough more than once first thing in the morning? Yes No
2. Do you usually cough more than once during the day? Yes No
3. Do you cough like this for as much as three months each year? Yes No
4. Did your cough first start with (1) Measles (2) Whooping Cough (3) Influenza (4) Pneumonia (5) Chest Cold (6) Sinus Trouble (7) Exposure to Dust (8) Chest Injury (9) Surgery (10) Hayfever (11) Smoking? Yes No

B—Phlegm

1. Do you usually bring up any phlegm from your chest first thing in the morning? Yes No
2. Do you usually bring up any phlegm from your chest during the day? Yes No
3. Do you bring up phlegm like this on most days (or nights) for as much as three months each year? Yes No
4. Have you ever coughed up any blood? Yes No

C—Breathlessness

1. Are you troubled by shortness of breath when (a) hurrying on level ground or (b) walking up a slight hill or (c) a flight of stairs? Yes No
2. Do you get short of breath walking with other people of your own age on level ground? Yes No
3. Do you have to stop for breath when walking at your own pace on level ground? Yes No

D—Wheezing (If Answer to 1 is No, Skip 2–5)

1. Has your chest ever sounded wheezing or whistling? Yes No
2. Is this wheezing only with colds? Yes No
3. Is this wheezing during the day, night, or both? Yes No
4. Is your breathing normal between attacks of wheezing? Yes No
5. Did this wheezing start after hard running, after exposure to pollen, dust or drugs, after chest cold, or for any other apparent cause? Yes No

Please Circle Below:

E—Weather

1. Does bad weather (rain, fog, cold) make your breathing hard or make you cough? Yes No
2. Has smog in the air ever affected your breathing? Yes No
3. Are you worse in any special seasons (a) Spring, (b) Summer, (c) Fall, (d) Winter? Yes No
4. Does dryness of air affect your breathing? Yes No
5. Does dry hot-air heat affect your breathing? Yes No

F—Nasal Catarrh

1. Do you usually have a stuffy nose or nasal drip? Yes No
2. Do you have this in any special season? Yes No
3. Do you have this on most days for as much as three months each year? Yes No

G—Chest Illness

1. In the past three years, have you had any chest illness which has kept you from work or school for as much as a week? Yes No
2. In the past three years, have you had increases of cough, phlegm or shortness of breath for at least a week without losing work or school? Yes No
3. Have you ever been told that you had: (1) Tuberculosis (2) Asthma (3) Allergy (4) Sinus Trouble (5) Bronchitis or bronchial trouble (6) Emphysema (7) any other chest or breathing trouble? Yes No

H—Tobacco Smoking

(a) Do you smoke now? (If answer is Yes, complete a and skip b) Yes No

1. Do you inhale this smoke? (1) slightly, (2) moderately, (3) deeply Yes No
2. How old were you when you started smoking regularly? under 16, 16–20, 21–25, 26–30, 31–35, 36–40, 40–45, 46–50, 50–55
3. How many cigarettes do you usually smoke per day? 1–10, 11–15, 15–20, 20–25, 25–30, 30–35, 36–40, over 40
4. How many packages of pipe tobacco do you smoke per week? 1, 2, 3, 4, 5
5. How many cigars do you smoke per day? 1, 2, 3, 4, 5, 6, 7, 8, 9

(b) If you do not smoke now, have you ever smoked? (If answer is Yes, complete the following) Yes No

1. How old were you when you started smoking regularly?

Please Circle Below:

under 16, 16–20, 21–25, 26–30, 31–35, 36–40, 41–45, 46–50, 50–55

2. How old were you when you last gave up smoking?
   under 16, 16–20, 21–25, 26–30, 31–35, 36–40, 41–45, 46–50, 50–55
3. How many cigarettes were you smoking per day before you gave up?
   1–10, 11–15, 16–20, 20–25, 26–30, 31–35, 36–40, over 40
4. How many packages of pipe tobacco were you smoking per week?
   1, 2, 3, 4, 5
5. How many cigars were you smoking per day?
   1, 2, 3, 4, 5, 6, 7, 8, 9

I—Occupation

1. Have you ever worked in a dusty job? Yes No
2. In a mine? Yes No
3. In a quarry? Yes No
4. In a foundry? Yes No
5. In a cotton, flax or hemp mill? Yes No
6. With asbestos? Yes No
7. Have you been exposed for a period of time to irritating gas or chemical fumes? Yes No
8. Have you ever been off work for a shift or longer following acute exposure to gases or fumes? Yes No

of C.O.L.D. and to determine how serious it is. Then the patient is given training in physical therapy over a three-week period and is taught how to operate nebulizers and other aids. The patient and his family consult with the physician, the social worker and the nursing staff for advice on a complete treatment program. Then the patient is followed at regular intervals of one, three, six and nine months, with reexamination and new tests and review of home activities.

Investigators in the program, Drs. Sumner Cohen, Ambrosio Medina, Frank Mount and John Kilfeher, are enthusiastic about what can be done in at-home treatment. They said that clinical improvement was found in more than 60 percent of patients who completed one year of the therapy program.

There are many things that can be done for emphysema and bronchitis, as shown in this community program and in others.

Bronchodilator drugs can be given to open up the airways. Steroids may be prescribed when bronchospasm is uncontrollable.

If there is any possibility that an infection may be complicating the situation, antibiotics can be given. The person with emphysema or bronchitis should take special precautions to avoid getting infections, and many physicians use antibiotics regularly as a prophylactic measure. As in infectious asthma, vaccines can be given against bacteria causing infections. Yearly influenza vaccines can be taken.

A water vaporizer and postural drainage can be used. Inhalation therapy may be prescribed, including a nebulizer, intermittent positive pressure breathing, and oxygen when indicated.

Simply increasing the amount of water intake and other fluids will be helpful to break up and thin out the mucus in the bronchi and the lungs. Special medicines containing iodides are effective. Other ways to enhance an expectorant action and increase the productiveness of a cough are drinking alcoholic beverages or using old-fashioned remedies like aromatic oils and balsam. A moist warm environment helps from a humidifier, a hot shower, a steam kettle or other device to produce steam. Hot drinks and hot soups will tend to relax throat muscles and reduce irritation. Gargling with salt or baking soda in hot water helps, as does hard candy, honey and sugar in drinks. Sometimes eating a cracker or cookie helps remove tickling sensations.

Occasionally just the cessation of cigarette smoking will be tremendously beneficial, reducing and almost eliminating symptoms.

It is important to eliminate as many irritants like dust in the house as possible. Moving out of a high air pollution area helps. A change in climate helps in about half of cases.

Sometimes patients with emphysema develop giant air cysts or blebs on their lungs, occasionally up to two dozen, and they may be so large that they fill half the chest cavity. Many patients get relief from symptoms when these air cysts are removed by surgery.

The person can be taught how to breathe better. Physical therapy helps with retraining in breathing and strengthening exercises to help build the person's general health. Doctors have found that people coming to them with breathing troubles almost always are not making the best possible use of breathing. Techniques of improving posture and increasing diaphragmatic breathing are outlined in the chapter on asthma.

One physician, Dr. Harry Bass, of Peter Bent Brigham Hospital in Boston, has been rehabilitating emphysema patients with bicycle exercise. He has trained men and women with severe emphysema to ride a stationary exercise bicycle on a schedule starting with three sessions a day of five to ten minutes each and gradually building up to thirty to forty-five minutes per session. "Before the study," Dr. Bass reports, "many of the patients were immobilized to the extent that they were confined to the house. Now they are out and back to work. . . . All of the patients feel better, do a lot more and lead a better life in general."

At six weeks patients showed definite improvement, he says, and this improvement reached a peak after about twelve weeks. To qualify for this program patients must have no serious illness other than their emphysema.

Many doctors advise emphysema patients to restrict their activity, says Dr. Bass, "But I tell them to do more, not less."

The important point with all these treatments is that they begin early in the disease before serious permanent damage occurs. Even a little treatment will help make breathing easier in a mild case. Having really complete treatment will usually slow down or prevent further downhill progress of the disease even in severe cases. And if the proper treatment is started early enough, the disease can even be reversed.

Chapter **8**

CIGARETTE SMOKING AND HOW TO CONQUER IT

One of the few things any person can do to prolong his life is to stop smoking. And if you have hayfever, asthma, emphysema or bronchitis, it is absolutely *essential* that you give up smoking completely to keep from hastening your steps into crippling disability.

Not only is it known that smoking cigarettes definitely worsens lung conditions, it has also been shown that the tobacco smoke can produce an allergy itself. It can have its effects when it is inhaled directly by your own smoking or even when it is simply breathed in from other people's smoke in the room. Children, for example, are greatly affected by the secondary inhalation of smoke in the air if their parents smoke.

You may have read the statistics that more than 100,000 physicians have already stopped smoking cigarettes. Sidelight to this—almost *no* pathologists or chest specialists smoke. Day after day they *see* those spotted lung x-rays and the polluted diseased lungs at autopsy and under the microscope.

To keep you from having those black sludgy lungs, the wracking morning cough and the aggravation to your allergic condition, we surveyed the American Cancer Society, the National Clearinghouse on Smoking and Health, the U.S. Public Health Service, smoking withdrawal clinics, and individual clinicians and psychiatrists to get their ideas on the best ways to give up smoking.

Here are the ideas we were given to pass on to you. Read them over. Think over whether group therapy or individual willpower is best for you. Decide whether cold turkey or gradual giving-up is your best approach. Choose the methods that suit you best, then work at them.

■ WHAT SMOKER TYPE ARE YOU?

One of the major things to help you will be to learn just what the particular reasons are for your smoking. Do you smoke for pleasure, and to enhance pleasure? Do you do it to help ease tensions when you are feeling depressed or tense? Do you mainly gain from the manipulation and procedures of smoking? Or do you smoke strictly from habit, hardly realizing that you light up? Psychiatrists and psychologists have learned that certain methods are best for "kicking" the habit, depending on which of the reasons predominate in any particular person.

The following tests have been developed by the National Clearinghouse for Smoking and Health of the United States Public Health Service, under the direction of Dr. Daniel Horn, to help you determine which smoker type you are. Read them now as a guide.

TEST 1

DO YOU WANT TO CHANGE YOUR SMOKING HABITS?

For each statement, circle the number that most accurately indicates how you feel. For example, if you completely agree with the statement, circle 4, if you agree somewhat, circle 3, etc.

Important: Answer every question.

	Completely Agree	*Somewhat Agree*	*Somewhat Disagree*	*Completely Disagree*
A. Cigarette smoking might give me a serious illness.	4	3	2	1
B. My cigarette smoking sets a bad example for others.	4	3	2	1

TEST 1 (*cont.*)

	Completely Agree	*Somewhat Agree*	*Somewhat Disagree*	*Completely Disagree*
C. I find cigarette smoking to be a messy kind of habit.	4	3	2	1
D. Controlling my cigarette smoking is a challenge to me.	4	3	2	1
E. Smoking causes shortness of breath.	4	3	2	1
F. If I quit smoking cigarettes it might influence others to stop.	4	3	2	1
G. Cigarettes cause damage to clothing and other personal property.	4	3	2	1
H. Quitting smoking would show that I have willpower.	4	3	2	1
I. My cigarette smoking will have a harmful effect on my health.	4	3	2	1
J. My cigarette smoking influences others close to me to take up or continue smoking.	4	3	2	1
K. If I quit smoking, my sense of taste or smell would improve.	4	3	2	1
L. I do not like the idea of feeling dependent on smoking.	4	3	2	1

HOW TO SCORE:

1. Enter the numbers you have circled to the Test 1 questions in the spaces below, putting the number you have circled to Question A over line A, to Question B over line B, etc.
2. Total the 3 scores across on each line to get your totals. For example, the sum of your scores over lines A, E, and I gives you your score on *Health*—lines B, F, and J gives the score on *Example,* etc.

							Totals
______	+	______	+	______	=	______	
A		E		I		Health	
______	+	______	+	______	=	______	
B		F		J		Example	
______	+	______	+	______	=	______	
C		G		K		Esthetics	
______	+	______	+	______	=	______	
D		H		L		Mastery	

Scores can vary from 3 to 12. Any score 9 and above is *high;* any score 6 and below is *low.*

INTERPRETATION

Four common reasons for wanting to quit smoking cigarettes are: Concern over the effects on *health;* desire to set an *example* for others; recognition of the unpleasant aspects (the *esthetics*) of smoking; and desire to exercise *self-control.*

The higher you score on any category, say *health,* the more important that reason is to you. A score of 9 or above in one of these categories indicates that this is one of the most important reasons why you may want to quit.

1. *Health*

Research during the past 10 or 15 years has shown that cigarette smoking can be harmful to health. Knowing this, many people have recently stopped smoking and many others are considering it. If your score on the HEALTH factor is 9 or above, the health hazards of smoking may be enough to make you want to quit now.

If your score on this factor is low (6 or less), look at your scores on Test 2. They tell how much you know about the health hazard. You may be lacking important information or may even have incorrect information. If so, health considerations are not playing the important role they should in your decision to keep on smoking or to quit.

2. *Example*

Some people stop smoking because they want to set a good example for others. Parents do it to make it easier for their children to resist starting to smoke; doctors do it to influence their patients; teachers want to help their students; sports stars want to set an example for their young fans; husbands want to influence their wives, and vice versa.

Such examples are an important influence on our behavior. Research shows that almost twice as many high school students smoke if both parents are smokers compared to those whose parents are nonsmokers or former smokers.

If your score is low (6 or less), it may mean that you are not interested in giving up smoking in order to set an example for others. Perhaps you do not appreciate how important your example could be.

3. *Esthetics* (*the unpleasant aspects*)

People who score high, that is, 9 or above, in this category, recognize and are disturbed by some of the unpleasant aspects of smoking. The smell of stale smoke on their clothing, bad breath, and stains on their fingers and teeth might be reason enough to consider breaking the habit.

4. *Mastery* (*self-control*)

If you score 9 or above on this factor, you are bothered by the knowledge that you cannot control your desire to smoke. You are not your own master. Awareness of this challenge to your self-control may make you want to quit.

TEST 2

WHAT DO YOU THINK THE EFFECTS OF SMOKING ARE?

For each statement, circle the number that shows how you feel about it. Do you strongly agree, mildly agree, mildly disagree, or strongly disagree?

Important: Answer every question.

	Strongly Agree	*Mildly Agree*	*Mildly Disagree*	*Strongly Disagree*
A. Cigarette smoking is not nearly as dangerous as many other health hazards.	1	2	3	4
B. I don't smoke enough to get any of the diseases that cigarette smoking is supposed to cause.	1	2	3	4
C. If a person has already smoked for many years, it probably won't do him much good to stop.	1	2	3	4
D. It would be hard for me to give up smoking cigarettes.	1	2	3	4
E. Cigarette smoking is enough of a health hazard for something to be done about it.	4	3	2	1
F. The kind of cigarette I smoke is much less likely than other kinds to give me any of the diseases that smoking is supposed to cause.	1	2	3	4
G. As soon as a person quits smoking cigarettes he begins to recover from much of the damage that smoking has caused.	4	3	2	1
H. It would be hard for me to cut down to half the number of cigarettes I now smoke.	1	2	3	4
I. The whole problem of cigarette smoking and health is a very minor one.	1	2	3	4
J. I haven't smoked long enough to worry about the diseases that cigarette smoking is supposed to cause.	1	2	3	4

TEST 2 (*cont.*)

	Strongly Agree	*Mildly Agree*	*Mildly Disagree*	*Strongly Disagree*
K. Quitting smoking helps a person to live longer.	4	3	2	1
L. It would be difficult for me to make any substantial change in my smoking habits.	1	2	3	4

HOW TO SCORE:

1. Enter the numbers you have circled to the Test 2 questions in the spaces below, putting the number you have circled to Question A over line A, to Question B over line B, etc.
2. Total the 3 scores across on each line to get your totals. For example, the sum of your scores over lines A, E, and I gives you your score on *Importance*—lines B, F, and J gives the score on *Personal Relevance,* etc.

						Totals
______	+	______	+	______	=	______
A		E		I		Importance
______	+	______	+	______	=	______
B		F		J		Personal Relevance
______	+	______	+	______	=	______
C		G		K		Value of Stopping
______	+	______	+	______	=	______
D		H		L		Capability for Stopping

Scores can vary from 3 to 12. Any score 9 and above is *high;* any score 6 and below is *low.*

INTERPRETATION

To attempt to give up smoking you must do more than simply acknowledge that "cigarette smoking may be harmful to your health." You must be aware that smoking is an *important* problem, that it has *personal* meaning for you, that there is *value* to be gained from stopping, and that people are *capable* of stopping. Test 2 measures the strength of your recognition of each of these factors.

If your score is 9 or above on any factor, that factor supports your desire to try to stop smoking. If your score is 6 or below, that factor will not help you, but note that you may have scored low because you lack correct information. For every factor for which you *do* have a low score, read the accompanying explanatory material with special care.

1. *Importance*

Cancer, heart disease, respiratory diseases—all related to smoking—are among the most serious to which man is exposed. You should not shrug off the growing evidence that they cause death and severe disability. Yet you may be doing this if your score is 6 or lower on the first part of Test 2.

Research has shown that one death in every three is an "extra" death among men who die between the ages of 35 and 60, because cigarette smokers have higher death rates than nonsmokers. One day of every five lost from work because of illness, 1 day in every 10 spent in bed because of illness, 1 day of every 8 days of restricted activity—all are "extra," because cigarette smokers suffer more disability than nonsmokers.

2. *Personal Relevance*

Some smokers kid themselves into thinking: "It can't happen to me—only to the other guy." If you score 6 or below, you may be one of these people.

Your reasoning may go something like this: "I don't really smoke enough to be hurt by it. It takes two packs a day over a period of many years before harmful effects show up."

Unfortunately, this is not true. Even people who smoke less than half a pack a day show significantly higher death rates than nonsmokers. Breathing capacity can diminish after only a very few years of regular smoking. Even what used to be considered light smoking, such as half a pack a day, can be harmful.

3. *Value of Stopping*

Evidence shows that there are benefits to health when you give up smoking—even if you have smoked for many years. A score of 6 or lower indicates that you do not realize this.

There are real advantages in giving up smoking even for long-term smokers; people who quit before any symptoms of illness or impairment occur suffer lower death rates than those who continue to smoke, and reduce the likelihood of serious illness.

People who have had heart attacks and those with stomach ulcers and chronic respiratory diseases should definitely give up smoking. It is difficult if not impossible to control such illnesses if they do not.

4. *Capability for Stopping*

If your score is 6 or lower on this part of the test, you believe that it will be hard for you to quit. But you may find encouragement in the fact that over 20 million adults are now successful ex-smokers. Of these, over 100,000 doctors, well over half of those who were ever cigarette smokers, have successfully quit.

In the following Test, No. 3, you will gain some insight into the reasons why you smoke. With this new knowledge, it may be easier for you to give up smoking than you thought it would be. At any rate, you must develop confidence that it is possible for you to control your smoking; if you do not, you are less likely to succeed in your attempt to quit.

TEST 3

WHY DO YOU SMOKE?

Here are some statements made by people to describe what they get out of smoking cigarettes. How *often* do you feel this way when smoking them? Circle one number for each statement.

Important: Answer every question.

	Always	*Fre-quently*	*Occa-sionally*	*Seldom*	*Never*
A. I smoke cigarettes in order to keep myself from slowing down.	5	4	3	2	1
B. Handling a cigarette is part of the enjoyment of smoking it.	5	4	3	2	1
C. Smoking cigarettes is pleasant and relaxing.	5	4	3	2	1
D. I light up a cigarette when I feel angry about something.	5	4	3	2	1
E. When I have run out of cigarettes I find it most unbearable until I can get them.	5	4	3	2	1
F. I smoke cigarettes automatically without even being aware of it.	5	4	3	2	1
G. I smoke cigarettes to stimulate me, to perk myself up.	5	4	3	2	1
H. Part of the enjoyment of smoking a cigarette comes from the steps I take to light up.	5	4	3	2	1
I. I find cigarettes pleasurable.	5	4	3	2	1
J. When I feel uncomfortable or upset about something, I light up a cigarette.	5	4	3	2	1
K. I am very much aware of the fact when I am not smoking a cigarette.	5	4	3	2	1
L. I light up a cigarette without realizing I still have one burning in the ashtray.	5	4	3	2	1
M. I smoke cigarettes to give me a "lift."	5	4	3	2	1
N. When I smoke a cigarette, part of the enjoyment is watching the smoke as I exhale it.	5	4	3	2	1

TEST 3 (*cont.*)

	Always	*Fre-quently*	*Occa-sionally*	*Seldom*	*Never*
O. I want a cigarette most when I am comfortable and relaxed.	5	4	3	2	1
P. When I feel "blue" or want to take my mind off cares and worries, I smoke cigarettes.	5	4	3	2	1
Q. I get a real gnawing hunger for a cigarette when I haven't smoked for a while.	5	4	3	2	1
R. I've found a cigarette in my mouth and didn't remember putting it there.	5	4	3	2	1

HOW TO SCORE:

1. Enter the numbers you have circled to the Test 3 questions in the spaces below, putting the number you have circled to Question A over line A, to Question B over line B, etc.
2. Total the 3 scores on each line to get your totals. For example, the sum of your scores over lines A, G, and M gives you your score on *Stimulation*—lines B, H, and N gives the score on *Handling*, etc.

						Totals
____ A	+	____ G	+	____ M	=	____ Stimulation
____ B	+	____ H	+	____ N	=	____ Handling
____ C	+	____ I	+	____ O	=	____ Pleasurable Relaxation
____ D	+	____ J	+	____ P	=	____ Crutch: Tension Reduction
____ E	+	____ K	+	____ Q	=	____ Craving: Psychological Addiction
____ F	+	____ L	+	____ R	=	____ Habit

Scores can vary from 3 to 15. Any score 11 and above is *high;* any score 7 and below is *low*.

INTERPRETATION

This test will help you identify what you use smoking for and what kind of satisfaction you think you get from smoking.

The six factors measured by this test describe one or another way of experiencing or managing certain kinds of feelings. Three of these feeling-states represent the *positive* feelings people get from smoking: (1) a sense of increased energy or *stimulation,* (2) the satisfaction of *handling* or manipulating things, and (3) the enhancing of *pleasurable feelings* accompanying a state of well being. The fourth is the *decreasing of negative feelings* by reducing a state of tension or feelings of anxiety, anger, shame, etc. The fifth is a complex pattern of increasing and decreasing "craving" for a cigarette representing a psychological *addiction* to cigarettes. The sixth is *habit* smoking which takes place in an absence of feeling—purely automatic smoking.

A score of 11 or above on any factor indicates that this factor is an important source of satisfaction for you. The higher your score (15 is the highest), the more important a particular factor is in your smoking and the more useful the discussion of that factor can be in your attempt to quit.

A few words of warning: If you give up smoking, you may have to learn to get along without the satisfactions that smoking gives you. Either that, or you will have to find some more acceptable way of getting this satisfaction. In either case, you need to know just what it is you get out of smoking before you can decide whether to forgo the satisfactions it gives you or to find another way to achieve them.

1. *Stimulation*

If you score high or fairly high on this factor, it means that you are one of those smokers who is stimulated by the cigarette—you feel that it helps wake you up, organize your energies, and keep you going. If you try to give up smoking, you may want a safe substitute: A brisk walk or modest exercise, for example, whenever you feel the urge to smoke.

2. *Handling*

Handling things can be satisfying, but there are many ways to keep hands busy without lighting up or playing with a cigarette. Why not toy with a pen or pencil? Or try doodling. Or play with a coin, a piece of jewelry, or some other harmless object.

There are plastic cigarettes to play with, or you might even use a real cigarette if you can trust yourself not to light it.

3. *Accentuation of Pleasure—Pleasurable Relaxation*

It is not always easy to find out whether you use the cigarette to feel *good,* that is, get real, honest pleasure out of smoking (Factor 3) or to keep from feeling so *bad* (Factor 4). About two-thirds of smokers score high or fairly high on *accentuation of pleasure,* and about half of those also score as high or higher on *reduction of negative feelings.*

Those who do get real pleasure out of smoking often find that an honest consideration of the harmful effects of their habit is enough to help them quit. They substitute eating, drinking, social activities, and physical activities—within reasonable bounds—and find they do not seriously miss their cigarettes.

4. *Reduction of Negative Feelings, or "Crutch"*

Many smokers use the cigarette as a kind of crutch in moments of stress or discomfort, and on occasion it may work; the cigarette is sometimes used as a tranquilizer. But the heavy smoker, the person who tries to handle severe personal problems by smoking many times a day, is apt to discover that cigarettes do not help him deal with his problems effectively.

When it comes to quitting, this kind of smoker may find it easy to stop when everything is going well, but may be tempted to start again in a time of crisis.

Again, physical exertion, eating, drinking, or social activity—in moderation—may serve as useful substitutes for cigarettes, even in times of tension. The choice of a substitute depends on what will achieve the same effect without having any appreciable risk.

5. *"Craving" or Psychological Addiction*

Quitting smoking is difficult for the person who scores high on this factor, that of *psychological addiction.* For him, the craving for the next cigarette begins to build up the moment he puts one out, so tapering off is not likely to work. He must go "cold turkey."

It may be helpful for him to smoke more than usual for a day or two, so that the taste for cigarettes is spoiled, and then isolate himself completely from cigarettes until the craving is gone. Giving up cigarettes may be so difficult and cause so much discomfort that once he does quit, he will find it easy to resist the temptation to go back to smoking because he knows that some day he will have to go through the same agony again.

6. *Habit*

This kind of smoker is no longer getting much satisfaction from his cigarettes. He just lights them frequently without even realizing he is doing so. He may find it easy to quit and stay off if he can break the habit patterns he has built up. Cutting down gradually may be quite effective if there is a change in the way the cigarettes are smoked and the conditions under which they are smoked. The key to success is becoming *aware* of each cigarette you smoke.

TEST 4

DOES THE WORLD AROUND YOU MAKE IT EASIER OR HARDER TO CHANGE YOUR SMOKING HABITS?

Indicate by circling the appropriate numbers whether you feel the following statements are true or false.

Important: Answer every question.

	true or mostly true	*false or mostly false*
A. Doctors have decreased or stopped their smoking of cigarettes in the past 10 years.	2	1
B. In recent years there seem to be more rules about where you are allowed to smoke.	2	1
C. Cigarette advertising makes smoking appear attractive to me.	1	2
D. Schools are trying to discourage children from smoking.	2	1
E. Doctors are trying to get their patients to stop smoking.	2	1
F. Someone has recently tried to persuade me to cut down or quit smoking cigarettes.	2	1

TEST 4 (*cont.*)

	true or mostly true	*false or mostly false*
G. The constant repetition of cigarette advertising makes it hard for me to quit smoking.	**1**	**2**
H. Both government and private health organizations are actively trying to discourage people from smoking.	**2**	**1**
I. A doctor has, at least once, talked to me about my smoking.	**2**	**1**
J. It seems as though an increasing number of people object to having someone smoke near them.	**2**	**1**
K. Some cigarette commercials on TV make me feel like smoking.	**1**	**2**
L. Congressmen and other legislators are showing concern with smoking and health.	**2**	**1**

M. The people around you, particularly those who are close to you (e.g., relatives, friends, office associates), may make it easier or more difficult for you to give up smoking by what they say or do. What about these people? Would you say they make giving up smoking or staying off cigarettes more difficult for you than it would be otherwise? (Circle the number to the left of the statement that best describes your situation.)

3 They make it much more difficult than it would be otherwise.
4 They make it somewhat more difficult than it would be otherwise.
5 They make it somewhat easier than it would be otherwise.
6 They make it much easier than it would be otherwise.

HOW TO SCORE:

1. Enter the numbers you have circled on the Test 4 questions in the spaces below, putting the number you have circled to Question A over line A, to Question B over line B, etc.
2. Total the 3 scores across on each line to get your totals. For example, the sum of your scores over lines A, E, and I gives you your score on *Doctors*—lines B, F, and J give the score on *General Climate*, etc.

							Totals
______ A	+	______ E	+	______ I	=	______	Doctors
______ B	+	______ F	+	______ J	=	______	General Climate
______ C	+	______ G	+	______ K	=	______	Advertising Influence
______ D	+	______ H	+	______ L	=	______	Key Group Influences
				______ M	=	______	Interpersonal Influences

Scores can vary from 3 to 6: 6 is *high;* 5, high middle; 4, low middle; 3, *low.*

INTERPRETATION

What will happen when you try to quit smoking? Aside from the problems that may arise within yourself because of the strength of the smoking habit and what you get out of it, to what extent will you get help from what is happening around you?

This test will help you identify which of five factors may be of particular importance to you in providing support to your efforts to quit smoking. A factor on which your score is 5 or 6 represents a part of your environment that can be a help to you. A factor on which your score is 3 or 4 indicates a situation that may hurt your chances of staying off cigarettes.

1. *Doctors*

Many people are influenced by what their physicians do and say about the smoking problem. We know that the overwhelming majority of doctors accept cigarette smoking as a serious health hazard and that well over half of the doctors who used to smoke have given it up. If you score 5 or 6 on this factor, talk to your doctor about smoking and get his support.

2. *General Climate*

A score of 3 or 4 on this factor indicates that the environment in which you live and work will not be very helpful in your effort to quit smoking. You may need to seek a more congenial environment. If so, make a point of talking to or associating with people who are trying to stop smoking or who have succeeded in doing so. Also, avoid places where smoking is permitted in favor of places where smoking is prohibited.

3. *Advertising Influence*

A score of 3 or 4 on this factor indicates that you are strongly influenced by cigarette advertising. You may have to avoid exposing yourself to these influences until you can withstand them.

4. *Key Group Influences*

Knowing the position taken by certain "key groups" can be very important for some people, and a score of 5 or 6 on this factor indicates that you are aware of the influence of such groups. Some people are strongly influenced by the actions of the federal government, some by public and private health agencies, others by schools. All these are on public record that smoking is harmful and all are engaged in programs to reduce cigarette smoking.

5. *Interpersonal Influences*

For most of us there are certain people who are particularly important to us. What these people think, do, and say can make a big difference in the way we behave. For some it is a husband or a wife. For others it is their children or their parents. For still others it is the people at work. Because there are so many possible influences, it is difficult to determine which ones are important to you through a simple set of questions. Your answer to Question M should serve as a guide in this area. If your score is 5 or 6, the people who are important to you are likely to be helpful in your effort to quit smoking. If, however, your score is 3 or 4, these important people may not be helpful unless you actively seek their support.

■ DOING IT YOURSELF

One health educator we know says that most people—if they try hard enough—can master giving up cigarette smoking by themselves. He feels that "nothing succeeds like a little willpower and a little blood in the sputum."

Actually you learned to be a smoker. You can reverse the process and learn to be a nonsmoker. If you want to do it on your own—and most people can make it this way—try the following recommendations.

Think over and actually list the reasons you should not smoke: the risk of disease, decrease in the taste of food, bad breath, morning-after ashtrays, effects on children, the fact that you may, if you continue smoking, lose six and a half years of life. Look over the list in the evening, just before you fall asleep.

Select Q Day for quitting and make preparations for it. Chart your smoking habits, making a daily record of how many cigarettes you smoke in each hour and under what circumstances. Rate those you like most, and those you need the least. You can discontinue some smoking right away by eliminating those cigarettes that are least desired. Or you may prefer the approach that has worked for some of increasing the number of cigarettes smoked before Q Day. They force themselves to increase their smoking from two packs up to four packs a day so their body is in revolt against the extra discomforts caused by smoking. Then stopping is a relief.

When Quitting Day comes you can quit gradually or go "cold turkey," a phrase used because when an addict withdraws from heroin he gets cold, sweaty, and has goose bumps all over, very much like a turkey just out from the freezer. Some people can stop this way; some people can't.

Giving up more gradually is usually easier. One gradual elimination system is to limit cigarettes at first to only one an hour. Or do it gradually by eliminating smoking between certain hours, and then extend the nonsmoking time by half an hour, an hour, two hours. Or cut in half the number of cigarettes you usually smoke in a week. Or smoke only one half of each cigarette. With any of these methods, the idea is to gradually cut down more and more and then to set a final target date after which you will *absolutely* not have any more!

In addition to pure willpower and schedules for quitting, there are other things you can do to help.

Switch from the cigarettes you like to ones that you find unpalatable and do not like.

Make it become a real effort to get to your cigarettes. Wrap them in several sheets of paper, or place them in a tightly covered box. Buy only one pack of cigarettes at a time; never buy a carton. Carry your cigarettes in a different place. At work, give them to your secretary or put them in another room. Leave your change at home so that you won't be able to use the cigarette machine. Give away your cigarettes and lighter. Put away the ashtrays.

Use substitutes. Drink frequent glasses of water and juices. Nibble fruit, celery, carrots, cookies, candy, clove, bits of ginger when you feel like reaching for a cigarette. Have something to reach for, something to do with your hands. The most helpful thing we have seen is to take four or five packages of gum in the morning, and every time you want a cigarette, chew a stick of gum.

Inhalers that clear sinuses may help you tide over the first few days. Take walks, brush your teeth frequently, use mouthwashes, lozenges and astringents.

If you can't quit completely, whether you are a man or a woman, try shifting to snuff, pipes or even cigars.

Breaking up the habit patterns and associative links to smoking is important. Avoid places, people and things that you usually connect with smoking. For the first difficult days spend as much time as possible in libraries or other places where smoking is forbidden. Don't ride in the smoker on the train. Go to the movies and the theater—in the no-smoking section—to pass a few hours. When possible, stay away from friends who are heavy smokers for the first two weeks. Some people find it easiest to give up smoking while on vacation when daily habits are not a factor.

Deep-breathing exercises often help because they serve the same purpose as smoking in giving a sense of pleasure in the chest. Take a deep breath, slowly but continuously for one to three seconds. Hold your breath. Hold it until you begin to feel uncomfortable. Then let your breath out very gradually and slowly. Do this ten or twelve times several times a day. To hold your breath even a little longer, try swallowing two or three times to keep from taking another breath.

During the withdrawal period frequently practice deep inhalations in front of an open window, or a single deep sigh once in a while will serve the same purpose. Learn to take a deep inhalation, then exhale slowly by keeping your lips together so you have to use a little force to let the air come out evenly.

Dr. Alton Ochsner, of New Orleans, says a patient of his, a prominent executive in a southern city, was a very heavy cigarette smoker. At age sixty, he felt he had to stop smoking. He tried to stop, but couldn't, and finally used self-hypnosis. He began thinking every time he took a cigarette about how horrible it tasted and how bad it smelled. Before long, he did not enjoy smoking and had no desire to begin smoking again.

■ GROUP THERAPY

Many people find giving up smoking is easier in a group situation and are helped by attending a smoking withdrawal clinic. Check on the clinics that are available in your community.

In Philadelphia every January the city has a special week devoted to smoking and health, and special withdrawal clinics are held at that time. Lung function tests are given, movies are shown, classes are held.

In New York the city runs a withdrawal clinic manned by a staff of volunteer ex-smokers.

The clinic is conducted in three phases over an eight-month period. All sessions in Phases I and II are held in a local high school in mid-Manhattan. Phase III takes place on an ad lib basis in homes, offices, restaurants, wherever small groups can find a place to gather.

Phase I begins with an evening lecture by the director of the city's Smoking Control Program and is followed by seven days of work from printed instructions. In this phase, the smoker begins the process of developing strong motivation, bringing the habit to a fully conscious level, gaining insight into some of the mechanisms supporting his smoking behavior.

Many who attend the opening session are discouraged or outright skeptical, but they are soon convinced that they possess the capacity to permanently free themselves of the habit and that withdrawal has the potential for being exciting and rewarding.

In Phase II, the withdrawal phase, smokers are placed in groups of fifteen with two volunteer ex-smokers assigned to each. These groups meet twice a week for four weeks, then once a week for an additional four weeks.

The smokers assist each other in building strong motivation and provide mutual guidance and support during and immediately following the period of withdrawal.

Sessions begin with smokers reporting on their progress (or lack thereof) since the last meeting. Each smoker's problems are presented in a "consultation session" where the group, through frank and open discussions, talk about the difficulties being encountered in withdrawal. When all have reported, the smokers develop plans for the next step in the elimination program. They work out their schedule of reduction for the next week and enter it on a smoking record card. Each smoker announces his pledge to the entire group; some smokers stop cold turkey; most choose to do it gradually.

A professional staff (three physicians, a clinical psychologist, and a public health social worker) circulate among the groups answering medical questions and assisting individuals with special problems.

Meetings are supplemented with fact sheets on smoking and health and lists of suggestions on techniques successful ex-smokers have found helpful in withstanding the urge to smoke.

In Phase III meetings are spaced at longer intervals, once a week for three to four weeks, then once every other week for five to six months. Groups meet in offices, homes, restaurants, bars, even in Central Park. The group reports to the program's central office by a large postal card on which they indicate the progress of each participant and the time and location of the next meeting. Once a month all participants join the program director for a brief talk followed by a question and answer period.

A questionnaire survey showed that in only two months following Phase II more than half the people were no longer smoking. Eighty-five percent had been cigarette-free for at least one month. Most of the others had reduced their smoking by 50 to 75 percent and had maintained this reduction.

Says former clinic director Dr. Donald Fredrickson: "As we see it—and we instruct our smokers accordingly—there are two attitude postures one can opt for during withdrawal. One is negative and basically self-defeating. The other is positive and can be powerfully self-reinforcing.

"When the smoker opts for the self-defeating attitude he tends to view withdrawal as an exercise in self-denial. He considers that an object of great value is being taken from him, one that may be a source of pleasure or a requirement for normal functioning. He feels that he is being put upon, being asked to suffer. Inevitably he feels sorry for himself, he suffers, and this suffering may become intense. The more he suffers the greater is the desire to smoke which, in turn, intensifies the suffering. This cycle results in the generation of intense negative effect that may prove too painful to tolerate."

On the other hand, he says, "When the smoker opts for the positive self-reinforcing posture, he looks upon withdrawal as an exercise in self-mastery. Rather than taking something away, he is adding to his life—a new dimension of self-control. He is teaching himself a more positive, constructive, self-fulfilling way to behave. There is evidence that, for some, development of control over cigarette smoking tends to generalize to other areas of behavior bringing, in turn, a renewed sense of one's ability and often what appears as an actual increase in one's capacity to deal more constructively with other problems of living. When experienced, this phenomenon can serve as a powerful incentive reinforcing nonsmoking behavior."

Many clinic physicians use drugs such as lobeline in addition to the techniques that the New York clinic uses; others do not. Some prescribe sedatives or stimulants, depending on the individual's need to take the edge off the initial difficult first three to four weeks. The medication is tapered off after the patient begins to get over the difficult initial period. Appetite depressants are sometimes helpful also.

Many private companies also have initiated group therapy programs to help their employees stop smoking. One company pays a ten-dollar bonus to each employee for each month that he refrains from using tobacco in any form. Another group called KICH (Kick the Idiotic Cigarette Habit) has weekly meetings with films and speakers, a ten-dollar award if you hold out for one month, a framed Nonsmoker Diploma at the end of five weeks, and a special drawing for a bonus trip to New York.

In some cities there is also an Ex-Smokers Association to help reinforce the new nonsmoking habit.

If you would like to start a club at your company or group sessions with your friends to help each other get rid of the habit, you can obtain material through local chapters of the American Heart Association, the National Tuberculosis Association, and the American Cancer Society or local medical associations. They have films, posters, payroll stuffers, and a list of physicians who will give free talks to your group.

■ SIDE EFFECTS TO WITHDRAWAL

There are a few temporary bad effects. As you withdraw from smoking or cut down, you may have constipation for a while or urinate frequently, or you may become shaky, tense, irritable or depressed. You may start to gain weight. Some people find that their coughing actually increases for the first week. Others have temporary shortness of breath, tightness in the chest, visual disturbances, sweats, headaches, gastrointestinal complaints. Don't let them alarm you. It simply is that your body is actively readjusting to the nonsmoking state.

In any event these symptoms all pass in a week or two, and are worth sweating through for the overall benefits.

Meanwhile keep reminding yourself of all the good effects. You are mastering the cigarettes, rather than letting them master you, which should give your ego and self-respect a good boost. Your appetite is better, your cough disappears, your sense of taste and sense of smell are improved. Skin circulation improves, with the facial complexion looking better almost immediately. You are less tired and are more alert during the day. You don't smell of tobacco. You usually have an increase in sexual energy. Your pulse rate goes down. You have more wind for running, tennis or other exercise, whatever it might be. Patients with chronic bronchitis, emphysema or asthma improve almost overnight and are able to breathe much more easily.

■ IF YOU SIMPLY CAN'T GIVE IT UP

Some people try sincerely to give up cigarette smoking, but simply cannot succeed. If they have been smoking a pack of cigarettes a day, they take about 60,000 puffs a year—60,000 times they repeat the same act, ingraining it into a behavior pattern hard to break. At one pack a day, in seventeen years they take a million puffs. It takes a lot of unlearning to break the habit.

If complete abstinence is too high a goal for you, there are several things—not as good as giving up completely, of course—but several things that will help a bit to cut down your risk of death and disability.

Here are the five basic steps to lowering your cigarette smoke intake recommended by the U.S. Public Health Service.

1. *Switch to a cigarette with less tar and nicotine.*

Learn the tar and nicotine content of your cigarette. The Federal Trade Commission gives the latest tar and nicotine ratings for all leading brands of cigarettes. See how your brand compares and reduce your tar and nicotine intake by switching to another brand.

2. *Don't smoke your cigarette all the way down.*

No matter which cigarette you smoke, the most tar and nicotine are found in the last few puffs. This is because the tobacco itself acts as a filter, retaining a portion of the tars and nicotine that pass through it. Thus, smoke from the first third of a cigarette yields only about 25 percent of the total tar and nicotine. But the last third yields 50 percent. So the sooner you put your cigarette out, the lower your dose of harmful ingredients.

3. *Take fewer draws on each cigarette.*

Reduce the number of times you puff on each cigarette. With practice, some people find they can substantially cut their actual smoking time without really missing it.

4. *Reduce your inhaling.*

It is the smoke that *enters your lungs* that does most of the damage. Cigar and pipe smokers are not so apt to inhale, which is probably the reason they are less likely to have lung cancer and many of the other diseases associated with cigarette smoking.

5. *Smoke fewer cigarettes per day.*

Pick a time of day when you promise yourself not to smoke. It may be before breakfast. Or while driving to work. Or after a certain hour each evening. It's always easier to postpone a cigarette if you know you will be having one later.

Maybe you're a pack-a-day smoker. Try buying your next pack an hour later each day. Stretch your supply by stretching the periods between each smoke. Carry your cigarettes in a different pocket, keep them in a drawer of your desk or in your locker, any place where you aren't able to reach for one automatically. The trick is to change the habit patterns you have established. Make a habit of asking yourself, "Do I really want this cigarette?" before you light up. You may be surprised at how many cigarettes you smoke that you don't really want.

Chapter 9

FOOD ALLERGIES

The great philosopher and mathematician Pythagoras was fleeing from pursuing Greek soldiers when he suddenly halted and said, "I will not cross this field of beans." He was overtaken and the soldiers killed him. Years later a group of his followers, the Pythagoreans, were fleeing the emperor Dionysius and they too halted at the border of a bean field and were slain. One man and wife were dragged before the emperor who demanded an explanation of the bean mystery. The husband chose death rather than explain the riddle, and the wife bit out her tongue and spat it at the emperor rather than "spill the beans."

Now, centuries later, it is known that many people are sensitive to the bean called the broad bean, which grew wild throughout the Mediterranean region. Sensitive individuals who eat the bean or who inhale its pollen may suffer from dizziness, nausea, vomiting and sometimes complete collapse. Apparently Pythagoras was one of the sensitive ones.

Food allergies existed long before we knew what they were. It wasn't until the eighteenth century that a doctor first wrote that an allergy from eating a particular food could cause asthma. Since that time it has become a cliché that one man's meat may be another man's poison.

Not only is allergy to food still with us, but many doctors feel it is much more important than ever realized. Food allergy is often ignored by both the lay public and the medical profession, they say, but more and more it is being recognized throughout the world as an important problem. It is generally understood that food allergies can cause gastrointestinal symptoms, but what is not always realized is that food allergies also may be a major cause of hayfever, asthma, headaches and many other persistent and puzzling illnesses.

Many people who have hayfever or asthma and get no relief with treatment against ragweed and other common inhalants often find that their allergy is really due to food. One allergist says that nearly every hayfever and asthma "failure" who comes to him can be clinically controlled by identification and elimination of the patient's food allergy.

Allergies to certain foods are rather common, and no age is exempt. Foods can cause allergy symptoms directly, or they can become additive to other allergic conditions already present, thus making them much worse.

If you have an allergy that just doesn't seem to respond to treatment, you should discuss with your physician whether it could be a food allergy.

■ SYMPTOMS FROM FOOD ALLERGIES

Food allergies can cause minor symptoms or major ones. One physician colleague knows when he goes to a clambake he can only have three crabs. After the fourth one, his lips swell. Nothing else. On the other hand, at Northwestern University Allergy Clinic in just one year, eight people were rushed in close to death from allergic reactions resulting from food.

Quite often the symptoms resulting from a troublemaking food are hives or digestive upset with nausea, vomiting, cramps, belching, constipation or diarrhea or abdominal distention.

However, food allergy may cause a wide variety of other symptoms as well. When you are sensitive to a food you eat, you may have asthma, stuffy nose, swelling of the face, eczema, headache, itchy eyes, canker sores, inflammation around the lips, or itching of the palms, head or other parts of the body. Or you may have dizziness, chronic ear symptoms, urinary tract symptoms, hoarseness, fatigue, "poor resistance," or even violent behavior disturbances. All of these have been proven by allergists as caused by food allergy.

These symptoms can be so confusing as to baffle even some competent physicians. For example, the migraine headache complex—one-sided headache, stomachache, nausea and spots before the eyes—is sometimes caused by food allergy, particularly in children. But sometimes these symptoms are so confusing and so severe that they are misdiagnosed as appendicitis, and only after removal of the perfectly normal appendix does the picture of food allergy emerge.

Allergy can also cause burning or pain on urination or a feeling of urgency, and if your doctor finds no signs of infection or obstruction, he would do well to check your diet for possible food allergies.

There are two distinct types of allergic reactions to food:

The immediate type is characterized by the rapid appearance of symptoms, often within minutes after the offending food is eaten. In fact some patients react even before the food is swallowed, while it is still in the mouth.

At other times there is a delayed type of allergic response. In such cases a number of hours or even a day or more may elapse after eating the food before symptoms appear. It is often difficult for patients and the physician consulted about this to relate the delayed type of allergy reaction to the foods causing it.

Allergists believe that in the case of the immediate type of reaction (such as hives appearing after eating strawberries or sea food), the offending allergen is the whole food protein, whereas with delayed reactions, the cause may be some product formed during the process of digestion of the food. This may explain why skin tests with whole extracts often fail to demonstrate the causes of food allergy.

■ TRACKING CLUES THROUGH SOUP AND NUTS

Food allergy has been frustrating to allergists. It is hard to diagnose, and no wonder. A tremendous number of foods can cause allergic reactions. Finding the guilty one or ones can be mighty difficult. Then, in addition, several factors confuse even the most observant doctor and patient. There is the delay in reactions that sometimes occurs. Ingredients of many foods are not known. A certain food may cause allergy symptoms at certain times, but not other times. Some symptoms occur only after the food has been eaten in large quantities, or only at times when the person's health is low or other stresses, both physical and psychological, are adding to the allergic tendency. Sensitivities to foods sometimes become more obvious during ragweed or mold seasons, and in many people symptoms appear only at these times because of the additive effects. The threshold factors of stress, weather change, infection, hormones, exertion and fatigue all fit into this same picture and add to the difficulty of unraveling the mystery of the food allergy.

Sometimes a person is so sensitive that he can have a reaction from the odors in a grocery store. Sometimes food sensitivities are transient, simply coming and going without apparent reason.

Sometimes foods that appear only in certain seasons will make a person think he has hayfever due to summer pollens. For example, peaches, plums, apricots and grapes become commercially available in the summertime. A person sensitive to them may sneeze and sniff and believe his symptoms are caused by grass pollens or ragweed.

Some patients have mild allergies to many foods, and may not have symptoms from one, but if they eat three or four of them at a single meal they would have symptoms. This is called a summation effect. It would be hard to tell what the guilty foods were.

Sometimes foods that cause no symptoms ordinarily will cause disturbances when taken with a cocktail. Cooking, too, can modify the allergenicity of a food. Both fruits and milk are less likely to cause allergy after they have been cooked. Dehydrated banana is less allergenic than raw banana.

On the other hand, a person may think he is allergic to a substance when it really is one tiny contaminant in that food that is causing the trouble. For example, a person may appear to be allergic to milk when it is really that the milk contains traces of penicillin or sulfa drugs that were used in treating a cow's infection. Allergists tell the story of English infants with eczema who were able to drink American evaporated milk, but found their eczema was made worse by English milk. Further investigation revealed that because of a wartime shortage of fodder, English cattle had been fed with a meal containing ground fish. The children were allergic to the fish protein that was carried over into the cow's milk.

One doctor thought he was allergic to dates for years, then discovered that when he washed them he had no symptoms. He had symptoms from the substance that was used to polish the dates.

Similarly, vegetable gums such as karaya, tragacanth and acacia are often used in the food industry to thicken foods. A person allergic to these gums may think he is allergic to candy, when actually he is sensitive to the gums in them. He would also react to the thickening in cheddar cheese, cream cheese, whipped cream cake, icing, toothpaste, commercial potato salad, mustard, Jello, wheat cake and many other foods, all of which would produce a confusing pattern of allergic reactions.

And in the other direction there are symptoms that suggest allergy that are really caused by other disorders. It is important that your doctor rule out diseases of the stomach, esophagus and intestines, as well as gallbladder and pancreas problems, as the possible causes of your symptoms. Emotional factors, drugs, fatigue or stress can also cause symptoms that could erroneously be interpreted as due to food allergy.

It is because of all this confusion that it is so important to work with your allergist in trying to determine the true causes of any allergy problems that you have.

SKIN TESTS

Two types of skin tests are used to test for food allergy—the scratch test and the intradermal test. Some allergists find the skin tests are good and helpful in making the diagnosis of clinical food sensitivities. Others feel that skin tests for food allergies frequently yield misleading or insufficient data, so they don't use them. Most allergists use the skin tests in combination with the patient's and their own clinical observations to point the finger at suspect foods. They may test the patient by eliminating the suspected food from the diet to see whether the symptoms stop. As a final proof some of the suspected foods are provocatively eaten to see if the symptoms return.

Children, whom allergists believe to have a greater degree of food sensitivity than adults, yield more significant results from skin tests than do adults.

One of the newer techniques of testing for food sensitivity is the provocative food test developed by Dr. H. Rinkel. This food test involves the intentional feeding for seven days in succession of suspected foods so that allergic symptoms may be produced.

Another new test has been developed by Dr. William T. K. Bryan and his wife Marian, of Washington University School of Medicine in St. Louis. The technique involves examining a patient's white blood cells under the microscope in the presence of different food allergens. If the patient is allergic to a specific food, his normally active white blood cells become sluggish and rounded when added to the allergen, and sometimes even disintegrate and explode.

FOOD DIARIES

The physician usually asks the patient to keep a food diary in a notebook or on printed sheets of paper. The person keeps track of every bit of food and drink and medicine he takes in a day, and then keeps a record of *all* symptoms that occur and at what specific times.

One doctor says if his patients have a positive skin test reaction to, say, five different foods, he has them avoid the suspected foods for a week or two. Then when the symptoms are gone, he has the patients eat a large amount of *one* of the foods and check for any reaction. If an allergic response flares up, he has the patient avoid the food for another week, then reintroduces it again. If an allergic response occurs three times in a row, he says it is reasonable to conclude that the patient is more than likely allergic to that particular food.

If there are no clues from skin testing, another approach often used is to put the patient on a basic low-allergen diet such as rice and lamb and then gradually add other foods one at a time so that the ones which are causing the trouble may be isolated and identified.

Occasionally if food diaries fail at home in discovering the guilty foods, the physician will hospitalize the patient. In the hospital the dietary intake can be more accurately controlled and the patient can be placed on various trial diets.

■ FOODS THAT ARE RELATED

One thing that will be helpful in your battle with food allergy is to be aware of foods in the same family as the one to which you are allergic. Because the foods within a family are chemically related, they often produce the same allergic symptom. For example, the person who is allergic to chocolate will also often be allergic to cola drinks, because cola and cocoa are related.

However, many foods thought of as being related are often not

SEVEN DAY FOOD DIARY

DATES / FOODS							
MORNING							
MIDDAY							
EVENING–AFTERNOON							
SYMPTOMS	TIME	TIME	TIME	TIME	TIME	TIME	TIME
MEDICATION	TIME	TIME	TIME	TIME	TIME	TIME	TIME

Enter every item of food and beverage consumed on each day of the week. *Also* list any symptoms that you had on those days and any medication you took for the reaction.

related at all. A person who cannot tolerate peanuts usually can eat cashews and walnuts, with no allergic reaction. But he will probably react to peas, lima beans, and soybeans, which are related legumes. Similarly, a strawberry-induced allergy does not indicate that a person will suffer an allergic reaction after eating all other berries. He will probably be unable to tolerate raspberries and other members of the rose family, but will not necessarily have trouble from blueberries, cranberries or gooseberries.

Similarly, cinnamon is not related to ginger, shrimp is not related to oysters, cabbage is not related to lettuce, potato to sweet potato, or wheat to buckwheat. Black pepper is not related to red pepper, crabs are not related to clams, raisins are not related to prunes, coffee is not related to tea.

However, there are other foods that *are* related that you might not think of as being related. For example, apples are related to pears, peaches are related to plums, peas and beans are related to peanuts, beets are related to spinach, onions and garlic are related to asparagus, cucumbers are related to melon, carrots are related to celery.

Sometimes these family relationships or unrelationships can lead to complications. One man was very allergic to tree nuts. When a girl friend saw him eat peanuts, which are unrelated, she decided that his allergy was all in his mind and ground a few English walnuts into a cake she was about to bake. He had only swallowed a few bites of the finished cake when his eyes began to close and his throat swelled. The doctor got there in time, but it could have been a deadly experiment.

We have taken care of several patients lately, all college students, who were in critical distress. They and their parents had always been careful in the past of their nut allergies, but recently flour with finely ground nuts in it has been used in commercial pastries. When these patients had only a small piece of such a cake, they became seriously ill in minutes, with giant hives and swelling of the tongue and throat. Luckily emergency help was available.

Cross-sensitivities are more frequently found in the plant kingdom than in the animal kingdom. So a patient sensitive to meats need not worry quite as much about reacting to other foods in the same family unless he is very sensitive. On the other hand, if a patient has an extreme sensitivity to fish, he not only needs to avoid other related fish, but should also avoid contact with fish odors and fish glue.

Knowing the biological relationships of foods is extremely important if a person has severe food reactions. If a child has had a very bad reaction from buckwheat, for example, he is very likely to end up in the hospital after he eats a related food—rhubarb.

In milder cases of food allergy, however, clinical symptoms may not be produced by related foods even when eaten in large quantities. If you really observe matters closely, then you can eat these related foods with some degree of impunity.

Many foods are related in other ways even though they may not belong to the same family groups. For example, many foods contain salicylates, and others have had salicylates added as flavoring. So anyone who is allergic to aspirin (acetylsalicylic acid) should not eat these foods: apricots, blackberries, strawberries, raspberries, currants, grapes, raisins, limes, vinegar, nectarines, peaches, plums, prunes, ice cream, bakery goods (except bread), chewing gum, soft drinks, jams, wintergreen flavors, candy, Jello.

If you know you are allergic to some particular food, the following list will alert you to other members of the same food family to be on the lookout for:

RELATED FOODS

APPLE FAMILY—Apple, pear, quince.

ASTER FAMILY—Lettuce, chicory, endive, escarole, artichoke, dandelion, celtuce, sunflower seeds, tarragon.

BEET FAMILY—Beet, spinach, chard, lamb's quarters.

BLUEBERRY FAMILY—Blueberry, huckleberry, cranberry.

BUCKWHEAT FAMILY—Buckwheat, rhubarb, garden sorrel.

CASHEW FAMILY—Cashew, pistachio, mango.

CHOCOLATE FAMILY—Both white and regular chocolate, cocoa and cola.

CITRUS FAMILY—Orange, lemon, grapefruit, lime, tangerine, kumquat, citron.

FUNGUS FAMILY—Mushroom, yeast, molds, antibiotics.

GINGER FAMILY—Ginger, cardamom, turmeric.

GOOSEBERRY FAMILY—Currant and gooseberry.

GRAPE—Raisin.

GRASS FAMILY—Wheat, corn, rice, oats, barley, rye, wildrice, cane, millet, sorghum, bamboo sprouts.

LAUREL FAMILY—Avocado, cinnamon, bay leaves, sassafras.

MALLOW FAMILY—Cottonseed and okra.

MELON (GOURD) FAMILY—Watermelon, cucumber, cantaloupe, pumpkin, squash, and other melons.

MUSTARD FAMILY—Mustard, turnip, radish, horse-radish, watercress, cabbage, kraut, Chinese cabbage, broccoli, cauliflower, Brussels sprouts, collards, kale, kohlrabi, rutabaga.

MYRTLE FAMILY—Allspice, guava, clove, pimento.

ONION FAMILY—Onion, garlic, asparagus, chives, leeks, sarsaparilla.

PALM FAMILY—Coconut and date.
PARSLEY FAMILY—Carrot, parsnip, celery, parsley, celeriac, anise, dill, fennel, angelica, celery seed, cumin, coriander, caraway.
PEA FAMILY—Peanuts, peas (green, field, blackeyed), beans (navy, lima, pinto, string, soy, etc.), licorice, acacia, tragacanth.
PLUM FAMILY—Plum, cherry, peach, apricot, nectarine, wild cherry, almond.
POTATO FAMILY—Potato, tomato, egg plant, peppers (including green pepper, red pepper, chili pepper, paprika, cayenne, capsicum, but not black and white pepper).
ROSE FAMILY—Strawberry, raspberry, blackberry, dewberry, loganberry, youngberry, boysenberry.
WALNUT FAMILY—English walnut, black walnut, pecan, hickory nut, butternut.
MOLLUSC FAMILY—Oyster, clam, abalone, mussel.
CRUSTACEAN FAMILY—Crab, lobster, shrimp.
FISH FAMILY—All true fish, either freshwater or saltwater, including tuna, sardine, catfish, trout, crappie.
BIRD FAMILY—All fowl and game birds including chicken, turkey, duck, goose, guinea, pigeon, quail, pheasant, eggs.
REPTILES—Turtle, rattlesnake, frog.
BEEF—Cow's milk.

■ IMPORTANT FOOD ALLERGIES

The most common causes of food allergy reactions are eggs, milk and wheat. Other major troublemakers are fish, shellfish, berries (especially strawberries), nuts, chocolate, peas, beans, potatoes, tomatoes, oranges, onions, pork, cabbage, fried foods, and condiments. And these are usually recognized by people as the basis for many allergic problems.

However, what is not always realized is that these foods are often hidden ingredients in other foods or food mixtures. A patient may think that he is allergic to eggs, but he is mystified as to why he also has allergic reactions after eating custards, pudding, ice cream, sherbet or some candy. The answer—all of these contain eggs in some form. In the same way there are eggs in almost all cakes, pancakes, muffins, egg noodles and salad dressing. And the white of egg is often brushed on bread, rolls and pretzels to provide a glazed appearance. All of these hidden ingredients can mystify the patient who is trying to track down and control his food allergy.

In the same way wheat-free bread often isn't really free of wheat, and many persons sensitive to wheat suffer after eating it. It often still contains gluten and other wheat proteins despite labeling that says otherwise.

And most people know that cottonseed oil is found in shortening, oleomargarines, salad oils, mayonnaise and salad dressings, but they aren't apt to know that cottonseed oil is used to polish fruits at fruit stands or that cottonseed and flaxseed are often fed to cattle and can be present in their milk, or that sardines may be packed in cottonseed oil, or that many cakes, bread, fish, popcorn, potato chips, candies, doughnuts and gin are made with it, or that olive oil is adulterated with it, or that it is used in cosmetics, fertilizer, animal feed and in the manufacture of paper, salt, machine tools, paint and varnish.

To help you find these hidden foods, we have listed at the end of this chapter the most common allergy-causing foods and the products you need to avoid if you are allergic to them.

■ MAJOR TROUBLEMAKERS

CORN ALLERGY

Many people are allergic to corn and do not realize it. It is used in the preparation of more kinds of food than any other single edible product. And because many times the patient does not realize that there is corn in a product, he doesn't know that corn is causing his allergy.

Sensitivity to corn is the most common cause of food allergy, and because of its prevalence it is the most difficult food to avoid. It can even cause allergic symptoms if you inhale the fumes of popping corn or the steam of corn on the cob boiling in the pot. You can also be exposed to it in body powders, in bath powders, and from the starch while ironing shirts.

Corn is found in shoes, as the sticky stuff on envelopes and stamps, as a diluting material in vitamins and other pills, in paper cups and paper plates. If you are allergic to corn, you can have a reaction simply from licking stamps, brushing your teeth or drinking milk out of a paper carton.

Dr. Kenneth J. Johnson, allergist of Bismarck, North Dakota, said that when he tested one series of patients for food allergy, half of the patients were found to be allergic to corn. The corn, he said, caused gastrointestinal symptoms, headache, respiratory problems, fatigue, runny nose, itchy eyes, skin reactions and salivary reactions.

Sometimes there is a difference in reactions to different forms of corn. Some people can eat fresh corn or succotash without having symptoms, but will have a reaction when they eat popped corn, hominy, corn oil or corn flour.

If you have corn allergy, you should completely eliminate corn and corn products and all foods containing any corn from your diet. This should be done until you are free of all symptoms. Even if certain forms of corn produce minor or subclinical reactions, if you continue to eat them you will tend to maintain a high degree of corn sensitivity.

CHOCOLATE SENSITIVITY

There is still a great deal of controversy about how much allergy is caused by chocolate. But Dr. Joseph H. Fries, pediatrician at the State University of New York Downstate Medical Center, feels that the evidence is strong that chocolate candy is a major cause of allergy, especially in children. And the effects of chocolate can add on to the effects of other allergies already present. As little as half a chocolate bar can set off an acute attack of wheezing, sneezing, skin rashes and abdominal upset in children with allergy to other substances.

White chocolate is just as allergenic as brown chocolate.

"I have findings on twenty-five children clearly showing that chocolate adds to the allergic youngster's already abundant trouble," says Dr. Fries. He explains that many children are slightly sensitive to chocolate, and do not always have clinical reactions to it, but do react from the added effect if chocolate is taken, for example, during some other particularly sensitive period such as the pollen season.

Other children have very severe reactions to chocolate. In children tested from age three to teen-age, one half to three chocolate bars caused symptoms that varied from rashes and hives to itching, redness around the mouth, weeping lesions, clogged-up noses, sneezing, coughing, wheezing, abdominal pains or vomiting. When chocolate was withdrawn the symptoms were dramatically reduced.

If you or your child loves chocolate you might try some chocolate substitutes. There are confections made from carob—known as St. John's bread—that mimic to a remarkable degree the texture and taste of chocolate.

Another answer is to take fairly large doses of vitamin E when you feel a deep craving for chocolate. Nutritionists have found that a person with vitamin E deficiency often craves chocolate, since chocolate is one of the few things in our diet that contains large quantities of vitamin E. Taking one therapeutic capsule daily for a week or so will generally restore your vitamin E supply and stop the craving.

MILK ALLERGY

Allergy to milk can occur in adults as well as in children. As a matter of fact, you can have an allergy to milk as an adult even though you were able to tolerate milk all through your childhood. Dr. James E. Stroh, of Seattle, Washington, reported one patient who had no problem with milk when she was a child, but in later life developed a severe sensitivity reaction to it. Every day she drank milk for breakfast, and about two hours later she had diarrhea, followed that afternoon by a runny nose and heavy mucus in her throat. About two days later the joints of her arms and legs became tender and swollen, and it took another three days before she was really well again. Dr. Stroh says she stays entirely well now by watching her diet and has not had an attack of asthma or other allergic symptoms since she learned of her milk sensitivity.

Dr. John Gerrard, of the University of Saskatchewan, urges that more people consider that they may have a milk allergy. He writes that one boy, only one year old, had had eight attacks of pneumonia. During the first six attacks he had required hospitalization, but during his seventh attack his mother merely took him off milk and dairy products, and he quickly recovered. Says Dr. Gerard, "In our part of Canada, there's an old wives' tale that claims: 'Milk makes mucus.' Being an old husband, I'm not inclined to believe old wives' tales, but I do think there is some truth in this one." He cited a father who had a persistent troublesome cough. He drank more than a quart of milk daily. When he stopped drinking milk and eating dairy products, within three weeks his coughing stopped.

One woman suffered from severe asthma for twenty-eight years. Nothing seemed to help. Finally by the use of trial and error and elimination of many foods in her diet, it was discovered that she was sensitive to milk. A quarter of a century of misery from asthma was ended as soon as she eliminated milk and milk products from her diet.

A large proportion of the world population may be intolerant to milk and a milk sugar called lactose, according to Dr. Theodore M. Bayless, of Johns Hopkins University. He reports that high percentages of both Oriental and Negro people cannot digest milk sugar and get cramps and diarrhea afterward. Caucasians have the problem less frequently. Often these people were able to tolerate milk as infants, says Dr. Bayless, and symptoms generally appeared in adolescence or early adulthood. In one study, nineteen out of every twenty healthy Oriental adults developed severe diarrhea after they drank the equivalent of one quart of milk. This condition involves an enzyme defect so that it is a milk intolerance rather than a milk allergy. The condition has widespread significance; sending milk as a source of nutrition for adults in underdeveloped countries may be a major mistake.

■ FOOD ADDITIVES IN ALLERGIC DISEASE

Food additives are being incriminated as a cause of an astoundingly large number of allergies. In fact at a recent meeting of the American College of Allergists in Washington, D.C., three separate speakers warned of the danger of additives in our food, and each of them individually reported hundreds of cases of allergy caused by additives.

The role of these additives in health has assumed such importance that the Food and Agriculture Organization of the United Nations and World Health Organization has established an international committee to investigate various aspects of this problem.

There are thousands of intentional food additives added during processing, and there are a great many unintentional additives, such as pesticides and antibiotics. There are also many secret formulas of which we know nothing about the additive agents.

In one recent year more than 660 million pounds of additives were used in this country, amounting to more than three pounds of food additives per person per year. Experts estimate that the use of food additives will climb to more than one *billion* pounds by 1975.

At the College of Allergists meeting, Dr. Ben Feingold, of San Francisco, chairman of a special roundtable discussion of the subject, reported two hundred cases of allergy in his own practice due to food additives. "Many cases of obscure diagnosis are probably due to the additives," he said, "and the cause is not generally recognized by either the profession or the public."

When the cause of a troublesome allergy cannot be identified, food additives should be given serious consideration, he said.

Some of the most important additives are food, drug and cosmetic colors which have a wide distribution in our food supply and also in medicines. Dr. Feingold said that almost all breakfast foods are dyed with red and yellow chemicals to produce a uniform color, as are Kool-Aid, Jello, and many vitamins and drugs.

There are some 2,112 chemicals that are added to foods for flavoring alone, he said, and he found over one hundred cases of sensitivity to the flavors in his practice. Symptoms ranged from runny nose, nasal polyps, cough, throat swelling, asthma, itching, skin lesions, hives, swollen tongue, belching, flatulence, constipation, canker sores, intestinal bleeding, headaches, swelling and pain in the joints to behavioral disturbances.

Major foods containing flavors are beverages, candy, chewing gum, ices, bakery goods, ice cream and condiments. "By eliminating these foods we were successful in controlling symptoms in a number of cases," he said.

Dr. Feingold talked about what he called the "pharmacology of violence," that the ingestion of chemicals can cause violent attitudes and behavioral problems.

He described one woman who complained of allergy symptoms and swelling of the forehead over her eyes. He found what was causing the trouble in her diet, changed the diet and she became free of her symptoms. A little later he got a call from a psychiatrist and learned that the woman had been under psychiatric care for years. "I don't know what you did," the psychiatrist said, "but since she came to you she has quieted down and all her psychiatric symptoms have disappeared."

"This has come up in many other cases in both adults and children," Dr. Feingold says. "As we manage the allergy, their personalities change. In approaching emotional problems we must look at these violent chemical factors as a cause of psychiatric disturbance." He questioned how much of today's violence could be due to chemicals in our food and environment.

The same kind of behavioral changes were described by Dr. Stephen D. Lockey, of Lancaster, Pennsylvania. One woman, he said, had developed a migraine headache every day after she took a vitamin pill and became very upset also after eating gelatin or yellow candy. When the vitamin tablet was washed off to get rid of the yellow dye before she took it, her symptoms disappeared.

"I have file drawers full of cases," Dr. Lockey says. "We must look into beverages and foods and drugs and the additives in them as a major cause of behavioral symptoms as well as a cause of more usual allergic symptoms." He reported that he has tracked down 30,000 additives so far in foods, beverages and drugs.

Artificial coloring that can cause allergy is found in gelatin desserts, maraschino cherries, orange skins, sausage casing, frozen desserts, ice cream, sherbets, carbonated beverages, dried drink powders, candy and confectionery products, bakery products, cereals, puddings, spaghetti, drug solutions, tablets, capsules, ointments, toothpastes, mouthwash, soaps, suntan oil, hair waving fluids, hair oils, shampoos, hair rinses, bath salts, nail lacquers, lipsticks, rouge, face powder and talcum.

A number of other allergists have documented the many mental symptoms and behavioral problems caused by food additives and food allergies. If mental illness caused by allergies were recognized more, and emotional factors not always sought to explain mental disturbances, a great deal of time and money could be saved, and patients' mental conditions eliminated. There are millions of patients enduring needless suffering. One can only guess at the number of major and minor tragedies that are enacted daily because of misinterpreted symptoms and inappropriate therapy.

■ SUBSTITUTES

There are many substitute foods manufactured for the person with difficult food allergies. For people allergic to milk, there are a variety of soybean substitutes, such as Mull-Soy, Sobee, Soyalac. Poi can substitute for cereal. Ry-Krisp crackers are wheat-free.

Many times rice flour can be used to substitute for other flour. It can be bought in most local groceries or dietetic or health food stores.

■ CORN-FREE DIET

FOODS YOU CANNOT HAVE

BEVERAGES—Ale, beer, soybean milk, instant tea, carbonated drinks, instant coffee, coffee substitutes, some fruit juices, gin, whiskey, anything in paper cartons.

BREADS—Biscuits, ready-mix pie crusts, doughnuts, pancake mixes, baking powder, batter for frying, some bleached wheat flour, confectioner's sugar, graham crackers, yeasts.

DESSERTS—Cakes, cookies, frostings, gelatin, ice cream, ices, Jello, creamed pies, puddings, custards, blancmange, sherbets, cream puffs.

DRUGS—Aspirin, dentifrices, various capsules and ointments containing corn, gelatin capsules, vitamins.

FRUITS AND VEGETABLES—Harvard beets, canned peas, canned and frozen string beans, creamed vegetables, confection dates, canned or frozen fruits or vegetables.

MEATS—Bacon, anything fried in corn batter, cured or tenderized hams, bologna, meats cooked with gravy, lunch ham, cooked sausages, weiners.

MISCELLANEOUS—Candies, cheeses, corn cereals, chili, chop suey, fried foods, Fritos, grits, hominy, chewing gum, popcorn, starch, jams, jellies, monosodium glutamate, peanut butter, coated rice, some salt, creamed or thickened soups, powdered sugar, commercially prepared syrups, tortillas, vanillin, vinegar, oleomargarine.

SAUCES—Gravies, catsup, French dressing, salad dressings, some sauces for sundaes.

OTHER THINGS TO BEWARE OF

Adhesives on envelopes, stamps, stickers, paper cups and other paper containers, bath powders, starch used on clothing, talcums, plastic food wrappers.

■ EGG-FREE DIET

FOODS YOU CANNOT HAVE

BAKING POWDER—Any that contains egg white or albumen.

BEVERAGES—Coffee, if egg white or shell has been used to clarify. Root beer, which may have had egg added to make it foam. Any prepared drink made with egg or from powders containing egg, dried egg or albumen. Malted cocoa drinks. Wine if cleared with egg white.

BREADED FOODS—If the breading mixture used contains eggs or crumbs that contain egg.

BREADS—Muffins, griddle cakes, waffles, gingerbreads, doughnuts and fancy nut and fruit breads. Commercial breads and rolls that have been brushed with egg white to glaze the top. Any homemade bread containing egg. Prepared mixes for pancakes, waffles, biscuits, muffins, doughnuts, breads and rolls unless the list of ingredients on the label shows no egg, egg powder, dried egg or albumen.

DESSERTS—Bavarian creams. Stirred or soft and baked custards, doughnuts, fritters, angel and sponge cakes, macaroons, meringues and whips. Pie filling containing egg, such as custard, lemon, coconut cream and pumpkin. Blancmanges, frostings, puddings, cakes, cookies, ice creams and sherbets unless made at home without egg or from a prepared mixture that does not contain egg, egg powder, dried egg or albumen.

EGG DISHES—Baked, coddled, creamed, deviled, scalloped, fried, poached, scrambled, shirred, hard or soft cooked eggs, egg drinks, egg sauces, egg meringues, souffles and omelets. Do not use dried or frozen eggs. Do not use any mixture that contains egg, egg powder, dried egg or albumen.

MEATS, POULTRY, GAME AND SEAFOOD—Sausages, loaves, croquettes or any meats using egg as a binding agent.

MISCELLANEOUS—Most noodles. French toast, fritters and timbales. Any prepared mix unless label shows it contains no egg, egg powder, dried egg or albumen. Pretzels.

SALAD DRESSINGS—All salad dressings except true French dressing unless homemade without egg or unless the list of ingredients on the label shows no egg, egg powder, dried egg or albumen.

SAUCES—Hollandaise, tartar and egg.

SOUPS—Mock turtle, alphabet and egg noodle soups. Consommés, bouillons, broths or any soup cleared with egg or containing ingredients made with egg. Dehydrated and canned soups if they contain egg, egg powder, dried egg or albumen.

SWEETS—Divinities. Any candy containing egg, egg powder, dried egg or albumen. (Many commercial candies made without eggs are brushed with egg white to give them luster.)

■ MILK-FREE DIET

FOODS YOU CANNOT HAVE

BEVERAGES—Made with milk or with chocolate, cocoa or preparations containing milk or milk products.

BREADED FOODS—If the breading mixture contains milk or crumbs from breads and crackers containing milk or milk products.

BREADS—Doughnuts, popovers, pancakes, waffles, rusks and crackers, except Ry-Krisp. Wheat, rice, rye, corn, graham, gluten, soybean breads and rolls made with milk or milk products. Most commercial breads and rolls contain milk or milk products.

DESSERTS—Cakes, cookies, puddings and pie crusts made or brushed with milk or milk products. Bavarian creams, blancmanges, custards, junkets, ice creams, mousses and milk sherbets. Prepared mixes containing milk or milk products.

FAT AND SALAD DRESSINGS—Butters and margarines. Salad dressings containing milk, cream, butter, margarine or cheese.

MEATS, POULTRY, GAME, FISH AND SEAFOOD—Dishes prepared with milk or milk products. Commercially prepared meats frequently contain milk or milk products. Most hamburgers, cooked sausage.

MILK AND MILK PRODUCTS—Fresh, whole and skim milks. Cultured and buttermilk. Creams. Condensed, evaporated, dried milk and milk solids. Casein and lactalbumin. Butters and margarines. Curds and wheys. Powdered and malted milks. All cheeses.

MISCELLANEOUS—Creamed and scalloped foods. Foods dipped in milk batter or fried in butter or margarine. Foods prepared au gratin (with cheese). Rarebits and timbales. Prepared mixes for biscuits, cakes, cookies, doughnuts, muffins, pie crusts and waffles if they contain milk or milk products.

SAUCES AND GRAVIES—White, cream, butter and hard sauces or any sauce or gravy made with milk or milk products. Any food using a hard, white or cream sauce in its preparation.

SOUPS—Canned and dehydrated soups containing milk or milk products or any soup made with milk or milk products.

SWEETS—Made with milk or milk products.

VEGETABLES—Creamed and scalloped vegetables, au gratin, or those prepared and served in any way with milk or milk products. Mashed potatoes.

■ SOYBEAN-FREE DIET

FOODS YOU CANNOT HAVE

BAKERY GOODS—Soybean flour and oil is now used by many bakers in their dough mixtures for breads, rolls, cakes and pastries. K-biscuits and several crackers have soybean flour in them.

CANDIES—Hard candies, nut candies and caramels. Lecithin is derived from soybean and is used in candies.

CEREALS—Sunlets, Cellu Soy Flakes.

MEATS—Many pork link sausage and lunch meats.

MILK SUBSTITUTES—Sobee, Mull-Soy. Some bakeries use soy milk instead of cow's milk.

SALAD DRESSING—Many salad dressings and mayonnaises contain soy oil, but only state on the label that they contain vegetable oil.

SAUCES—Oriental Show You Sauce, La Choy Sauce, Lea & Perrins Sauce, Heinz Worcestershire Sauce.

MISCELLANEOUS—Soups, coffee substitutes, Chinese dishes, nuts (soys are roasted, salted and used instead of peanuts), soybean noodles, macaroni and spaghetti. Reezon seasoning, Crisco, Spry and other shortenings, oleomargarine and butter substitutes. Cheese Tufu, Natto and Miso and some others.

OTHER CONTACTS TO AVOID—Varnish, paints, enamels, printing ink, candles, celluloid, massage creams, linoleum, paper sizing, adhesives, fertilizer, nitroglycerine, paper finishes, blankets, urease, Gro-Pup dog food, French's fish food, soap, automobile parts, fodder, glycerine, textile dressing, lubricating oil, illuminating oil, some plastic window frames, steering wheels, gear shift knobs, distributors and other car parts, upholstery fabric, rubber substitutes, lecithin in leaded gasoline.

■ WHEAT-FREE DIET

FOODS YOU CANNOT HAVE

BEVERAGES—Coffee substitutes, Ovaltine, cocomalt, most beer, gin, malted milk, whiskey.

BREADED FOODS—In which breading mixture contains wheat products.

BREADS—Whole wheat, graham, gluten and white breads, rolls, muffins and biscuits. Doughnuts, popovers, sweet rolls, johnnycake, pancakes, waffles, rusks, pretzels, zwieback and crackers (except Ry-Krisp). Prepared mixes for pancakes, waffles, biscuits, muffins, doughnuts, breads and rolls. Rice, potato and soybean breads, rolls, muffins and biscuits; corn and rye bread, rolls and muffins unless made at home without wheat flour.

SWEETS—Commercial candies that contain wheat products.

VEGETABLES—Any vegetable prepared or served with a sauce thickened with wheat flour or those prepared and served in any way with wheat products.

■ YEAST-FREE DIET

FOODS YOU CANNOT HAVE

BREADS—Buns, rolls, cookies, crackers, biscuits, pastries, cake and cake mix, pretzels, flour enriched with vitamins from yeast, flour and enrichment wafers, meat fried in cracker crumbs, salt-rising bread, all cereals fortified with thiamin, niacin, riboflavin, and other vitamins, some cereals.

BEVERAGES—Whiskey, wine, brandy, gin, rum, vodka, root beer, ginger ale, all citrus fruit juices, either frozen or canned (only home squeezed are yeast free). Black tea.

CEREALS—Wheat cereals and wheat or wheat products, white bread, all-purpose flour, cake, pastry, graham, wheat germ, bran, farina, semolina, cracker meal, bread crumbs and malt.

DESSERTS—Cakes, doughnuts, dumplings, pastries and ice cream cones. Custard, cookies, pies and puddings made with wheat products. Prepared mixes for cakes, cookies, ice creams, puddings and pie crusts, unless the list of ingredients on the label shows no wheat products.

MALTED PRODUCTS—All cereals, candy and milk drinks which have been malted.

MEATS, POULTRY, GAME, FISH AND SEAFOOD—Swiss steak. Bread and cracker stuffings. Chili con carne, croquettes, fish and meat patties and loaves, unless made at home without wheat products. Meat fried in frying fat which has been used to fry meats rolled in flour, particularly in restaurants. Most cooked sausages (weiners, bologna, liverwurst), lunch ham, hamburger.

MISCELLANEOUS—Dormison rest capsules, dried fruits (prunes, raisins, dates), penicillin, mycin drugs, chloromycetin, tetracyclines, lincocin, and other drugs derived from mold cultures; milk fortified with vitamins, mushrooms, truffles, cheeses of all kinds including cottage cheese, buttermilk, sour cream, most vitamins, matzos, synthetic pepper, yeasts. Dumplings, noodles, spaghetti, macaroni, ravioli, mostaccioli, vermicelli, soup rings, alphabets and kindred products. Vinegar, olives, pickles, chili peppers, sauerkraut, mince pie.

SALAD DRESSING—Some mayonnaise, condiments, horseradish, French dressing, any salad dressing thickened with wheat flour.

SAUCES AND GRAVIES—Soy sauce, gravies, butter sauces, cream and white sauces unless homemade without wheat flour. Catsup, barbecue sauce, tomato sauce.

SOUPS—Cream, unless made at home without wheat flour. Vegetable and meat soups, chowders and bisques if thickened with wheat products.

Chapter 10

SKIN ALLERGIES

Allergies have been the subject of much conjecture and writing throughout the centuries, and skin allergies have been written about the most.

The Bible refers to a plague of boils that occurred in Egypt thousands of years ago. Scientists now believe that it was actually a plague of skin allergies caused by tiny particles of dust landing on the skin from the ashes of the furnaces in operation at that time.

And there has been poetry:

"There was a young lady from Natchez,
Whose clothes were always in patches,
When comment arose,
As to the state of her clothes,
She replied, 'When Ah itchez, Ah scratchez.' "

And Ogden Nash once wrote:

"One bliss for which
There is no match
Is when you itch
To up and scratch."

There are many current stories concerning skin allergies, too. You may have read about the actress who was allergic to her false eyelashes, the cowboy sensitive to his horse's blanket, and the bank teller allergic to the ink on dollar bills.

Skin allergies have been with us through the ages, but there have never been as many factors to cause them as we have with us today.

All of us are today surrounded by a sea of substances that can cause allergies. Our technological explosion has brought thousands of new chemicals and substances into the home, the garden, industry and the playpen. From the moment you put your shoes on in the morning until you crawl under a wool blanket at night you are in contact with at least 700 or 800 different substances in your own private sea of matter. And any one of them could cause you trouble.

■ DIFFERENT TYPES OF SKIN ALLERGIES

The marvelous envelope that holds together our muscles, bones and flesh is exquisitely sensitive to heat and cold and touch and is also sensitive to allergy-producing substances.

You no doubt know by now that how a substance you are allergic to gets into your body doesn't have much to do with the final destination at which the allergic reaction takes place. Your skin can react from something touching it or from some food or medicine that you take into your stomach or, less often, from something you inhale.

And, as in other allergies, multiple factors are involved in making the symptoms more or less severe—fatigue, nutrition, systemic infection and other allergies all influence the allergic response.

There are also many special things that govern the sensitivity of your skin. Race is a factor. In general, the darker the skin, the less the susceptibility to irritants, with fair skin being the most susceptible to irritating substances. Women's skin is more sensitive and more susceptible to skin irritants than men's. A sweaty skin is more sensitive because the perspiration makes many substances more irritating as they become moistened.

We have become aware that there are many genetic factors in skin allergies. Parents sensitive to substances that cause allergic dermatitis have children who tend to be equally sensitive.

And psychological attitudes can sometimes play a role. This is especially noted in individuals wo have had bad episodes of hives brought on or aggravated by excitement or emotional upsets.

Skin allergy for an individual may be slight or severe. It may appear at any age level. It can come on suddenly and disappear in a few months. It may change gradually over the years or may last a lifetime. You may have skin symptoms from just one substance, or your skin may become sensitized not only to that substance but to many closely related substances.

Skin allergies can take many forms. There may be individual hives or in clusters. The itchy hives may come and go, may last several hours or several days or even longer.

Or the skin allergy may be a fine rash or a solid redness (called erythema). The diffuse redness may cover the entire body or just a small area. It may subside without any side effects or may terminate in an ugly peeling process (called exfoliative dermatitis).

There may be swelling (angioedema) of the eyelids, the tongue, the mouth, hands or feet, or the entire body. If the swelling is intense and occurs in the larynx, the person may have a great deal of trouble breathing, or suffocation may occur so quickly that a physician cannot reach them before they die.

There may be bleeding into the skin, causing reddish-purple bruise-like markings (called purpura).

Sometimes the reaction is a strange one. A reaction can occur as a result of a drug, with a single isolated rash breaking out in one spot, perhaps on the face or on one wrist or some other part of the body. Then weirdly, the eruption breaks out in that some single sensitized spot repeatedly each time the drug is used. Then after several appearances, a new location pops up for the eruption.

Allergic skin reactions can also arise in distant parts of the body from an infection present somewhere else in the body. This reaction often occurs with mold infections such as ringworm, athlete's foot or gym itch. One woman had hives for nine years that turned out to be due to chronically infected molar teeth. When the teeth were pulled, the hives disappeared.

One of the most common skin reactions is eczema. In infants it often appears on the cheek, scalp, the wrists, in the elbows and behind the knees. In teen-agers and adults the eczema is usually more severe, sometimes covering greater parts of the body, often with a thickening of the skin. Because the rash is so irritatingly itchy, the person usually scratches and rubs at it, making it worse, and it often thickens, cracks or weeps with moisture, crusting as the moisture dries.

The most common skin allergy is contact dermatitis, and we will spend most of this chapter discussing it. Contact dermatitis is a reaction of the skin, not to something that you eat, or drink, or breathe, but to something that you touch, to something with which the skin is in direct contact. The skin that has come in contact with the offending substance itches and becomes red, often swells or may have little bumps or blisters. The blisters may break and form crusts and scales.

There are also numerous cases of dermatitis due to a primary irritation and injury of the skin from alkalies, acids, other chemicals or rough materials. For example, "detergent burn" of housewives is not a true allergy, but a simple irritation.

■ CONTACT DERMATITIS: TRACKING DOWN THE CAUSES

Determining the cause of a contact dermatitis can be one of the most intriguing detective games in the whole gamut of allergy. So many thousands of things can be the cause of this type of allergy.

And any one substance can be found in such a strange variety of places. Flaxseed, for example, can cause a reaction when it is eaten as food, when it is inhaled as a dust, or by direct contact. It is found in cereal, flaxseed tea, some cough medicines and laxatives, in cattle and poultry feed and in milk of cows who have been fed flaxseed. It can also be found in setting lotion, shampoos, hair tonics, bird lime, furniture polish, flaxseed poultices, carron oils, linseed oil, paints, varnishes, linoleum, printers' ink, soft soap, depilatories, linens, damask, huckaback, oilcloth, thread, insulating plaster, flax rugs, straw mats, wax paper, fiberboard, and the stuffing material for furniture and cushions.

It takes an alert physician and observant patient to review the clues from this many areas and put them together to find the guilty troublemaker.

The detective game is made more difficult because sometimes a person's habits can cause skin rashes that resemble contact allergy but really are not. For example, many children unconsciously suck their lips and the surrounding area, causing redness or even scaling or fissuring.

As you work with your doctor in tracking down the factor involved in your skin allergy, it is important for you to keep a regular check of the specific times and under what circumstances the rash appears. Try to figure out whether the rash occurs as a general reaction after some food or medicine you take, or whether it is a dermatitis from something you touch. Analyze whether you did anything different during the day the rash appeared or during the three or four days before that. Think of whether you have had contact with some of the things that are frequent causes of skin allergies, such as black or brown dyes, leather, furs, gloves, soaps, fingernail polish, hairsetting fluids, hairsprays, lacquers, nickel, chromium, rubber or plastics.

Think of things you handle where you work, in the car, in the bedroom, kitchen, bathroom and living room at home, at the grocery store, church, clubs, in the garden or other outdoor areas.

Sometimes your physician or members of your family may notice a nervous habit that may be contributing to the dermatitis, such as rubbing a coin or a metal object, rubbing your hands through your hair with hairdressing on it, twirling your watch or glasses or toying with a keychain.

One objective method to help determine the cause of a contact dermatitis is by a patch test. A small amount of a suspected substance is applied to a small piece of gauze and kept taped to the skin of the arm or back for twenty-four hours. Then the patch is removed. If you are allergic to the substance, your skin will show a reaction. Usually the reaction takes about twelve to forty-eight hours to appear, but in a few rare cases it may occur even ten days later.

Sometimes you can be exposed to a substance for many years and then suddenly, for some unknown reason, become sensitive to it, developing a dermatitis. So all contactants, both old and new, need to be considered.

Regular skin tests are usually not used in cases of contact dermatitis, although they are used in cases of eczema caused by allergy from sources other than contact.

At the recent 25th Congress of the American College of Allergists a commemorative medal was distributed in honor of the group's silver anniversary. Instead of being round, the medal might well have been in the shape of a detective badge, judging from the Sherlock Holmes type yarns that kept occurring in scientific reports and corridor conversation.

One allergist, for example, was talking about a woman who came in with blistered and itchy lips. He investigated various foods and drugs but did not find any answer; then he did patch tests with common allergy-producing substances, and found out that she was sensitive to nickel. But that didn't really give any answers until she came

LOCATION OF RASH AS A CLUE TO ITS CAUSE

BOTH SEXES

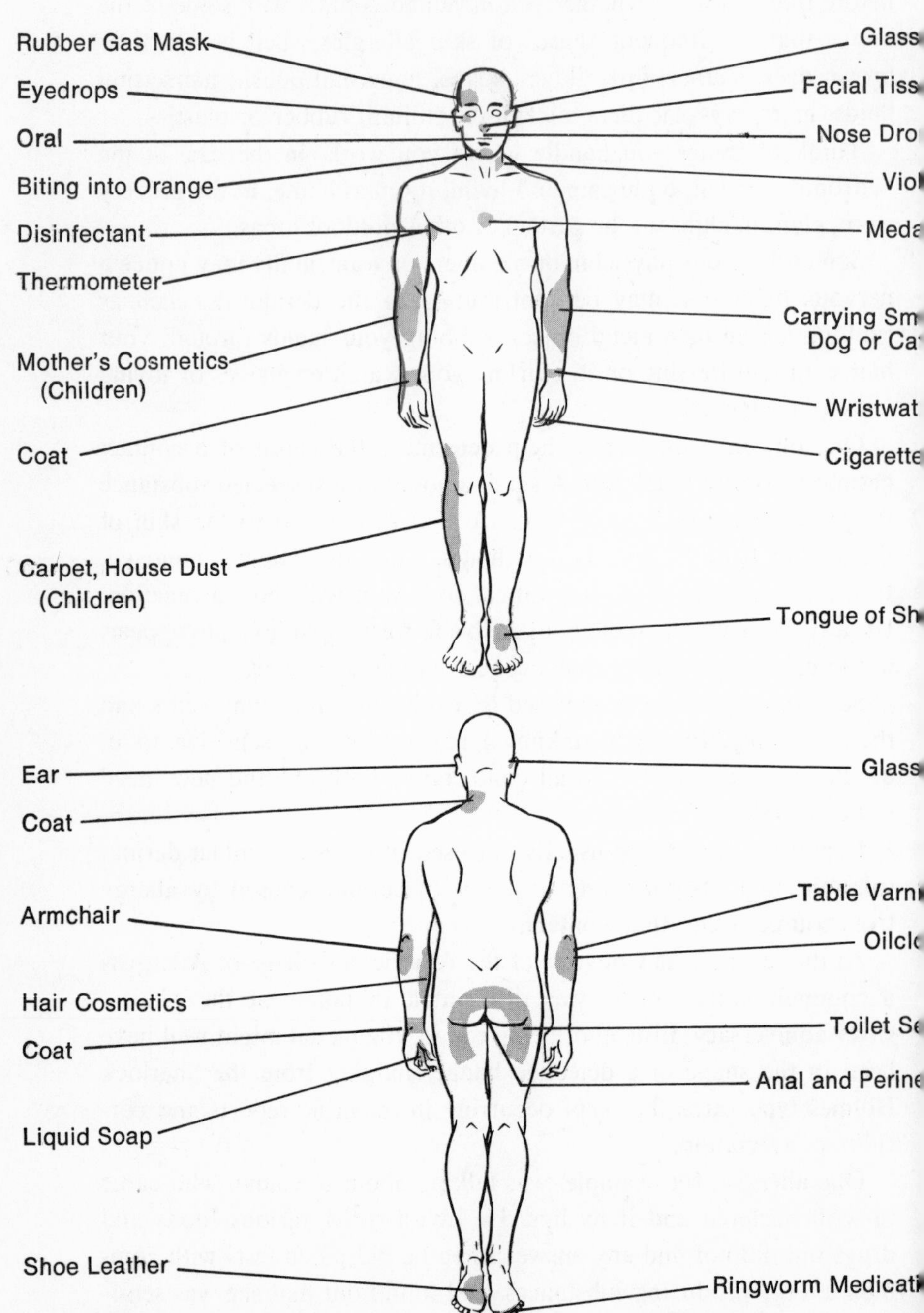

ADAPTED FROM DRAWINGS BY GEORGE WALDBOTT, M.D., HARPER HOSPITAL, DETROIT, MICHIGAN

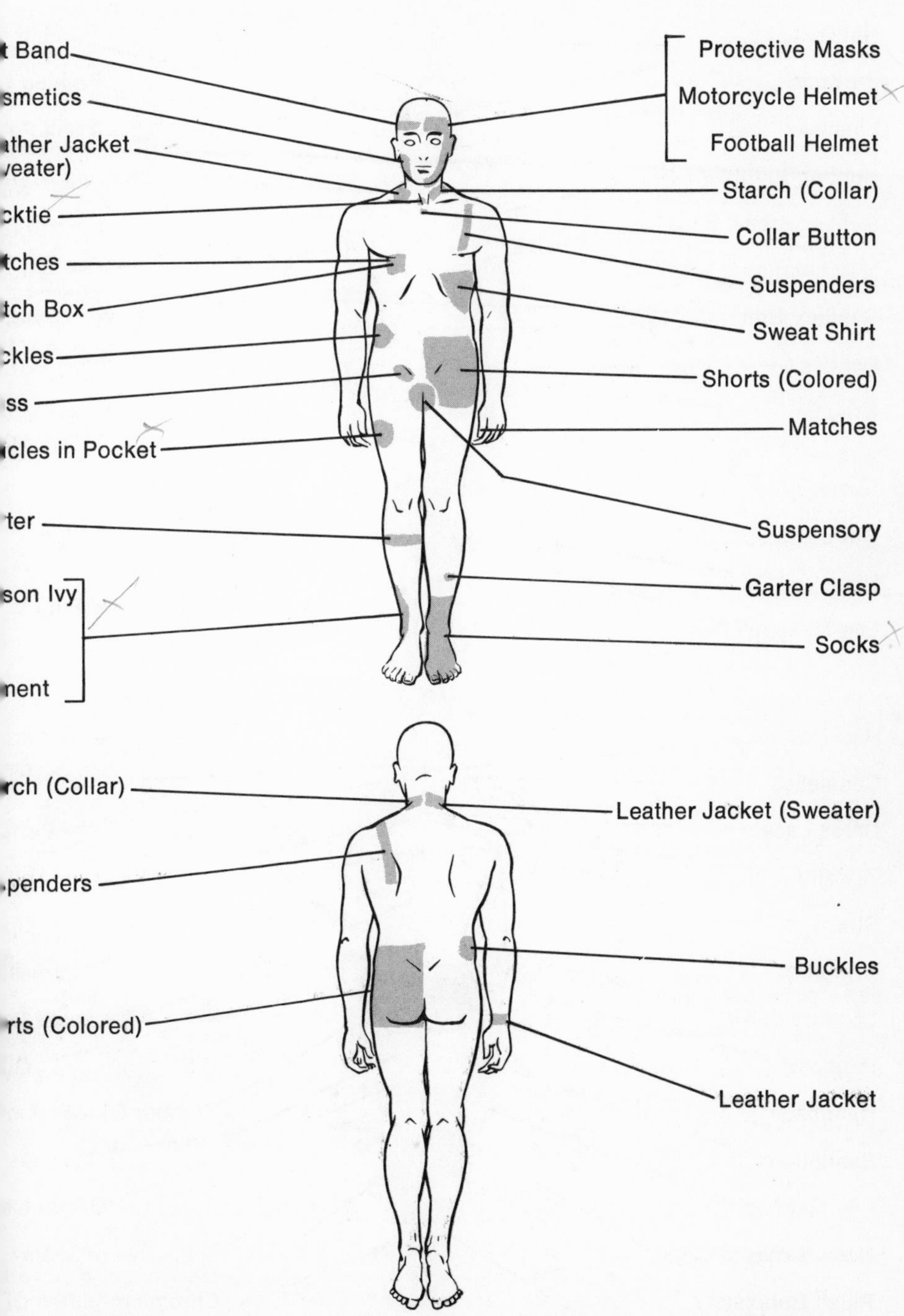
MEN
t Band
smetics
ather Jacket
veater)
cktie
tches
tch Box
ckles
ss
cles in Pocket
ter
son Ivy
nent
Protective Masks
Motorcycle Helmet
Football Helmet
Starch (Collar)
Collar Button
Suspenders
Sweat Shirt
Shorts (Colored)
Matches
Suspensory
Garter Clasp
Socks
rch (Collar)
penders
rts (Colored)
Leather Jacket (Sweater)
Buckles
Leather Jacket

WOMEN

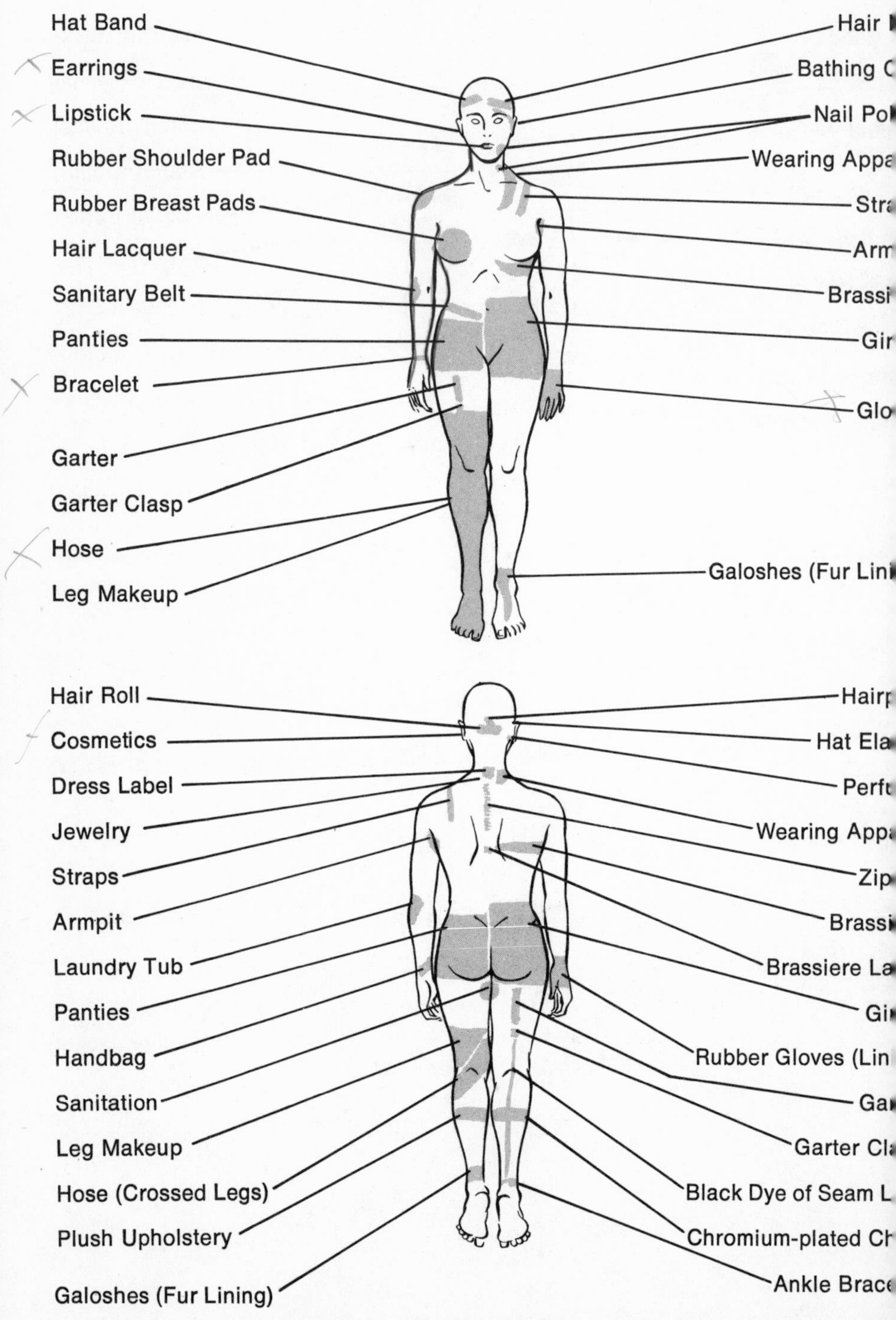
Hat Band
Earrings
Lipstick
Rubber Shoulder Pad
Rubber Breast Pads
Hair Lacquer
Sanitary Belt
Panties
Bracelet
Garter
Garter Clasp
Hose
Leg Makeup
Hair
Bathing
Nail Po
Wearing App
Stra
Arm
Brassi
Gir
Glo
Galoshes (Fur Lin
Hair Roll
Cosmetics
Dress Label
Jewelry
Straps
Armpit
Laundry Tub
Panties
Handbag
Sanitation
Leg Makeup
Hose (Crossed Legs)
Plush Upholstery
Galoshes (Fur Lining)
Hair
Hat Ela
Perf
Wearing App
Zip
Brassi
Brassiere La
Gi
Rubber Gloves (Lin
Ga
Garter Cl
Black Dye of Seam L
Chromium-plated Ch
Ankle Brac

in one day with her hair messed up from the wind, and tried to fix it. The allergist noticed that she held some nickel-plated hairpins in her mouth before she stuck them in her hair.

Another patient came in with a red and painful big toe. Was it gout? Was it infection? Why only one toe on one foot? A patch test showed that he was allergic to rubber. The answer—a cloth lining in one shoe had worn away, exposing rubber underneath. The patient threw away his shoes, and his toe healed.

One of the most important clues to finding the cause of a contact dermatitis is the pattern that the rash forms—where it occurs on your body and in what specific shape. For example, if you have a streaked rash below your eye, the rash may be caused by eyedrops. If you have vertical streaks extending down from your neck, it might be dye from a fur that you were wearing that became wet from the rain. If the folds of your skin are free from dermatitis, then a solid object is suspected. Fluid or semifluid materials will tend to gather in the folds and creases. A rash between your fingers could mean allergy to cigarettes you are smoking or to the smoke.

The following lists indicate some of the intriguing patterns and hint at some of the factors that can be the causes.

FINGERS ONLY

Fingertips

Button or starter of a car
Radio pushbutton
Light switch
Wristwatch clasp
Dial
Matches lighted with the fingernail
Hairpins
Musical instruments
Hair cosmetics (scratching head, massaging scalp)
Rosin on violin strings
Creams and liquids around the nails
Eyedrops or ointments
Polish on piano keys
Oil on typewriter keys
Cash register
Cedar wood of pencil

Finger Grip Type

Metal or plastic buttons
Knobs on furniture, office equipment, kitchen cupboards
Jewelry
Lipstick container
Pills and tablets
Food (popcorn, peanuts, olives)
Medicine dropper
Chain or cord
Coins
Tulip bulbs
Lacquered hairpins
Rubber hair curlers
Pins
Knitting needles
Crochet hook
Florist's wire

FINGERS ONLY (cont.)

Finger Turn

Knob on radio dial
Knob on a bottle brush
Small screwdriver
Cap of a bottle or tube
Hair cosmetics (from twisting hair)
Rolling cigarettes
Zipper
Comb
Toothpaste tube
Gear shift
Nozzle of enema or douche bag
Handle of a safety razor
Flicking pages of book, carbon paper
Pipe
Radiator valve

Finger Band

Rings
Creams or soap beneath ring
Hair cosmetics (curling hair around finger)
Elastic bands
Knitting yarn
Rubber electric cord
Scissors
Manila twine on mailbag

Finger Caps

Thimble
Finger cot
Contraceptive pills and jellies
Dipping fingers into fluid (oils, detergents, disinfectants)
Bowling ball
Hypodermic injections
Mucilage
Telephone dial

Lateral Finger

Pens and pencils
Cigarettes and cigarette holder
Metal instruments (dentist's drill)
Poison ivy
Billiard cue
Book cover (leather)
Plastic playing cards
Manila folder
Rotogravure newspaper
Leather billfold or spectacle case
Shoelaces
Armrest
Bridge table

FINGERS AND PALM

Ball Types

Football
Grapefruit
Rubber ball
Cocktail shaker
Colored labels of tin cans
Heel of riding boot (shoe polish)
Shoe box
Orange, lemon, lime
Atomizer bulb
Sponge
Pocketknife
Leather key case
Electric razor
Match box
Water faucet
Douche bulb
Door knob

FINGERS AND PALM (cont.)

Bar Types

Stair railing
Athlete's bar
Dog leash
Briefcase
Tray
Bridle strap
Handle of a baby carriage
Handle of a lawnmower
Handle of a kitchen drawer
Thick handle of a knife
Leather handbag strap
Handle of a handbag, luggage
Handle of bucket
Clothes brush
Rope
Book
Insulating wire
Comb
Handrail in bus
Golf clubs
Saw handle
Tennis racket
Trowel handle
Rubber hose
Bicycle grip
Hairbrush
Vacuum cleaner
Steering wheel
Flashlight
Refrigerator handle
Electric iron handle
Telephone receiver
Handle of a jumping rope
Dumb waiter (cable)
Handles of pots and pans

Palm Types

Knob of a cane
Vitamin tablets
Toothbrush
Bricks
Aspirin
Medicine bottle
Barroom tap
Vacuum cleaner
Handle of a frying pan
Knob of a whiskbroom
Old-fashioned gearshift
Eraser of a small pencil
Knob of a fluid soap dispenser
Tooth powder, toothpaste, creams, cosmetics, pills
Certain foods (held in palm)
Cleaning dentures (anise oil in cleaner)
Rolling cotton on wooden applicators
Rolling pin handle
Small screwdriver
Grating horseradish
Cleaning carrots, celery
Scaling fish
Hand mirror handle
Umbrella handle
Wooden mixing spoon
Hedge clippers
Handle of a grease gun
Handle of a gasoline hose
Leather insert of cloth glove
Shells (explosive powder)

PATTERNS INVOLVING FINGERWEBS

Thumb Index Area

Lacquered cash box
Plastic manicure tray
Plastic ashtray
Leather wastepaper basket
Paper bag
Rubber balloon
Dictaphone mouthpiece
Rubber shower appliance
Gate of office partition
Switchboard plug
Spilled medicine on bottle

PATTERNS INVOLVING FINGERWEBS (cont.)

Flat Object Design

Plastic playing cards
Gripping newspaper, magazine, book

Other Web Spaces

Golf tee
Drawing dyed wool through fingers
Leather keycase
X-shaped water faucet
Keychain

WRIST

Leather desk pad
Drawing paper
Sewing machine cover
Furniture polish
Hand lying on skirt (dye)
Leather armchair
Oil cloth or plastic cloth
Handbag
Handbag strap
Wristwatch
Bracelet
Leather wrist strap
Cuff of gloves
Cuffs (starch, dye, leather, fur)

DORSAL PATTERNS

Reaching into:
- box of filing cards
- stacked diapers
- stacked wooden food trays
- paper cartons
- box of cleansing tissues
- tucking in bedding
- woman's handbag
- trouser pocket
- coat pocket

Chalk (erasing from blackboard)
"Pitcher's dermatitis"
Tucking shirt into trousers
Contact with cow udder
Gunpowder from pistol shooting
Mending clothing
Pastes applied to snuffbox area by printers and lithographers
Dog hair (leading dog by collar)
Cotton gloves with leather back

NICKEL

Dermatitis from nickel is very common. People get nickel allergy from handling coins, as well as from wearing jewelry or wristwatches with nickel alloys.

Whenever ears are pierced for earrings, solid gold posts should be used since other earrings often contain nickel alloys. Two doctors in Monroe, Wisconsin, reported that seventeen young women came in with what appeared to be a chronic bacterial infection of the earlobe with swelling, draining and an eczemalike rash. They had all had their ears pierced and were allergic to the nickel in their earrings.

Medallions, identification tags and necklaces can cause nickel dermatitis on the upper chest and back. Hairpins, curlers and bobby-pins can cause it on the face and scalp. Thimbles, needles, scissors, coins and pens can affect the fingers. Nickel buckles, grips, garters, zippers and metal clips on the straps of slips can cause reactions. If you are allergic to nickel, you can buy zippers, clips and garters in nylon instead of metal.

A woman may find she's sensitive to the nickel in costume jewelry or garter grips in the summer, getting an itchy, prickly sensation, but she does not have the problem in the winter. This is because perspiration in the summertime increases the symptoms. If this is your problem, try applying talcum or absorbent powder to the skin under the metal to minimize the sweat.

Soaps or detergents can also collect underneath jewelry and cause allergy.

Recently doctors have also been reporting dermatitis produced by jewelry made from gold contaminated by radioactivity.

RUBBER DERMATITIS

Rubber products frequently cause allergic contact dermatitis. One New York clinic alone reports some two hundred cases every year. It's not so much the rubber causing the trouble as the chemicals that have been added in manufacturing.

Rubber products can be found in many places: rubber padding in dress shields, rubber baby panties, rubber adhesives used on false eyelashes, rubber edges of eyelash curlers, rubber gloves.

Easiest solution to a rubber allergy is to find proper substitutes. Stretchable garments can now be found of synthetic fibers called spandex that serve the same purpose in foundation garments, swimming suits, support hose, etc., without causing the rubber sensitivity.

CHROMATE

People may be exposed to chromate in leather, matches, paints, disinfectants, bleaches and glues. Occupational exposure is common in many industries, including automobile, welding, foundry, cement, railroad and building industries. Chromate often occurs in leather dye and often causes dermatitis of the feet. Some matchheads contain chromates, and perspiring fingers that touch matches can become contaminated and then touch other parts of the body. Some people who clean or scratch their ears with matches produce itching and irritation of the ear canal from even the small amount of contamination.

SYNTHETIC RESINS

For some thirty-five years textile finishing agents have consisted chiefly of natural gums, starches, minerals and vegetable oils, and they usually washed out in the first laundering or dry cleaning. Now synthetic resins make possible wash-and-wear and drip-dry clothes, but they also bring with them many allergies. One allergist of Detroit, Michigan, reports a "marked increase" of patients complaining of pimply eruptions on their legs and derriere. The eruptions were due to wash-and-wear garments that contained formaldehyde as a finishing treatment.

This formaldehyde can cause problems in the workers manufacturing the clothing too. The Environmental Control Committee of the Department of Health, Education, and Welfare released a report on several permanent press clothing manufacturing plants using formaldehyde gas to finish fabrics. They found one out of ten employees had to seek medical attention for dermatitis, respiratory complaints, eye irritation, fatigue or depression due to the formaldehyde.

You can often detect formaldehyde in newly purchased clothing by a "laboratory" type of odor.

Besides being used in cloth fibers, synthetic resins are also used in plastic jewelry and accessories, watchbands, fungicides, mirroring, tanning materials, rubber, glossy paper, cigarette packages, photographic plates and embalming fluid.

CLOTHES

Many people have specific allergies to wool or silk. Many times though, it is not the material itself that causes skin inflammation, but the dye. People also may have simple physical irritation from the roughness of a fabric.

And many people have irritations from underwear, not because of the fabric, but because it has been laundered in the same wash as fabrics made with glass fibers. This is not an allergic reaction, but simply a physical and mechanical irritation of skin by the fibers. The situation is being helped by glass fibers manufactured in different diameters that do not cause irritation. As improvements are made, the newer fiberglass fabric will probably be used for bedspreads, sheets and clothing, since it is flameproof.

DERMATITIS OF THE FEET

Many skin eruptions of the feet are mistakenly attributed to athlete's foot and other infections when they are really due to allergy. Shoes are the chief source of trouble, not necessarily because of leather, but also because of various rubber and synthetic materials, unfriendly dyes and adhesives and materials used in the tanning. Sometimes it is the felt, the asphalt filler, the dye or glue used in the insoles and linings.

Usually the irritation first appears where the skin is thin and delicate between the toes, and the irritation is worst where the pressure from shoes is the strongest. A person with sweaty feet often has the worst problem, for perspiration tends to extract the chemicals.

If shoe dermatitis is your problem, there are many things you can do besides go barefoot. If it is the rubber in the box toe you are allergic to, buy shoes with plastic box toes. If the dye is causing your problem, buy undyed shoes or those colored with pure vegetable dyes. If the tanning chemical is the cause, buy shoes made of vegetable-tanned leather, fabric or plastic. If it is the leather itself, buy some of the modern plastic shoes.

Sometimes foot rashes are caused by the dye in socks. Wear white ones, even if they're not stylish.

DRUGS

Many skin problems can be caused by drug allergies. Here are the major reactions and the drugs that commonly cause them.

1. Hives	Organ extracts, penicillin, streptomycin, salicylates, sera, food adulterated with coloring, flavoring and preservative agents of coal tar origin
2. Eczema	Sulfonamides, penicillin, mercurials, arsenicals, local anesthetics, quinacrine, quinine, aniline dyes, arsphenamine
3. Fixed eruptions	Barbiturates, phenolphthalein, quinacrine, sulfonamides, gold, phenacetin, antipyrine

4. Red rashes and nodules	Bromides, iodides, salicylates, phenacetin, sulfonamides, penicillin, phenolphthalein
5. Purpura	Barbiturates, gold salts, iodides, sulfonamides, arsphenamine
6. Eruptions	Barbiturates, sulfonamides, heavy metals, arsenic, salicylates, foods adulterated with coloring, flavoring and preservative agents of coal tar origin, penicillin
7. Blister eruptions	Iodides, gold, salicylates, sulfonamides, phenolphthalein
8. Peeling or scaly dermatitis	Arsenicals, barbiturates, gold salts, mercurials, quinacrine, belladonna

SOAP PHOTOALLERGY

Several commercial soaps and other products contain bithionol, hexachlorophene and halogenated salicylanilides. All of these compounds are incorporated in the soaps to reduce the number of bacteria on the skin and thus to minimize body odor. Some people are photosensitive to the substances; that is, after using them if they go out into the sun, they have an allergic skin reaction.

Photodermatitis is often noted after the weekend when the person has exposed himself to sunlight. Parts exposed to the sunlight become especially red—the face, backs of the hands, ears.

If such a photoallergy is suspected, special patch tests are done. An ointment of the substance is put on the back, with the patch remaining up to twenty-four hours; then the patch is removed and the skin is irradiated with ultraviolet light.

Treatment is to switch to a soap or compound that does not contain the troublemaking agent. Sometimes a phenomenon known as "persistent positive reactor" occurs, in which the patient continues to have difficulty for several months following withdrawal of the offending agent. However, it finally does go away.

■ OCCUPATIONAL DERMATITIS

The term "occupational dermatitis" refers to any skin condition caused by what you do at work. It's a very significant factor that costs industry an estimated $200,000,000 every year and affects tens of thousands of workers.

Many of the substances producing occupational dermatitis are the same substances found in the home, but many others are found only in the work environment. Plastic manufacturers, farmers, refiners, bakers, laboratory workers, brewers, hairdressers, fur dyers, chemists, sausage makers, woodworkers, wool handlers, all have their own materials they work with and their own set of skin allergies. Cobalt workers have the cobalt itch. Bakers get baker's dermatitis. Fur and leather workers develop reactions to many dyes. Pharmaceutical workers develop dermatitis from handling penicillin.

Other substances used in industry sometimes cause hives.

Castor oil used in jet engines and soaps and printing inks can cause asthma as well as dermatitis. Farmers can get asthma and dermatitis from using the ground-up castor beans as fertilizer, and families of both the factory workers and farmers have developed symptoms from exposure to contaminated workclothes, and garbage collectors have developed symptoms from handling old burlap bags which had been contaminated by the beans.

Asthma and dermatitis can be produced by substances in epoxy resins and in substances used in the manufacture of plastic foams.

A typical story is the one of twelve people working at a nursery who got a dermatitis after making cuttings of the tops of chrysanthemum plants for replanting. They had burning and itching of the arms, face, neck and abdomen. The cause was that the plants had been sprayed with an insecticide just before the cutting operation. The problem was solved for the future by not exposing workers to plants for at least several hours after insecticides were applied.

Occasionally a condition appears to be due to an allergy but in the final analysis is the result of a low-grade irritation. For example, some 3 to 7 percent of workers in corn processing plants get a corn dermatitis known as corn rash or corn itch. It's especially common in people who have their skin wet for long periods when handling corn. Patch tests are negative. They generally solve the problem by wearing protective gloves or creams on their hands.

PREVENTING OCCUPATIONAL DERMATITIS

Much can be done by the employer to reduce occupational dermatitis. Exhaust ventilation should be installed in areas where there is mixing of resin or other irritating procedures or where there is dust generated by sanding fiberglass or plastics. Special housing with vacuum cleaner lines can be attached to sanders and routers. Paper containers can minimize contact in cleanup.

You can also do many things yourself to reduce occupational dermatitis. Wear protective clothing, including gloves and aprons. Use the protective ointments that your physician recommends. Removal of resins with solvents should always be followed by soap and water washing and application of a cream to minimize drying and chapping.

PRINCIPAL CONTACT AGENTS IN VARIOUS OCCUPATIONS

The following is a list of possible causes of contact dermatitis by occupation that may provide clues in tracking down any offending chemicals:

AGRICULTURAL LABORERS AND MARKET GARDENERS—Poisonous plants and woods; artificial fertilizers, insecticides; animal hair.

ARTISTS—Turpentine, thinner, calcium sulfate, lead, oxalic acid, linseed oil, camel's-hair brushes.

AVIATORS—Insecticides sprayed by planes; lead, arsenic, toxic gas, gasoline.

BAKERS—Spices, sugar, vanilla, lemon, cinnamon, wheat flour conditioners. Consider flare-ups from simultaneous sensitivity to these foods.

BARBERS, BEAUTICIANS—Soaps, shampoo preparations, dyes, hydrogen peroxide, rubber gloves, permanent-wave setting solution, colocynth used as denaturant in alcohol.

BOOKBINDING INDUSTRY—Glue, shellac, inks, coloring materials.

BOOT AND SHOE MANUFACTURERS—Organic dust, ammonia, amyl acetate, benzene, benzol, mercury paste, nitrobenzene.

BROOMS AND BRUSHES—Various kinds of woods, celluloid, metals, lead bleaching materials.

BUILDING CONSTRUCTION—Earthy bases of calcium, sulfuric acid, lime dust, cement, aniline dyes, chromium compounds, arsenic, lead, ammonia, turpentine. ROAD BUILDERS—Tar, asphalt, bitumen, coal tar, cement.

BUTCHERING, SLAUGHTERING AND MEAT PACKING—Animal hair, dermatomycoses.

BUTTON MANUFACTURING—Ivory and horn dust, calcium carbonate, wood, brass, nickel, iron, gold, silver, paper, celluloid.

CANDY MANUFACTURING—Starch; foil and paper; cord; granulated sugar; oils used in flavoring: oil of cassia, peppermint, orange peel, lemon peel, anise, cloves; oil of birch; extract of vanilla; citric acid; tartaric acid; chocolate; pineapple; citrus fruits; cashew nuts; calcium chloride.

CANNING AND FOOD PRESERVING INDUSTRIES—Irritating juices and essential oils, dyes, preservatives, insecticides, kerosene, soaps, mustard, vinegar, lead, rubber, resin, benzene, lacquer, gasoline, sulfurous acid, copper sulfate.

CEMENT WORKER—Chromium, alkali.

CLERKS AND OFFICE WORKERS—Aniline-colored pencils, glue, carbon paper, typewriter ribbon, dust, desk pads.

DAIRY WORKERS—Primrose rash, ragweed (handling udders of cows), cow hair, borax, alkaline substances.

DENTISTS—Procaine, metals, sulfa, benzocaine, eugenol.

DIESEL MOTORS—Sodium bichromate in radiator fluid.

DISINFECTANTS AND FUMIGANTS—Acetaldehyde, alum, aluminum chloride, ammonia, aniline colors, bromines, calcium chloride, chlorine, cresol, creosote, essential oils, formaldehyde, hydrochloric acid, hydrocyanic acid, lead, methylated spirits, mercuric chloride, nitronaphthalene, phenol, picric acid, pitch, resin, sodium carbonate, sulfur dioxide, sulfuric acid, tannin, tar, tar oil, turpentine, zinc chloride, zinc sulfate.

DOCK LABORERS AND WAREHOUSE MEN—Pads between shoulder blades (leather dye), dusts from grain, minerals, coal, lead, manganese, arsenic, calamine, artificial fertilizers.

DOLLS, TOYS, AND ADVERTISING NOVELTIES—Resin, glue, lead, lacquer, enamel, aniline colors, excelsior, amyl acetate and other solvents, wood, iron, copper, nickel, bronze, paper, Bakelite, leather, fur, rubber.

DRY CLEANING INDUSTRY—Glycerine, oleic acid, glacial acetic acid, petroleum, ether, chloroform, hydrofluoric acid, oxalic acid, denatured alcohol, benzene, naphtha gasoline, turpentine, trichlorethylene, carbolic acid, nitrobenzene, amyl acetate, carbon tetrachloride, strong alkali, benzene soap, ammonia.

ELECTRIC APPARATUS MANUFACTURER—Carbon monoxide, sulfur, arsenic, Bakelite, rubber, acetone, benzene, benzone, hydrochloric acid, lacquer, mercury, resin, sulfuric acid. ELECTRIC LAMP MANUFACTURER—Mercury, ether, amyl acetate, methyl alcohol, nitric acid, hydrofluoric acid, copper, nickel, lime.

EXTERMINATORS—DDT, arsenic, formalin, sodium fluoride, lead.

FEATHER INDUSTRY—Aniline dyes, arsenic, glue, sulfur dioxide, hydrogen peroxide, soap, benzene, turpentine, methyl alcohol.

FIREPROOFING—Copper, brass, glue, resin, benzene, sharp dust particles, chlorinated naphthalene, tar, lime.

FISH INDUSTRY—Fish scales.

FLORISTS—Plants, manures, fertilizers, insecticides, dyes of ribbons and other decorative articles. ARTIFICIAL FLOWER INDUSTRY—Lead chromates, arsenic, picric acid, methyl alcohol, benzene, carbon tetrachloride, chrome colors, rubber solution, varnishes.

FLOUR AND GRAIN INDUSTRY—Dust, sulfur dioxide, chlorine.

FURRIERS—Arsenic, dyes, chromium.

GARAGES, AUTOMOBILE REPAIR SHOP, CHAUFFEURS—Oil, grease, kerosene, benzene, gasoline, lead, tetraethyl, potassium cyanide, impure petroleum, antifreeze.

GARMENT AND MILLINERY INDUSTRIES—Dyes, iron, tin, antimony, aluminum, lead, zinc, copper, turpentine, benzene, methyl alcohol, carbon tetrachloride, salts of chromium.

GLUE MANUFACTURER—Hydrochloric acid, nitric acid, sulfur dioxide, formaldehyde, bichromates, resin, shellac, benzene, acetone, turpentine, ammonia, lime, caustic soda, alum, borax, tannic acid, glycerine, shale oil, zinc sulfate, lead, nitrous and other acid fumes, fatty acids, arseniuretted and sulfuretted hydrogen, mercaptan.

GROCERIES AND DELICATESSENS—Dyes of labels, citrus fruit rinds, insecticides, insect sprays, cardboard boxes, paper bags, dry ice.

HOTELS, RESTAURANTS—Boric acid, sulfurous acid, sulfites, borax, salicylic acid, formaldehyde, disinfectants, fungicides, insecticides, irritant oils, fruit juices, vegetables (asparagus, celery), caustic soaps, grease.

ICE CREAM MAKING—Fruits, nuts, flavoring and coloring materials, sugar.

INK—Aniline dye, turpentine, cashew nut oil, chromates.

JANITORS—Polishing materials, arsenic, thallium, lead, benzene, hydrocyanic acid, oxalic acid, soap.

JEWELRY AND ALLIED INDUSTRIES—Platinum, ammonium hydroxide, nickel, nitric acid, hydrochloric acid, sulfuric acid, potassium cyanide, lead, shellac, resin, amyl acetate, chrome, enamel lacquer, alkalies, nitrous fumes, soap, soda, trichlorethylene, radioactive substances, mahogany, ebony, walnut (in watches and clocks).

LAUNDRY WORKERS AND WASH WOMEN—Coconut oil soaps, starch, bleaching powder.

LUMBER AND WOODWORKING INDUSTRIES—Brazilian walnut, creosote, zinc chloride, mercury chloride, chlorphenols, plaster of Paris, diphenyl, tar oil, creosote oil, aniline colors, cocobolo wood, glue, diphenylchlorarsine, arsenic, amyl acetate, oxalic acid, varnish, lead, boxwood.

MACHINERY MANUFACTURE—Oil, cyanogen compounds, nitric acid, yellow ochre, Viennese chalk, oxide of iron, putty powder, methyl alcohol, benzene, turpentine, slaked lime, hydrochloric acid, oxalic acid, nickel sulfate, potassium cynanide, zinc chloride, chromates, beryllium.

MATCH AND MATCH BOX INDUSTRY—Phosphorus, chlorate, red lead, chromium compounds.

MEDICAL AND ALLIED PROFESSIONS—Novocain, pantocaine, formalin, rubber, plaster of Paris, cocaine, procaine hydrochloride, mercury, formaldehyde, phenol, cresol, thymol, wood alcohol, ethyl silicate, Apothesine, borax, epinephrine, mercury, chromates, arsenic salts, sulfur, carbon tetrachloride, phenylhydrazine, strychnine, atropine, morphine, codeine, opium, quinine, emetine, cantharides, hydrogen peroxide, iodine.

MIRRORS—Ammonia, formaldehyde, essential oils of cloves, thyme, chamomile, glucose, resins.

MUSICAL INSTRUMENTS AND MUSICIANS—Irritating woods, lead, hydrogen peroxide, sulfuric acid, sodium peroxide, calcium chloride, glacial acetic acid, benzene, methyl alcohol, turpentine, resin-pitch mixture.

PASTRY COOKS—Glucose, oils of citrus fruits, vanilla, cashew nut oil, nitrobenzol, angelic acid, cinnamon.

PENCIL AND CRAYON MANUFACTURE—Aniline and chromium compounds, sawdust of red cedar wood, waxes, gums, glue.

PHOTOGRAPHERS—Pyrogallol, chromates, aniline dyes, lacquers.

PLUMBING, GAS, AND STEAM FITTINGS—Lead, hydrochloric acid, zinc chloride, tetraline.

POTTERY WORKERS—Cobalt, alkali.

PRINTERS—Arsenic, chromate, artificial coloring and hydrocarbons in inks.

PULP PAPER AND PAPER PRODUCTS—Arsenic compounds, sulfuretted hydrogen, chlorine, formaldehyde, hydrochloric acid, sodium hydroxide, sulfur dioxide, sulfuric acid. PAPER BOX MANUFACTURE—Moist glues and paste.

PUTTY MANUFACTURE—Lead, linseed oil, benzene, benzol, carbon disulfide, antimony sulfide.

ROPE AND CORDAGE MANUFACTURE—Sodium hydroxide, potassium hydroxide, dust, impure oils, dyes.

SHEET METAL, STAMPED AND ENAMEL WARE—Amyl acetate, antimony, arsenic, benzene, carbon disulfide, chromium, hydrochloric acid, lead, manganese, naphtha, nitrous gases and nitric acid, quicklime, sulfuric acid, tetrachlorethane, turpentine.

SPICES AND FLAVORING MANUFACTURE—Cinnamon, pepper, ginger, oil of anise, mustard, vanilla, oils of citrus fruits, oil of bitter almonds.

SPORTING GOODS—Lead, rubber, nickel, chrome, leather, leather dyes.

STONE WORKERS—Limestone, lime, stone dust, oxalic acid.

TANNERS—Bichromate, hydrochloric acid.

TAXIDERMY—Lysol, arsenious oxide, chloride of lime, mercury chloride, tannin, calcined alum, gasoline.

THEATRICAL PROFESSION AND MOTION PICTURE INDUSTRY—Cosmetics, assorted woods, developer, dyes.

TRUCK DEALERS AND WRECKERS—Lead, brass, bronze, zinc, benzene, sulfuric acid, lime, cement, lead, tar, creosote.

UNDERTAKERS AND EMBALMERS—Formaldehyde and other embalming fluids, mercury, carbolic acid, oil of cinnamon, oil of cloves, thymol.

WATERPROOFING—Resin, sodium carbonate, rubber, chrome, glue, alum, potassium bichromate, chromium fluoride, chrome alum, turpentine, yellow wax, groundnut oil, iron sulfate, essence of thyme, shellac, amyl acetate, creosote oil.

WINDOW SHADES AND VENETIAN BLINDS—Benzene, paint, shellac.

WOOL—Alkali solutions, black dye, mineral oil, wool.

■ POISON IVY AND OTHER PLANT PROBLEMS

Of all the plants that can cause contact dermatitis, poison ivy is the most common. You can get it after petting a dog who has brushed through the weed or from touching contaminated clothes or being exposed to the fumes of burning poison ivy plants. You can get it in the winter by brushing the twigs as well as in the summer by touching the leaves. Sometimes children even eat the berries, causing an allergic reaction in the mouth or in the rectal area when the plant is excreted.

The plants have long been a source of misery. In fact the American Indians told the early settlers about the ill effects of the plant, and Captain John Smith described them in his journal in the early days of American colonization.

It is estimated that sensitivity occurs to poison ivy and its relatives poison oak and poison sumac in approximately 70 percent of all people. On the other hand, some people seem to possess a natural immunity to the effects of the plants and do not get a rash no matter how much exposure they have, even if they rub the leaves directly on the skin.

ALL THESE PLANTS CAN CAUSE ALLERGIC REACTIONS.

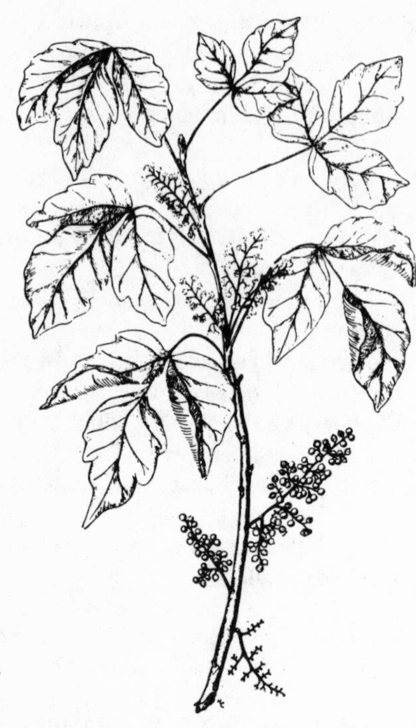

Poison Ivy
Toxicodendron radicans

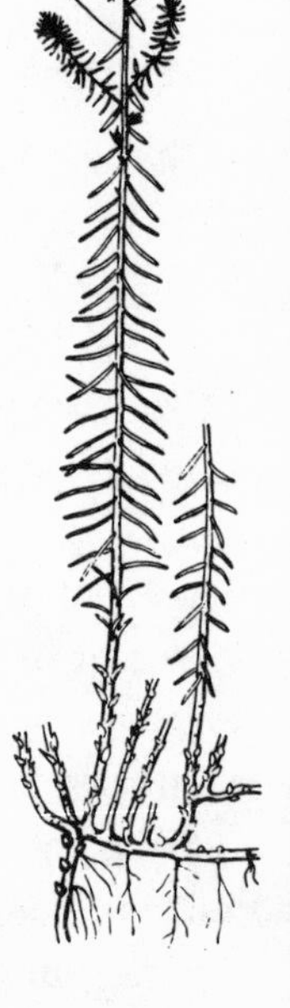

Cypress Spurge
Euphorbia cyparissias

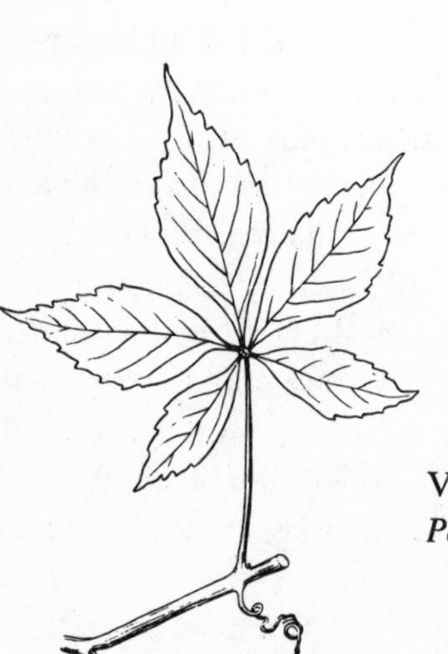

Virginia Creeper –
Parthenocissus quinquefolia

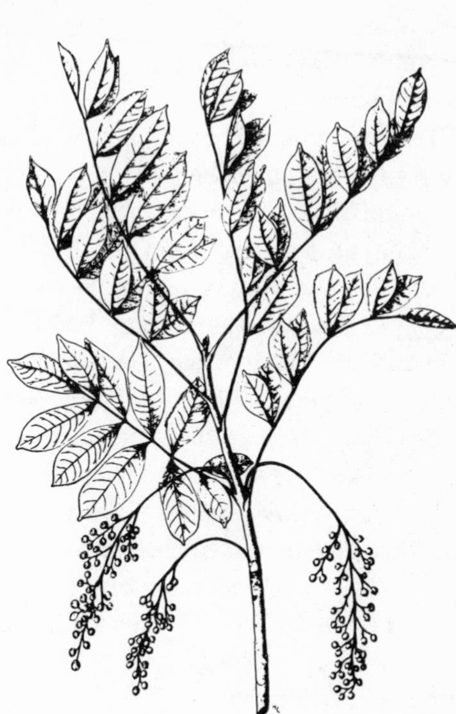

Poison Sumac
Toxicodendron vernix

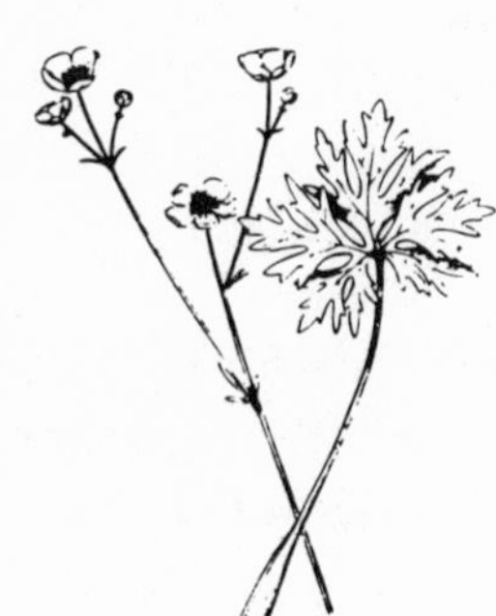

Tall Field Buttercup
Ranunculus acris

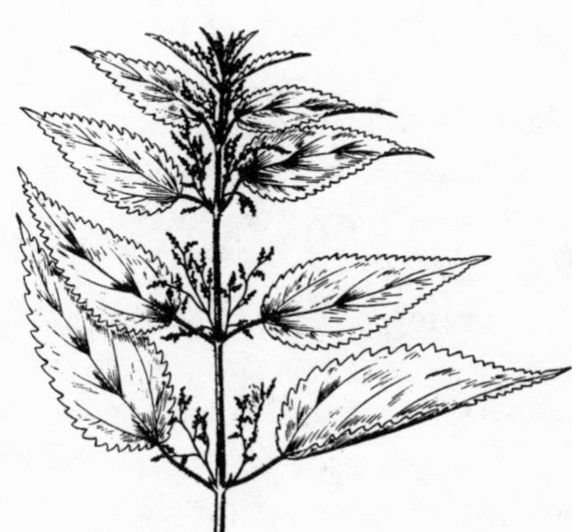

Stinging Nettle
Urtica dioica

The latent period between contact with the plant and appearance of the rash may vary from a few hours to ten days or longer. The rash usually lasts, on the average, two to three weeks.

A plant is most poisonous when it contains the most sap; this is generally in the spring and early summer. The dry sap maintains its potency for many months.

Besides the usual formation of water blisters that any country boy can recognize immediately, there is another form of eruption that can be caused. The skin turns white, then later turns black, and in eight to ten days a scab may form which is sloughed off.

Avoiding the plant is the best protection. When you expect to come in contact with the plant, wear long sleeves, long trousers and gloves. You can also apply protective ointment to the skin before working around the plant. When you know you have been in contact with poison ivy, change clothes immediately and wash with a strong laundry soap. Give your pet a bath also if he has been in it.

Poison ivy, oak or sumac rash will usually clear quickly by itself, but there are some medicines that will help dry the rash and relieve the itching. Calamine lotion and Ivy-dry are helpful. Oral antihistamines can help diminish the itching. Check your doctor for other drugs, such as prednisone when the rash is very severe and will not respond to treatment.

Some physicians recommend injections of poison oak and poison ivy extract to prevent the disease. However, the desensitization must be maintained on a booster basis; otherwise it does not last very long, so is worthwhile only for people who are very sensitive. Another method of hyposensitization is by taking capsules of the extract by mouth before the worst part of the poison ivy season. The easiest way is to learn to recognize the plants and stay away from them.

In cases where a patient has a very severe attack, he can sometimes be treated by being given small doses of extract at frequent intervals, usually every day or every other day, until the symptoms have subsided.

To destroy poison ivy and oak, the United States Department of Agriculture recommends the use of herbicides such as amitrole, Ammate, and 2,4,5,-D, which are sold under a variety of brand names. If you grub out the plants, put them in plastic bags rather than leaving them uncovered for the unsuspecting trash collectors.

OTHER PLANTS THAT CAN CAUSE DERMATITIS

Many outdoor and indoor plants beside poison ivy, poison oak and poison sumac can cause allergy. Known troublemakers are gaillardia, krameria, tumbleweed, buttercups, primroses, may apples, poinsettias, chrysanthemums, philodendron, pines, daisies and tulips. Even dried plants that a hunter brushes against in the field can cause dermatitis, as can handling houseplants, tulip bulbs or orange peels.

In Europe the main outdoor plant causing contact allergy is the primrose. In Japan a lacquer tree contains an oil that is related to poison ivy. Fishermen often get a rash from using lacquer fishing gear manufactured in Japan. Voodoo dolls imported from Haiti and drink stirring sticks made from cashew nuts may produce a poison-ivylike dermatitis, as will the rind of a mango.

In India, ink from the marking-nut tree is sometimes used to mark laundry, and underwear marked with it can sometimes cause dermatitis.

Irritation of the skin by stinging nettles, mullen plants, and leaves of beans is purely physical, not allergic. Raw potato peelings, green raw tomatoes and tomato stems can induce a rash as well, but this is because of a toxic substance, not because of allergy.

■ ALLERGIES TO COSMETICS

Allergy to cosmetics affects both men and women and occurs much more often than generally realized. It is estimated that more than 3,000,000 men and women in the United States are allergic to some form of cosmetics, and that some 85 percent of these don't even realize what it is that is causing their trouble. About 9 percent of women have drying and cracking of their lips after using certain lipsticks, and 10 percent have a respiratory or skin allergy to perfumes.

No statistics have been compiled on men yet, but as they use more lotions and cosmetics, the cases of allergy are increasing. And many men have allergies to their wife's or date's perfume, lipstick, hairspray or powder. More than one romance has taken a turn for the worse when the boyfriend developed swollen lips every time he kissed his girl. One man who sold women's shoes had to change his job because the perfumes that most of his customers wore gave him asthma.

Babies, too, can be allergic to their mother's cosmetics. And even dogs have been known to get hives from their owner's face powder or talcum powder.

The vast increase in allergy to cosmetics is due to several factors: hairsprays, eye makeup, perfumes and other cosmetics are being used more, manufacturers are increasing the amount of indelible dyes used in lipsticks to make them more permanent and smearproof, and medicines and exotic new chemicals are being developed and incorporated into cosmetics. All of these factors mean more opportunity for allergic reactions.

The kinds of symptoms caused by cosmetic allergies are the same as those of other allergens. Contact dermatitis is the usual symptom with redness and itching, scaling, puffiness or eczema. The constant irritation to the skin from the symptoms can also lead to aging and drying effects over the years. There can also be hives or respiratory symptoms.

A lipstick can cause dryness of the lips or severe cracking, puffiness and scaling. If the person is also photosensitive, the condition can be made even worse by exposure to the sun. Redness and itching of the eyelids may be due to mascara, eyeshadow, eyeliner or adhesive on false eyelashes, and can also be due to soap or hair dye or to nail polish from rubbing your eyes. Dermatitis of the scalp can be caused by shampoos, hair tonics, hair dyes, permanent wave solutions, or hairsprays.

Sometimes cosmetics do not seem to give any problem ordinarily, but do cause a problem during hayfever season. This is due to the two allergic factors added together; the allergic threshold is breached and the person has symptoms.

A reaction may appear after you have changed to a new type of cosmetic or when a new ingredient is added to your regular brand, or it may suddenly and unexplainedly appear with the continued use of the same cosmetic even after years of use. Some women are allergic to substances only when they are pregnant. Other women lose their allergies when they are pregnant.

Allergy to cosmetics is not always easy to recognize. One woman had a stuffy nose, then for two months had an inflamed pharynx and bad sinus trouble, then she had a burning tongue for several days. For what was supposed to be a severe cold and sinusitis several weeks later, she took antihistamines, throat lozenges, nasal sprays, antibiotics, nasal packings, and infrared treatments. Finally a new indelible lipstick was incriminated. The woman was told to discontinue it and was free of all symptoms in four days.

Another woman had a severe eyelid dermatitis, with puffy and reddened lids. She also complained of burning and itching of the neck, under the chin, under the arms and on the abdomen. It seemed to be an allergy, but to what? The doctor was nonplussed until she mentioned her symptoms were most severe the day after her weekly visit to the beauty shop for a shampoo and manicure. Patch tests for the shampoo were negative, but the nail polish provided an instantaneous reaction. The symptoms on the neck, arms and abdomen? The nail polish touched there when she rubbed her eyes, fiddled with her necklace and scratched her abdomen after taking off her girdle.

When one Chicago doctor sent questionnaires to dermatologists throughout the nation to find out what the most common cosmetic troublemakers were, he found that hair products led all other cosmetics and toiletries as causes of reactions. The other most common complaints involved reactions to antibacterial soaps, nail polishes, perfumes, face and eye products, deodorants and antiperspirants.

Two of the major offenders in cosmetics are orris root and karaya gum. They are found in face powder, shaving cream, facial cream, sunburn lotion, shampoo, rouge, perfume, lipstick, soap, hair tonic and also in items such as sachets, teething rings, toothpaste, dental adhesive powders, and some drugs and diabetic foods. Karaya gum is also found in junket, certain brands of gelatin, ices, ice cream, some salad dressings, factory-made pies, gumdrops and similar candies.

Recently substances called paraben esters have also been incriminated as causative factors in inducing allergic illness. They are found in most cosmetic creams and lotions and also in many medical ointments. Many times the very ointments that are being used to try to clear up a dermatitis contain paraben, which makes it worse. Paraben is also found in some foods and dentifrices and in suppositories.

Dr. William F. Schorr, a Wisconsin dermatologist, writes in the *Journal of the American Medical Association* that parabens may be the cause of long-standing progressive dermatitis and the diagnosis is often missed, partly because patch tests for it are often negative unless the test is done with a high concentration of paraben.

One of the recent surprising causes of allergies has been pesticides found in cosmetics. Traces of DDT, dieldrin and other pesticides have been found in a vast number of cosmetics because they contain lanolin from sheep treated for parasites.

Another troublemaker in people who dye their hair is a substance called para-phenylenediamine (PPDA), which is found mostly in dyes that require mixing with peroxide before application. If a person is sensitive to PPDA, he is usually also sensitive to other hair dyes and clothing dyes and certain medicines. Semipermanent hair dyes that do not require oxidation and rinses can usually be used safely. Patch tests should be done behind the ear before using any hair dye. People allergic to PPDA should also beware of local anesthetics such as procaine, benzocaine, xylocaine and carbocaine, all of which are related to PPDA.

HYPOALLERGENIC COSMETICS

A few decades ago beauty products were far from pure. In fact, a government exhibit called the "Chamber of Horrors" showed pictures of such disfigurements as a woman permanently blinded from using an eyelash dye. Now, since the Food, Drug and Cosmetic Act of 1938, most American makeups are safe and pure. However, they still contain many substances that, even though they are safe for most people, can cause allergic reactions in others.

Hypoallergenic cosmetics were first introduced in 1932 by Philip Blazer, who became interested in them when his wife developed a skin condition attributed to impure cosmetics. Mr. Blazer produced a line of cosmetics that eliminated many allergy-causing substances. These products were originally called nonallergenic cosmetics. However, it was soon recognized that there is no such thing as a 100 percent allergy-proof substance, and the name "hypoallergenic" was coined. These are cosmetics designed to have as few as possible of the ingredients that most frequently cause allergies.

Hypoallergenic cosmetics are not in any sense medicated. It's not anything that's added, it's what's left out that counts. And it's not a matter of purity. All cosmetics must be made with pure materials. But hypoallergenic cosmetics have none of the indelible dyes, perfumes, lanolin and other substances that so often cause allergic reactions in the hypersensitive individual. One manufacturer of hypoallergenic cosmetics says their company has eliminated more than sixty ingredients that are ordinarily contained in cosmetics. The hypoallergenic cosmetics are available in the usual up-to-date variety of fashion colors.

Most of the hypoallergenic cosmetics can be found in drugstores.

If your physician or drugstore cannot supply them, write to any of the companies who make the cosmetics: Ar-Ex Products Company, 1036 West Van Buren Street, Chicago, Illinois 60607; Almay Cosmetics, Schieffelin & Co., 41 East 42nd Street, New York, New York 10017; Marcelle Hypo-Allergenic Cosmetics, The Borden Company, 350 Madison Avenue, New York, New York 10017.

These companies make free and full disclosure of all the ingredients used in their cosmetics. Many times if a patient is still having symptoms, even with a hypoallergenic cosmetic, the manufacturer will cooperate with him to try to find out exactly what ingredient is causing the trouble. Sometimes they will even, on special request, furnish cosmetics without that specific ingredient.

Many people use hypoallergenic cosmetics only during hayfever season and find that their symptoms are minimized.

If you are sensitive to cosmetics and switch to hypoallergenic ones, don't forget to discard your old powder puff. Also remind your barber or hairdresser not to use any powder or any other allergy-causing preparations on you.

The following list (adapted from a report prepared by Ar-Ex Products Co.) should help you in working with your physician to find any cosmetics you might be sensitive to.

COMMON COSMETIC IRRITANTS AND ALLERGENS

Ingredients used in cosmetic manufacture reported to cause allergic reactions

Substance	*Commonly Found In*	*Symptoms*
ACETONE	Nail polish removers	Peeling and splitting of the nails Dermatitis of the fingers
ALMOND OIL	Cosmetic creams Perfumes Soaps	Stuffy nose Contact dermatitis
ALUM	Astringent lotions Anhidrotics	Contact dermatitis
ALUMINUM	Astringent lotions Anhidrotics Deodorants	Contact dermatitis

COMMON COSMETIC IRRITANTS AND ALLERGENS (*cont.*)

Substance	*Commonly Found In*	*Symptoms*
AMMONIUM CARBONATE	Permanent wave solutions	Dermatitis of the scalp, forehead, and hands
ANTIMONY COMPOUNDS	Hair dyes	Contact dermatitis
ARROW ROOT	Dusting powder Dry shampoos	Stuffy nose Inflamed eyes
ARSENIC COMPOUNDS	Hair tonics Hair dyes	Contact dermatitis
BALSAM OF PERU	Perfumes	Contact dermatitis Stuffy nose
BARIUM SULFIDE	Depilatories	Contact dermatitis
BENZALDEHYDE	Cosmetic creams Lotions	Contact dermatitis
BETANAPHTHOL	Hair dyes Skin peeling preparations	Contact dermatitis
BISMUTH COMPOUNDS	Bleaching creams Freckle creams	Contact dermatitis
CALCIUM SULFIDE	Depilatories	Contact dermatitis
CORNSTARCH	Dusting powders Face powders	Inflamed eyes Stuffy nose Perennial hayfever
DIBROMFLUORESCEIN	Indelible lipsticks	Inflamed eyes often with respiratory symptoms and dermatitis Gastrointestinal symptoms
GUM ARABIC	Wave sets Rouge and powder compacts as a binder	Hayfever Dermatitis Gastrointestinal distress Asthma
GUM KARAYA	Wave sets Toothpaste Denture adhesive powder	Hayfever Dermatitis Gastrointestinal distress
GUM KARAYA	Hand lotions Rouge and powder compacts as a binder	Asthma

COMMON COSMETIC IRRITANTS AND ALLERGENS (cont.)

Substance	*Commonly Found In*	*Symptoms*
GUM TRAGACANTH	Wave sets Hand lotions Rouge and powder compacts as a binder	Hayfever Dermatitis Gastrointestinal distress Asthma
LANOLIN	Cosmetic creams Lotions Shampoos Ointment bases	Contact dermatitis
LEAD COMPOUNDS	Hair dyes	Contact dermatitis
LYCOPODIUM	Dusting powders	Stuffy nose Hayfever
MERCURY COMPOUNDS	Bleaching creams Freckle creams Hair tonics Medicated soaps	Contact dermatitis
METHYL HEPTINE CARBONATE	Perfumes Toilet waters Perfumed cosmetics	Stuffy nose Hayfever Dermatitis
OIL OF BERGAMOT OIL OF CANANGA OIL OF CORIANDER OIL OF GERANIOL OIL OF HELIOTROPINE OIL OF LAVENDER OIL OF LEMON OIL OF LEMONGRASS OIL OF LINALOOL OIL OF NEROLI OIL OF ORANGEPEEL OIL OF ORIGANUM OIL OF ORRIS OIL OF YLANG YLANG	Perfumes Toilet waters Perfumed cosmetics	Stuffy nose Hayfever Asthma Dermatitis Photosensitivity
OIL OF CASSIA (CLOVE) OIL OF PEPPERMINT OIL OF SPEARMINT OIL OF WINTERGREEN	Perfumes Toilet waters Perfumed cosmetics Toothpaste Toothpowder	Stuffy nose Hayfever Asthma Dermatitis

COMMON COSMETIC IRRITANTS AND ALLERGENS (cont.)

Substance	*Commonly Found In*	*Symptoms*
OIL OF CITRONELLA	Perfumes Toilet waters Perfumed cosmetics Mosquito repellant creams	Stuffy nose Hayfever Asthma Dermatitis
ORRIS ROOT POWDER	Toothpaste Dry shampoos Sachets Formerly contained in most face powders but now only rarely used	Infantile eczema Hayfever Stuffy nose Conjunctivitis Asthma
PHENOL	Hand lotions	Contact dermatitis
POTASSIUM CARBONATE POTASSIUM SULFITE	Permanent wave solutions	Dermatitis of the scalp, forehead, and hands
PYROGALLOL	Hair dyes	Contact dermatitis
QUININE SULFATE	Hair tonics	Contact dermatitis
RESORCINOL	Hair tonics	Contact dermatitis
RICE STARCH	Face powder Dusting powder	Conjunctivitis Stuffy nose Hayfever
ROSIN	Hair lacquers	Contact dermatitis
SALICYLIC ACID	Deodorants Hair tonics	Contact dermatitis
SODIUM CARBONATE	Permanent wave solutions	Dermatitis of the scalp, forehead, and hands
STRONTIUM SULFIDE	Depilatories	Contact dermatitis
TETRABROM-FLUORESCEIN	Indelible lipsticks	Inflamed lip often with respiratory symptoms and dermatitis Gastrointestinal symptoms
THIOGLYCOLLIC ACID SALTS	Cold permanent wave preparations	Contact dermatitis
WHEAT STARCH	Dusting powders Face powders	Conjunctivitis Stuffy nose
ZINC	Astringent lotions	Contact dermatitis

■ WHAT TO DO FOR THE DERMATITIS

The first thing to do in treating a dermatitis is find out what is causing it. Work both on your own and with your doctor to discover the guilty substance. Then use the list at the end of this chapter to find out all the relatives of that substance, so that you can eliminate them from your environment.

Learn to read labels. Manufacturers don't always list the ingredients on the labels, sometimes having secret formulas, but they do it often enough to make label reading worthwhile.

Experiment with different brands. You may often have a reaction to one brand of something but not to another. Even something as simple as adhesive tape will have different substances in different brands, so that you may react to one but not another.

REDUCING IRRITANTS

There are also things you can do to reduce other irritating factors that can add to the dermatitis.

If you tend to get "housewife eczema," protect your hands with cotton-lined plastic or rubber gloves while working. (Unlined ones will cause sweating and irritate the hands even more.) For non-wet work, use light cotton gloves. Don't use large amounts of soap and detergents. They are not usually particularly irritating when used in the proper amounts, but people tend to forget that modern materials are more effective than they used to be. Usually a tiny capful of liquid detergent will do a whole sink full of dishes. Use mild soaps rather than strong ones.

Do not use wool clothing or blankets. Keep your child from playing on wool rugs or coming in contact with adult wool, silk or fur clothing. Special precautions must be taken around the wrists, ankles and neck to prevent contact of wool with these areas.

Cut down on use of water. Do not stay in the bath over eight minutes. Add oil preparations to the bathwater. Take fewer baths. Unless the weather is terribly hot, babies need a bath only twice a week, not every day.

Keep as cool as possible; excess perspiration may cause a flare-up of the rash or irritate the skin.

Cover rash areas at bedtime with long-leg or long-sleeve pajamas.

Avoid pressure of garments over rash, such as tight clothes, rings and watch bands.

Avoid marked temperature changes and fatigue, nervousness or emotional upsets which could increase the irritation.

Great care should be taken to rinse thoroughly all the soap from clothes.

Don't hand wash diapers and baby clothes. They get a great deal cleaner and are rinsed better if you do them in the washing machine.

If a baby reacts to baby lotion, try simple salad oils or shortenings.

OTHER CONDITIONS

If there are associated conditions, treat them also. If you have overactive oil glands, shampoo hair daily until cleared; then shampoo two to three times per week as necessary.

If you have rough, dry skin use special bath oils and creams to moisten skin. If you have overactive sweat glands, particularly of the feet, keep them dry with frequent change of cotton socks.

If the eczema becomes secondarily infected, see your doctor for medication.

Do not apply oils, lotions or medications other than those prescribed.

If you have winter itch, take fewer baths, lower the heat in your home and increase the humidity by putting pans of water on the stoves and radiators or buying a humidifier. Use creams and lotions to retard evaporation of moisture. Use a lubricating body lotion after bath or shower and before bedtime. Wear a foundation cream under makeup.

SPECIAL PRECAUTIONS

Patients with eczema should *not* have smallpox vaccination while they have an active rash, nor should any other members of the family living with them be vaccinated. Contact of the vaccine material on an eczema lesion can produce a very serious, often fatal disease called vaccinia.

However, there is a new live attenuated smallpox vaccine which may prove to make vaccination safe in those with eczema.

ALLEVIATING SYMPTOMS

Despite your diligence, there are going to be times when you cannot avoid your allergy waterloos. Here are some means of alleviating dermatitis symptoms.

Many people find it helps to relieve itching if they soak their hands in cool water and let the water evaporate without rubbing with a towel.

If you have blisters, do not apply lotion or salve unless your doctor tells you to. They usually prevent the blisters from healing. After the skin has returned to normal, however, regular use of lotion may help prevent further recurrences.

There are many medications that can be of help. Some effective ones are hydrocortisone, fluocinolone, triamcinolone, coal tars and antihistamines. (If coal tar or a derivative is used, it may cause photosensitivity. Stay out of the sun or your skin may become permanently discolored and rough.)

If a lesion is oozing, hot saltwater dressings should be used continuously for two days, allowing the skin to air-dry for thirty minutes about every twelve hours. As the dermatitis subsides, the dressings should be applied four times a day for an hour each. A topical steroid hormone is used after each wet dressing.

Sometimes it helps to put something like plastic wrap around the ointment to increase the rate of diffusion from the medicine into the skin. However, no tight dressing should be kept on longer than twelve hours, and the skin should be watched carefully because in some people this kind of dressing may aggravate the disease.

Systemic corticosteroids should be given only as a last resort. When you do use the corticosteroids, the lesions usually clear up dramatically, but using these hormones for prolonged periods is dangerous. Under *no* circumstances whatsoever should you ever have prescriptions refilled without consulting your doctor.

Any time an ointment is used on a rash, both the patient and the physician should be aware of the fact that the medicine—if you happen to be sensitive to it—can make the skin lesion even worse. The dermatitis gets worse and spreads, not despite the treatment, but *because* of it. It can present a baffling situation. When the medication is stopped, the rash clears up. Be especially alert for medicines containing lanolin, antibiotics or parabens. Also watch out for medicines that have metallic compounds in them, or phenol, salicylate or tannic acid. Antihistamines in salves can sometimes cause problems.

Several doctors are reporting excellent results in treating chronic dermatitis in both children and adults by having them discontinue the use of all soaps and baths, cleaning the skin instead with a lipid-free lotion (Cerephil) and then applying the medication of fluocinolone acetonide in a nonlipid base. About 85 percent of patients with chronic eczema are having a good to excellent response so far. All patients were very pleased despite the fact that they have had to give up baths completely. After the skin remained clear for several months, then brief baths about once or twice a month were allowed.

In other recent research heparin has been found to be an excellent local application for weeping eczema. The heparin counteracts histamine in the skin cells that causes the cells to swell and burst. The solution that seems best so far is a 5 percent solution applied in a wet pack in combination with cortisone and an antibiotic. Dr. David Dolowitz, of the University of Utah, also reports that heparin taken orally during an acute attack alleviates symptoms of asthma and spasms of the larynx and bronchitis; however, this work is still experimental and has not yet been substantiated.

EMOTIONAL ASPECTS

Emotional factors must be considered also. Consider the child with a skin allergy. His skin itches and he scratches, aggravating the lesions and making them itch the more. Resulting nervousness and tension cause sweating and other stress reactions, which increase the itchiness and the scratching.

If a person's condition is unsightly, he may have an acute anxiety, which becomes a major factor in the persistence of the illness. The psychological damage may be lasting, even if there is little or no permanent physical disfigurement.

Also in considering emotional factors, parents of a child with skin allergies should be careful not to give him too much attention when he gets the rash or when he accidentally gouges his lesions. They should also be careful not to overstimulate and overmanipulate the child's skin. Overstroking the skin can overstimulate the pain receptors and cause perpetuation of the lesions.

In an adult or child, emotions can increase the amount of histamine and thus help bring on or worsen allergy episodes, so emotional excitement should be minimized as much as possible.

■ POSSIBLE SOURCES OF CONTACT DERMATITIS

One of the problems in avoiding the substance that causes a specific dermatitis is knowing all the places that substance is found. The following is a list of common causers of contact dermatitis and where they are often found. Every brand in a category will not necessarily contain the substance—i.e., all adhesives do not contain zinc oxide—but many do, so you can be on the alert for it there if you are sensitive to zinc oxide, and if one brand causes you trouble, you can try other brands.

ACETANILIDE—Cellulose ester varnishes, medication, dye manufacture.

ALDOL—Rubber vulcanizing.

ALIZAN—Coal tar, synthetic dyes, red paints, hair dyes.

ALUMINUM ACETATE—Fur dye, fabric finishing, waterproofing, dye compounds, disinfectant by embalmers.

ANILINE BLUE—Cosmetics, carbons, fur dyeing, hair dyes, nail polish, rubber, photographics, inks, colored pencils and crayons.

ANISE SEED OIL—Flavoring in liqueurs, confectioneries, perfumes, soaps.

ANTHRAQUINONE—Starter in the manufacture of vat dyes, used on seed to make them distasteful to birds.

ASPIRIN—Medications.

BALSAM OF PERU—Hair tonics, perfumes, china painting, oil painting, laboratory work.

BEESWAX—Adhesives, church candles, ointments, modeling wax, wax polishes, lithographing inks, carbons, cleansing cream, some paints, typewriter ribbon inks.

BENZOCAINE—Local anesthetic, tincture of benzoin.

BERGAMOT OIL—Cologne, hair tonics, china painting, ceramics, perfumes.

BERYLLIUM NITRATE—Electroplating, fluorescent and neon light, special ceramics.

BISMARCK BROWN—Dyeing silk, wool, leather.

CAMEL HAIR—Rugs, fabrics.

CAMPHOR OIL—Horn-rim glasses, nail polish, plasticizer for cellulose esters, lacquers, varnishes, moth repellent, embalming fluid, explosives, pharmaceutical preservative.

CANADA BALSAM—Cement for lenses, fine lacquers, mounting slides.

CARAWAY SEED AND OIL—Spice in baking, liqueurs, soaps, candy, cheese, condiments, perfume, rye bread, sausage.

CARBON PAPER—Office work, lithographing, art, blueprinting.

CASTOR BEAN—Fertilizers, some lipstick and rouge.

CAT HAIR—Animals, toys, caps, ear muffs, imitation furs, gloves, rug pads.

CATTLE HAIR—Blankets, brushes, ozite, rugs, rug pads.

CHLORAL HYDRATE—Manufacture of DDT, hair tonic, anesthetic for animals and poultry.

CHROMIUM SULFATE—Textile inks, paints, varnishes, leather processing, lithographing, fur dyeing, electroplating, blueprinting.

CINNAMON AND OIL—Beverages, flavorings, food, medication, bubble gum, toothpaste, confections, condiments.

CITRONELLA OIL— Liniment, cologne, perfume, insect repellent.

CLOVE OIL—Mucilage (postage stamps), perfume, condiment, flavoring, toothache treatment, dental surgery, chewing gum.

COAL TAR—Adhesives, creosotes, insecticides, phenols, woodworking, preservation of food.

COBALT SULFATE—Alloys, dyeing, lacquers, glass paints, some inks, oilcloth colors.

COCOA—Cosmetics, chocolate, flavoring, toilet preparations.

COCONUT OIL—Oleomargarine, cooking fat, baking, confections, soaps and detergents and anything washed in them.

COPPER SULFATE—Insecticides, fungicides, food processing, fertilizers, fur dyeing.

CORN—Adhesives on envelopes, stamps, stickers, tapes, aspirin and other tablets, bacon, baking mixes, baking powders, bath powders, batters for frying, some flours, bologna, bourbon and other whiskies, breads and pastries, cakes, candy, carbonated beverages, catsups, cheeses, chili, chop suey, cookies, confectioner's sugar, corn flakes and other corn cereals, corn flour, cornmeal, corn sugar, corn syrup, cough syrups, cream pies, cream puffs, excipients or diluents in capsules, lozenges, ointments, suppositories, tablets and vitamins, french dressing, fritters, Fritos, frostings, canned or frozen fruits, fruit juices, frying fats, gelatin capsules, gelatin dessert, glucose products, graham crackers, gravies, grits, gum, gin, hams, harvard beets, hominy, hot dogs, ices, ice cream, jams, jellies, Jello, drinks in paper cartons, monosodium glutamate, Mull-Soy, Nabisco, Nescafe, oleomargarine, pablum, paper containers, peanut butter, canned peas, plastic food wrappers, popcorn, powdered sugar, preserves, puddings, some salt, salad dressings, sandwich spreads, sauces, sausages, sherbets, stringbeans (canned or frozen), creamed soups, soybean milks, starched clothes, succotash, talcums, instant teas, toothpaste, tortillas, canned, creamed or frozen vegetables, vinegar, yeasts.

COTTONSEED—Cotton wadding or batting in cushions, comforters, mattresses and upholstery, varnishes, fertilizer, animal feed, gin, xylose, most salad oils, most oleomargarines, lard substitutes, sardines packed in cottonseed oil, most commercial fried and baked cakes, breads, fish, popcorn, potato chips and doughnuts, candies, olive oil, liniments, salves, camphorated oil, miner's and altar lamp oil, manufacture of paper, salt, machine tools and paint; cosmetics; used to polish fruit.

DDT—Insecticide, agricultural sprays.

DIHYDROXYACETONE—Some suntanning preparations.

DOG HAIR—Chinese rugs.

FEATHERS—Food, fertilizer, mattresses, pillows.

FERRIC CHROMATE—Pigment in paints, varnishes, watercolors.

FISH GLUE—Bookbindings, envelopes, furniture manufacture, labels, rug sizing, shipping tapes, straw hats.

FLAX—Fertilizers, linoleum, linseed flaxseed oils, poultices, cereals, roman meal, flaxseed extracts in cough remedies, flaxseed tea, bird lime, carron oil, some depilatories, fertilizers, furniture polish, some hair tonics, linoleum dust, linseed oil, lithographers' ink, meal for cattle and poultry, paints, poultices, printers' ink, some shampoos, soft soap, varnishes, wave sets, some cloth, insulating plaster, flax rug, straw mats, paper, wax paper, upholstery, chair seats, cushions, fiberboard, insulating material in refrigerators.

FORMALDEHYDE—Cosmetic industry, disinfectant, nail polish, soap, preservative in food, synthetic gum, synthetic resins, waterproofing, tanning leather, some fabrics, antiseptic, fungicide.

FURACIN—Medication.

GARLIC—Dressings, meat sauce, cold meats, pickles, salad dressings.

GELATIN—Confections, foods, Jello, capsules, ice creams, marshmallows.

GINGER OIL—Condiments, confections, medication.

GLUE—Manufacture of furniture, shoes, books, model toys, etc., waterproofing.

GOAT HAIR—Rug pads, protective padding, some rugs.

GREEN SOAP—Shampoo, hospitals, factories.

GUM ARABIC—Cake icings, candy fillings, some diabetic foods, printers' drying spray, pharmaceuticals, mucilage, pastries, ice cream, adhesive agent in finishing fabrics, ink, matches, lithographing.

GUM TRAGACANTH—Candies, cheese (processed), cheese spreads, chewing gum, creams, some gravies, salad dressings, wrappings for cigars, ointments, salad dressings.

HENNA—Hair coloring.

HOG HAIR—Brushes, rug pads.

HORSE HAIR AND DANDER—Binder in plaster, brushes, clothing, gloves, violin bows, hats, mattresses, wigs, horse serum used in some injected medicines.

JUTE—Sacks, twine, furniture manufacture.

KAPOK—Furniture upholstery, life jackets, mattresses, pillows.

KARAYA GUM—Dental adhesive powders, diabetic foods, laxatives, wave set, hair-fixing solutions, Karabim, Karaba, Kara Jel, Mucara, many mineral oils, some toothpastes, hand lotions, flavoring, some gelatins, gumdrops and similar candies, ices, some ice creams, some factory-made pie fillings, lemon, custard, salad dressings, adhesives, printing inks.

LANOLIN—Adhesives, cosmetics, hairsprays, hair tonics, ointments.

LAVENDER OIL—Cologne, cosmetics, soap, ceramics, china painting.

LEAD ACETATE—Dyeing and printing cottons, weighing silks, laboratory determinations.

LEAD ARSENATE—Fungicide, insecticide.

LEAD CHLORIDE—Fur processing, felt processing, calico printing, solder, flux.

LINSEED OIL—Paints, varnishes, sculpturing, furniture polishes, refinishing waxes.

MANGANESE OXIDE—Pigment in rubber goods, alloy in iron and steel, manufacture of dry batteries, coloring in brick and pottery, dyeing industry, drying paints, varnishes, glass making, printing and dyeing textiles.

MERCURY BICHLORIDE—Processing artificial silk, bronzing, dental laboratories, electric wiring, electroplating, paints, reagents, electric batteries, embalming fluid, fur processing, felt processing, engraving, printing, thermometers, metal work, mirror finishing, lamp bulbs, photography, insecticides.

METHYLAMINOPHENOL SULFATE—Photographic developer, dyeing furs.

METHYL ORANGE—Indicator.

MOHAIR, GOAT HAIR—Furniture and automobile upholstery.

MOLDS—May occur in soil, on awnings, window shades, wallpaper, upholstered furniture, kapok, food, decaying grass and plant life.

MUSTARD OIL—Oleomargarine, salad oil, condiment, liniment, drying oil, contaminant in linseed oil, soap making.

NICKEL SULFATE—Costume jewelry, electric wiring, garters and supporters, hair dyes and bleaches, eyeglass frames, silver work, telephone wiring, mordant in dyes, insecticide, fungicide, nickel plating.

NICOTINE SULFATE—Agricultural sprays, insecticides.

NOVOCAINE—Local anesthetic.

NUTMEG OIL—Condiment, cooking, Mace.

NUTS—Almonds, margarine, peanut butter, peanut oil, pecans, pistachios, salad oils, walnuts.

NYLON—Clothing, draperies, rugs, shoes, upholstery, fishing tackle, surgical sutures.

OIL RED—Dye used in cheap cosmetics and lipsticks.

OLIVE OIL—Creams, salad oils, soaps.

ONIONS—Cold meats, pastry.

ORRIS ROOT—Dentifrices, perfumes, cosmetics, adhesives, teething rings, bath salts, face powders, facial creams, hair tonics, lipstick, rouges, sachets, shampoos, shaving cream, scented soaps, sunburn lotion, toothpaste, tooth powder.

PARA-PHENYLENEDIAMINE—Fur processing, hair dyes and bleaches, leather processing, photographic and photogravure work, lithographing, vulcanizing, fabric dye.

PHENYL SALICYLATE—Polymer for plastics, lacquers, adhesives, waxes, polishes, suntan oil.

PINEAPPLE JUICE—Used to tenderize casings for sausages.

POTASSIUM DICHROMATE—Adhesives, bleaches, blueprinting, dry colors for paints, fur processing, glass, glues, inks, lithographing, match making, wool dyeing, military paints, photographic reagents, metal plating, printing, tanning, varnishes, wood stains, anti-rust compounds.

POTASSIUM IODIDE—Photographic emulsions, animal and poultry feed, table salt, medication.

PYRETHRUM—Insecticides, plant sprays, cut flowers, chrysanthemums, moth proofing.

RABBIT HAIR—Gloves, lined clothing, imitation fur.

REDWOOD—Red color in dyeing manufacture, red inks, woodworking.

RESORCINOL—Tanning process, explosives, manufacture of resins, dyes, cosmetics, freckle cream, dyeing and printing textiles.

RICE POWDER—Cosmetics, drying agent.

SESAME SEED—Bakery goods, flavoring.

SISAL—Furniture and twine.

SILVER BROMIDE—Photographic processing, mirror finishing.

SODIUM ARSENATE—Arsenical soaps, insecticides, hair tonics.

SOYBEANS—Bakery goods, candies, cereals, some shortenings, ice cream, pork sausage, lunch meats, milk substitutes, nuts, oleomargarine, some salad dressing, some sauces, soups, adhesives, automobile parts, blankets, candles, celluloid, cloth, coffee substitute, custards, enamels, fertilizer, fodder, French's fish food, glycerine, Gro-Pup dog food, illuminating oil, linoleum, lubricating oil, massage creams, nitroglycerine, paints, paper finishes, paper sizing, printing ink, soap, textile dressing, urease, varnish.

SUDAN RED—Coloring oils, stain, dye for waxes and resins.

SULFUR—Ointments, hair medications, shampoos, sizing and dyeing socks, gunpowder, matches, bleaches, insecticide, fungicide.

SURFACAINE—Surface anesthetic.

TANNIC ACID—Mordant in dyes, sizing paper and silk, polished fabrics, manufacturing tortoise shell frames, coagulant in rubber manufacturing, tanning leather, photography.

TOBACCO—Directly or in smoke.

TOLUENE—Solvent, manufacturing rubber and adhesives, manufacturing dyes and perfumes.

TOMATO—Catsup, chili sauce, pickles, steak sauce, salad dressings, salads, soups.

TRAGACANTH—Compact powder, candy manufacture, calico printing, drying agent, drug filler, sizing paper, printing, wave setting fluid.

TURPENTINE—Manufacture of synthetic resins, shoes, stoves and furniture polishes, solvents for waxes, cleaning fluid, insecticides, paint solvents, medicinal.

YEAST—Bread, crackers, beer, wine.

ZINC OXIDE—Adhesives, sock and hosiery manufacture, paints, galvanizing, zinc plating, drying agent, dental cement, automobile tires, white glue, white inks, medicinal ointments and powders.

Chapter 1

ALLERGIES TO INSECTS

Millions of insects are swarming the earth and they have found many ways to bug us. One of their sneakiest ways is through allergies. They can cause allergies by biting you or stinging you, or you can have an allergic reaction from touching them, inhaling bits of dust from their wings, or eating them.

Depending on your sensitivity, your reaction can be many things: a slight case of hives, or swelling and pain, or hayfever and asthma symptoms, or even death.

The first allergic reaction to an insect was recorded nearly three thousand years before Christ on the tomb of the Egyptian King Menes. In typical Egyptian two-dimensional style the tomb drawings depict the details of the demise of the tomb's occupant from a fatal wasp sting.

The wasps and other bugs have been at it ever since, and today's roster of insects that can cause allergy by one means or another include bees, wasps, ants, mosquitoes, flies, fleas, lice, beetles, moths, spiders, ticks, mites, scorpions and caterpillars.

Severe reactions are common. The Insect Committee of the American Academy of Allergy analyzed the data on more than 2,500 persons who had allergic reactions to insect bites or stings over a three-year period. One out of every four had had reactions serious enough to be considered life-threatening.

This study showed not only how frequent and dangerous insect stings are but also that these life-threatening generalized reactions can occur without any previous unusual reactions taking place as a warning! Nearly 400 of the people involved said that they did not recall being stung before or, if so, they had only had very mild local reactions.

"It has been stated that bees kill more people in this country than any other venomous animal, including the rattlesnake," says Dr. Claude A. Frazier, North Carolina allergist. "This is a medical problem deserving concentrated attention." He cites an example in the literature of a forty-two-year-old man in excellent health who was stung on the forehead, the neck and under the arms by yellow jackets. Within three minutes he was unconscious, with frothy blood drooling from his mouth; within five minutes, he was dead. About three weeks previously a sting in the arm had resulted in massive swelling of the whole arm. Despite this evidence the cause of death was given by the local coroner as "natural, cause unknown."

So many times relatives or physicians pay no attention to insect stings, thinking the sting is only accidental to someone's dying. Because of this, quite often deaths really due to insect stings are reported as being due to a heart attack or some unknown cause.

Says Dr. Frazier: "Many people, of whom this coroner was one, still cannot believe that a little thing like a few insect stings can possibly cause death."

■ STINGING INSECTS

Sometimes swarms of bees or wasps attack in hordes.

"A man in Africa was walking along a river bank when without warning or provocation, a swarm of bees attacked and covered the upper half of his body in a layer about three inches thick. They began to sting him and he felt an intense burning sensation as though he were on fire. He dived into the river and must have lost consciousness, for his next recollection was of finding himself standing in backwater, without his shirt, vomiting and having diarrhea ~~so persistent that he~~

was incontinent and the bees were still upon him and around him, stinging repeatedly.

"He moved toward deeper water, sat down and put his shorts over his head to try to protect himself, but the bees continued to sting through the material. He then plastered his shorts with mud, but every time his arms came above the water to do this he received more stings. He eventually completed this task but had to leave a hole for air which the bees found. When they landed to sting, he tried to brush them away, but this exposed more of him to be stung and he found that the best thing to do was to keep his mouth close to the hole and bite the bees with his teeth. Many of these bees he had to swallow and he maintained that they passed right through him.

"Throughout this time, he was suffering headache, diarrhea and a continuous burning pain in his stomach, but at no time did he have any trouble with respiration.

"He was in the water for about four and a half hours before he was found at dusk, the bees having dispersed."

This is an actual report from a medical journal (*West Virginia Medical Journal*). More than 200 stingers were removed just from the man's eyelids, lips and the inside of his mouth. He lived after his terrifying experience. Yet other people have died after one sting.

There appear to be more and more severe reactions occurring. You read or hear about typical cases. A neighbor painting his house is stung by yellow jackets and is taken to the hospital in a coma. A woman on a picnic is stung by a bee and dies in minutes. A child running through the garden is stung and falls to the ground unconscious. To people like these, venturing outdoors during the seasons when stinging insects are abroad can be a fear-filled and alarming experience.

Bees, wasps, hornets and yellow jackets can all cause serious reactions in the person who is sensitive to their venom. It is not easy to avoid them, there being more than 100,000 different species of these insects. In fact, there are some 10,000 different species of just bees.

Some insects with stingers are aggressive and some are not. The solitary bees—those who live alone and not in colonies—do not sting very often, and the results are usually mild. The serious cases of beestings are usually due to the social bees, those who live in organized colonies, such as the honeybee and bumblebees. In wasps also the community livers are more vicious than the solitary dwellers, and are particularly aggressive in the vicinity of their nests.

ALL THESE INSECTS CAN CAUSE SEVERE ALLERGIC REACTIONS.

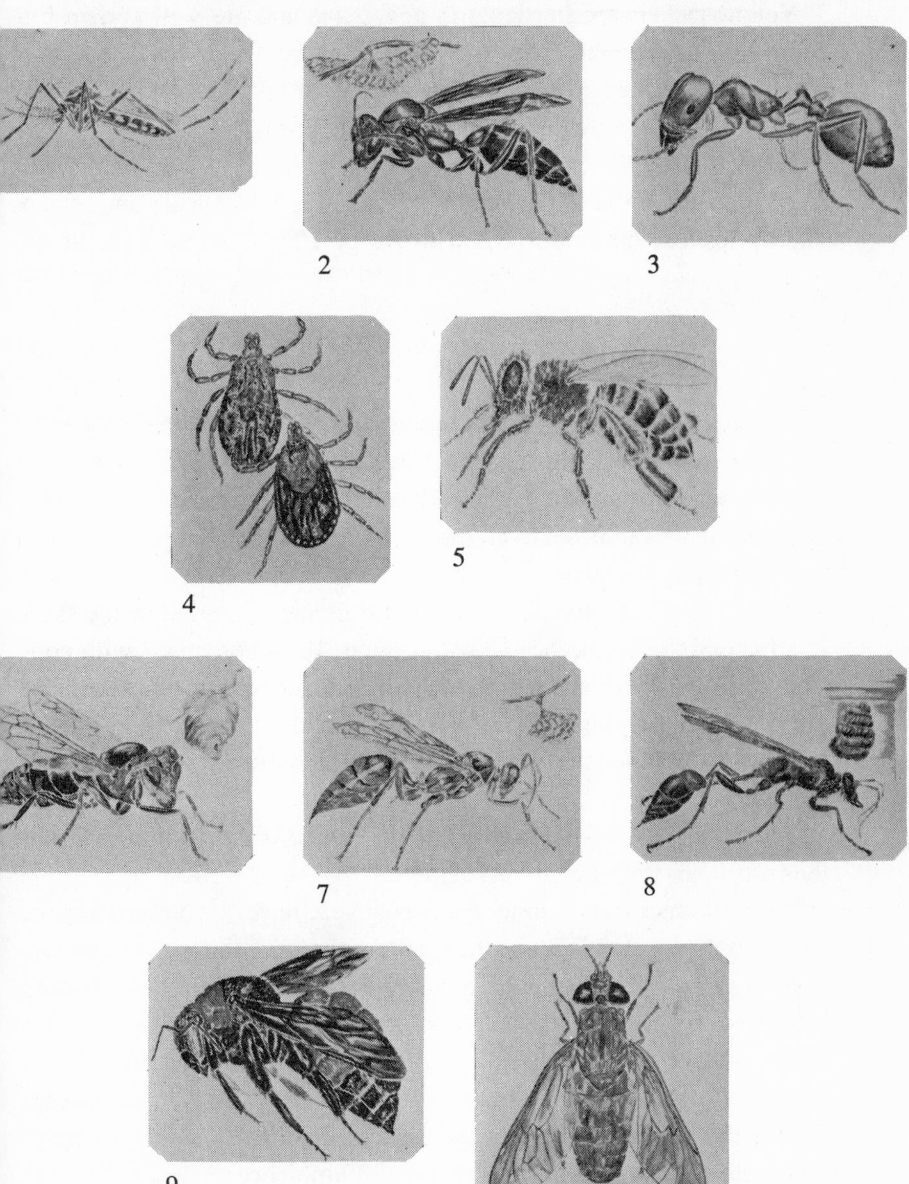

1. mosquito
2. wasp
3. large red ant
4. dog ticks (male and female)
5. honeybee
6. bald-faced hornet
7. yellow jacket
8. mud dauber
9. bumblebee
10. deerfly

COURTESY OF CENTER LABORATORIES, PORT WASHINGTON, N.Y.

Yellow jackets are particularly aggressive and are well known for being easy to provoke. They are especially nasty in orchards because they eat the fermented fruits and get crazy drunk. To top it off, they do double damage by biting you before they sting you.

Hornets are the most ferocious when their nests are disturbed. Sometimes the hornets' nest will be as much as a foot wide and, when slightly jostled, may pour out a drove of 10,000 hornets intent on revenge.

TYPES OF STINGS

An insect stinger usually lies hidden inside the tip of the abdomen. It's like a hollow needle split lengthwise into three pieces. When the insect is ready to attack, he extrudes the stinger, jams it into his victim and the venom flows from the poison sac in the abdomen through the needle into the skin.

A bee stinger is barbed, and once it becomes anchored in the skin, it is impossible for the bee to withdraw it. He is convulsed with contractions that thrust the stinger deeper and deeper into the skin, and the contractions pump the venom through the stinger. In the bee's struggle to escape, his whole stinging apparatus is pulled off and he dies.

The wasp stinger is not barbed, so it can be withdrawn at will and the insect can sting again and again.

Bees, wasps, hornets and yellow jackets have a combination of from four to six chemicals in their venom that can cause allergic reactions. Some of these chemicals are common to all four of these stinging insects so that a person sensitive to one of these is probably sensitive to the sting of the other members of the group. However, bumblebee venom doesn't seem to be related to any of the other venoms except that of the honeybee, so that the person sensitive to a yellow jacket would not necessarily be sensitive to a bumblebee.

If at all possible, it is helpful to know what kind of insect stung you and to tell your doctor so that he will know what type of injections to give you to protect you in the future.

TYPES OF REACTIONS

Symptoms from a sting may last for a few hours or may continue for days. A reaction may occur within seconds or minutes after the sting, or it may not appear until several days after the sting, making it almost impossible to connect the two events. The reaction can be local, occurring in the area of the sting, or can be systemic, involving the whole body.

Getting stung several times over the years may result in a naturally acquired immunity, as some beekeepers report, or it may produce increased sensitivity so that any later encounter with an insect can be severe or fatal.

The usual response to the sting is a feeling of a sharp pinprick followed by rather severe pain. Within a few minutes a small red area appears and is gradually surrounded by a white ring. There is swelling, which gradually subsides within the next few hours; then there are itching, irritation and heat. Usually all phases of the sting reaction disappear within twenty-four to forty-eight hours.

But when a person is sensitive to insect stings the symptoms can be serious.

When a generalized allergic reaction is taking place, it may first be indicated by a dry hacking cough, a sense of constriction in the throat or chest, swelling or itching about the eyes, huge hives all over the body, sneezing, wheezing, an increased pulse rate, a drop in blood pressure, a reddening or sometimes paling of the skin, a sense of uneasiness and impending disaster or sense of approaching death. These symptoms usually appear within two or three minutes of the sting.

If death occurs, it usually occurs within the first twenty minutes.

Sometimes the site of the sting seems to make a difference. When stung on the arm or leg, a person may simply remove the stinger and go on working. The same person, when stung on the neck or head, turns red, becomes weak and has to lie down.

If the sting penetrates a vein or artery, the reaction is extremely quick and severe.

There can be complications, too, even to a local reaction sting. Infection of the site may develop several hours after the sting or even several days later. At least three cases have been reported of men and women who have died from infection that occurred after they were stung on the neck.

Stings around the eyes are particularly dangerous and can result in cataracts, abscesses, glaucoma, or puncturing of the eyeball. Sometimes a sting on the eyelid will injure the eye months or years later after the stinger has worked its way through the lid.

SUMMER STRATEGIES FOR PREVENTING INSECT STINGS

If you are sensitive to insect stings, knowing how to keep yourself from being stung can be lifesaving.

One commonsense measure is to avoid situations that attract insects. Especially in the autumn stay clear of areas covered with fallen leaves on humid days. There is something about this combination that drives yellow jackets almost mad. Avoid picnic areas or orchards when trees are in blossom or fruit is fermenting.

Stay away from bird baths on a hot summer day because there will be a steady procession of wasps stopping by for a drink.

The odor of perspiration is irritating to stinging insects so try to keep from getting hot and sweaty, and if you do, change your clothes and take a shower.

Watch where you are going. If you see more than two yellow jackets or bumblebees close to the ground, watch them. If they continue to fly about, they are merely hunting and will not bother you; but if they suddenly vanish into the fallen leaves or grass, it means that is where their nest is located. Stay at least three feet away, because when their nest is threatened, their attack is fast and vicious.

Spray picnic areas with a repellent chemical before spreading food. Keep food covered until the moment it is served. Any food will attract yellow jackets and bees: they will gather where there is outdoor cooking, where pets are being fed, or will even follow the dribble from a child's popsicle.

Keep the garbage can area meticulously clean for the same reason. Always keep the cans covered, and spray regularly with an insecticide around the area.

Make sure there is adequate screening on your windows and doors.

Garden cautiously. A trowel penetrating a bumblebees' nest will cause serious trouble, as will running a power mower over a lawn where yellow jackets have a nest. The vibrations from a power mower will send a yellow jacket into a rage. Anyone who is sensitive to insect stings should not use electric hedge clippers, tractors or power mowers. Teach children not to go around kicking dead logs when they are on a hike or in the woods. This also sends vibrations into the ground. Teach them the old rattlesnake technique of inspecting any object for bees or wasps before they touch it, sit on it or step on it. Yellow jackets often are on wagon handles or toys where fingers sticky with food have been.

Do not apply anything to your body that has a sweet odor such as hairspray, suntan lotion or perfume. They often contain sweet or floral odors that attract bees and wasps.

Wear long trousers and long-sleeved shirts. When in insect areas, avoid dark clothing, bright colors or flowered prints. It seems to infuriate them. Wear white, light green, tan, which apparently do not antagonize them. Avoid wearing leather, tweed, flannel or other clothing that has a rough texture or natural odor. Women should wear a scarf or hat over their hair to prevent bees from being accidentally entangled. Wear shoes.

If you're buzzed by a bee or wasp or one lands on your skin or clothing, don't flail at it. Instead, hold still or keep walking slowly. Stinging insects are more apt to attack a fast-moving object than a stationary one. They are very sensitive to air movements and sudden motion.

Carry an insecticide bomb in the glove compartment of the car for spraying any stray insects that may fly in, or keep a large handkerchief or rag on the seat so you may grab the intruder and throw him out the window instead of flailing at the insect and losing control.

Use repellents. They will not lessen the determination of an angry insect intent on attacking, but they will discourage insects who are only looking for food.

One way to keep bugs of all kinds away from you or your children was told to us by Dr. Jack Cooperman, New York nutritionist. He says if you take a vitamin B capsule daily on the days that you are going to be outside, you will seldom have a bug bite or sting. The extra vitamin B in the body is secreted through the sweat and causes a slight odor on the skin which stinging insects and other bugs find offensive.

DESTROYING HIVES

If you notice an unusual number of wasps, yellow jackets or bees around your yard, look around carefully for evidence of hives. Once you have located them it is best to call an exterminator and let him remove the hives. They know the proper techniques and have strong industrial chemicals. Under no circumstances whatsoever should you remove the hives yourself if you are sensitive. It could kill you.

If you simply cannot find an exterminator, then have someone who is not allergic use the following guide to locating and eliminating the hives around your home.

Wasps build open comb nests under eaves, in carports, behind shutters, in shrubs—in almost any protected place. These nests can be destroyed by hosing them down or knocking them down with a stick or broom handle; or scrape or clip them into a jar and cover it quickly. Let the completely sealed container stand for several days until all insects have suffocated. The area should be sprayed with insecticide once daily for three days thereafter.

Yellow jackets build in the ground, emerging through small holes. This outlet should be marked during daylight with a stick. At dusk when all the insects have returned for the night, gasoline or kerosene should be poured down the hole. It need not be lighted. Lye may be used in the same way. The entire operation should be repeated the following evening. Water should never be sprayed at the hole, for this will cause the insects to swarm over the person holding the hose and sting him unmercifully.

Hornets usually build gray football-shaped hives in shrubs or trees, often high or far out on a branch. If a nest cannot be reached by a flaming torch or cannot be clipped into a covered container, then an exterminator should be called, or the fire department with the aid of ladders may succeed in removing it.

Honeybees, whether swarming on a twig or nesting in a hollow, may be removed by some of these same methods or by a beekeeper, who frequently is delighted to have an extra colony for his trouble.

■ OTHER STINGING, BITING OR BLOOD-SUCKING CREATURES

There are many other forms of animal life that can cause reactions. Nearly anything that looks dangerous is—except perhaps the ferocious-looking dragon or damsel fly, which neither stings nor bites.

ANTS

The bites and stings of most ants are rarely more than a temporary annoyance, but occasionally they do lead to an allergic reaction. There are two ants that are particularly aggressive and poisonous: the harvester ant and the fire ant.

The harvester or agricultural ants are vicious and attack both men and animals. They live in dry, warm, sandy places where they excavate their nests to form low mounds of dirt. Their name comes from the fact that they cut seed from grasses and weeds and grind them up with their powerful jaws. They have been known to kill small farm animals that have blundered into their nests.

Fire ants are called that because of the burning pain that comes with their bite. They are found in the southern United States and in the tropics. They make their nests in tunnels sometimes running eighty feet long just a quarter of an inch below the surface of the ground. They eat bees, bird eggs and young birds, especially quail. They sometimes infest homes, devouring every bit of unprotected food and eating holes in clothes. When their nest is disturbed, they teem forth by the thousands and within a few seconds administer some three to five thousand stings to the unfortunate person who stumbled upon them.

They puncture the skin and hold on with their jaw, then while holding on, sting once or several times. Fluid-filled bumps (vesicles) form, remaining for several days, then forming a crust and scar tissue. Reactions can be severe and death can occur. So far no local treatment has been found effective.

Red ants, prevalent in southern states, can cause the same reactions.

BLOOD-SUCKING FLIES

The bite of a fly is really not a bite but a stabbing with a bayonet-like proboscis. Then the fly injects fluid from his salivary glands that breaks down tissues and make it easier for him to obtain and digest your body fluids.

Many of these flies, such as the horsefly and deerfly, travel from animal to animal and are highly suspected as carriers of many diseases in both animals and man. It has already been shown that they can transmit anthrax and tularemia.

Blackflies only come out during daylight. They may be found by the millions where flowing water is present. You don't usually feel a blackfly when it first bites, but within an hour there is extreme pain accompanied by itching and local swelling; then either eczema-like patches or rough bumps may appear. Death can occur either from poisoning or an allergic reaction.

Sand flies or tiny blood-sucking gnats are so small that they can usually penetrate any netting or screen. The females hide in dark corners and crevices and come out looking for blood at night.

Biting midges are tiny blood-sucking scavengers that live and thrive around water, moist earth or trees. They fly in swarms, forming dense clouds, dancing as the sun goes down. This is the special time of their attack on humans.

Any time you are bitten by flies, it is important to clean the area around the bite because of the great likelihood of infection resulting from these filthy disease carriers. Sometimes antibiotic-steroid ointments are used to treat the bites. If secondary infections occur, systemic antibiotics prescribed by your physician may be necessary. Sometimes even hospitalization is required.

FLEAS

Allergy to flea bites is quite common and is an irritating problem in many areas. Besides the local reaction, there is usually a delayed reaction. Generalized hives over the body frequently occur with a number of flea bites, but not with a single flea bite. Some allergists find that it helps a patient to have desensitization to flea bites; others say it doesn't.

MOSQUITOES

Allergic reactions to mosquito bites can take the form of severe swelling, redness and pain at the site of the bite, or there can be widespread hives or eczema.

If you are sensitive to mosquito bites, you should be aware that certain factors make a person more attractive to mosquitoes. You are most likely to be bitten under the following conditions:

If you have a dark complexion. In experiments at the University of Western Ontario, naturally dark-skinned persons attracted 22 percent more mosquitoes than light-skinned persons. Orientals attracted 27 percent more mosquitoes than Caucasians, and Negroes attracted 60 percent more than white persons.

If you are warm-skinned. The average internal temperature of healthy humans doesn't vary much from 98.6°F, but there is a considerable variation in skin temperatures. Experiments showed that warm-skinned persons attracted 30 percent more mosquitoes than those with cooler skins.

If you are in good health. Researchers at Union Carbide Corporation have discovered that mosquitoes put the bite on healthy people more frequently than on persons in poor health.

If you perspire greatly. The more a person perspires, the higher his "attractivity index" to mosquitoes.

If you breathe heavily. Apparently the carbon dioxide in expired air helps guide the mosquito to its target.

If you are highly active. The energetic person constantly on the move is the one who attracts the mosquito's attention, possibly because of the motion, possibly because of the body heat.

If you wear perfume, cologne or after-shave lotion. Anything with a noticeable odor seems to invite the mosquitoes to bite.

If you wear dark clothing. The less light a material reflects and the duller it is, the more attractive it is to mosquitoes. They are attracted to black, dark reds and dark blues, so you should wear white, yellows and light greens, which they dislike most.

If you are taking steroid sex hormones. If this drug is secreted through the skin it tends to attract mosquitoes.

You can help protect yourself with repellents. According to the U.S. Department of Agriculture the best all-purpose insect repellent is *N,N*-diethyl-*m*-toluamide (commonly known as DEET). It comes in liquid, foam, pressurized sprays, stick, cream and wipe-on forms.

The best method of prevention is to see that all mosquitoes are destroyed in your immediate vicinity. Most mosquitoes travel no more than two or three blocks during their lives, so if the people in your area eliminate breeding spots such as pools of stagnant water, old automobile tires, open cans and fish ponds, it wlil greatly reduce the problem of mosquito bites.

SPIDERS

The two most dangerous spiders to man in the United States are the black widow spider and the brown recluse spider, both of which can be killers. Reactions have also been reported to the running spider and to the black and yellow garden spider.

The black widow is found everywhere in the United States except Alaska and is especially prevalent in the southern states, the Ohio Valley and along the West Coast. It has the familiar shiny black body and the red hourglass mark on the underside of the abdomen. As is so often the case, it is only the female that bites. Often a person does not know that he has been bitten, feeling only a sharp pinprick followed by a dull pain. But soon there is more local pain and often excruciating abdominal pain and rigidity of the abdominal muscles or pain in the back and chest with each breath. In a few hours the muscle pains progressively involve all the muscles of the thighs, legs, chest, shoulders, arms and back. Sometimes the person also has cold sweats, dizziness, convulsions, paralysis, delirium, shock, cyanosis, nausea and vomiting.

The brown recluse spider is light to dark brown with a band of dark color extending back from the eyes, of which there are three pairs in a semicircle. The brown recluse is sometimes found outdoors under stones or leaves, but is usually found inside in storage closets, attics, garages or outhouses. The local reaction to the bite may produce mild to severe pain; and a week or two later, a series of skin changes occurs, often resulting in a nasty open ulcer that usually heals in about three weeks but sometimes requires skin grafting. The bite can also cause serious systemic reactions with chills and fever, weakness, nausea and vomiting, and pain in the joints and often eruptions all over the body within twenty-four to forty-eight hours. There are severe blood changes, and sometimes blood clots form and lodge in the heart or lungs, causing death.

Many people believe that spider bites should be treated like snakebites, using a tourniquet and making an incision and drawing out the venom. However, most authorities in this field say this only adds to the discomfort and increases tissue injury. What you should do, they say, is to apply ice packs to reduce local pain and slow down the rate of absorption of the venom. Then go to a doctor who will prescribe certain muscle relaxants that are helpful for spider bites, such as calcium gluconate and methocarbamol. In severe reactions the physician may prescribe steroids, antihistamines and antibiotics. The best treatment, when it is available, is antivenin, which is made from the serum of horses immunized with spider venom.

MITES

There are several types of mites that attack man, including the mite that causes scabies, poultry mites, rodent mites, straw mites and chigger mites.

The chigger is unique because it feeds on man only during the larval stage. The tiny, dot-sized red chigger crawls around on grasses and bushes looking for an animal on which to lodge. When you brush against it, it runs along your skin until it finds a soft spot or is stopped by some tight clothing such as a belt, garter or bra strap. It pierces skin, releases a liquid that digests skin cells, then sucks the liquid up, at the same time gradually tunneling into the skin. Patting the chigger bump with witch hazel or calamine lotion is often enough to stop the itching, but if the bite is very annoying, a medicine called Kwell (designed to treat scabies) will help immensely.

TICKS

Ticks eagerly attack man and other warm-blooded animals in all three stages: larval, nymph and adult. It can take from four to twenty-one days for the tick to suck enough blood to be completely engorged. The reaction is usually immediate, but delayed skin lesions may appear days or even months after the tick bite. In rare cases an acute tic paralysis occurs. The patient becomes very irritable and tired; then numbness and pain start in the legs and gradually work up the body. As the paralysis reaches the higher regions of the body, the patient may die of respiratory failure. Once the tic is removed, the paralysis clears up quickly.

When tics attach themselves to the skin, they fasten on with their teeth and then reinforce the attachment by a cementlike secretion. Any attempt at pulling out the tic will usually leave the mouth parts imbedded, and the squeezing during the attempt will inject more toxin into the wound. Instead of trying to detach the tic manually, one should drop gasoline or ether on its head or touch the hot tip of a cigarette or match to it, then allow about ten minutes for it to voluntarily detach itself.

WHEEL BUG

The wheel bug usually eats caterpillars and June bugs, but when accidentally encountered by man will, in self-defense, stab with its beak to inflict a painful laceration. The pain is usually temporary, but more severe reactions can occur.

KISSING BUG

This insect, also called an assassin bug or a *Triatoma,* resembles a bedbug.

Usually it lives under logs or in nests and obtains its blood from opossums, skunks, armadillos, rats and other small animals. Sometimes, however, it takes up residence in the house, living in crevices, emerging at night to feed on its sleeping victim. It often stands on the bedclothes and extends its proboscis to contact the skin and then sinks its hollow stiletto into the skin. One tube carries saliva into the drill hole to serve as an anesthetic, and the other tube is for sucking blood. It may feed from three to thirty minutes. It seldom wakes its victim and may go for five or fifteen days before feeding again.

The bites usually are multiple, with as many as fifteen in a group, and they often occur in vascular areas such as the eyelids or lips.

It is the saliva that causes the allergic response. Usually the bite causes bumps slightly larger than that of a mosquito or chigger, but there may also be huge swellings, asthma or severe anaphylactic shock. Fear of the bite sometimes makes it almost impossible for the people who are sensitive to this bug to fall asleep.

The patient should make a meticulous search of his bed, mattress and bedcovers, and all cracks and crevices in the bedroom. Repeated spraying of insecticides should be done in the room, including mattresses, bedframes, walls, baseboards and carpets.

Patients who are severely allergic to these *Triatoma* bites should carry emergency supplies of antihistamines and should consider desensitization injections. Several allergists have reported using extracts made from the insects for desensitization, which decreases the severity of the reactions.

SCORPIONS

During the day, scorpions remain hidden under stones, banks, piles of lumber or in closets, attics and cozy places like shoes. During the night they come out seeking water and food. Some scorpions have a comparatively mild venom that usually causes only local reactions of burning, swelling and discoloration. Others have a very powerful venom that poisons the nervous system. When you are stung by the highly poisonous variety, there is a sharp pain, then a pins-and-needles sensation in the bite area which rapidly extends up the arm or leg. As it spreads, numbness and drowsiness set in. Then you develop itching of the nose, mouth and throat, speech becomes impaired, and the muscles of the lower jaw are often so contracted that it becomes difficult to give oral medication. The patient begins to twitch involuntarily, then has severe muscle spasms with pain, nausea, vomiting, incontinence and convulsions. Death often results from respiratory or circulatory failure.

At any time you are stung by a scorpion, prompt action during the first few minutes is important. Ice should be applied immediately. A tourniquet should be placed above the site of the sting, then the entire limb should be placed in ice water. The tourniquet may be removed after the limb has been immersed in the ice water for at least five minutes, but the limb should remain in the ice water for about two hours. The rest of the body should be kept warm. A specific antivenin is available for many species of scorpions, but not all. If given early enough, it can be lifesaving.

PORTUGUESE MAN-OF-WAR

The Portuguese man-of-war and the jellyfish can both inflict severe stings. So can sea anemones and corals. In one Philadelphia study a review was made of four hundred stingings reported in four days along the coast of New York and Connecticut. Five persons were hospitalized, forty required emergency care and two had severe shock and respiratory distress.

A typical reaction is severe hives followed by pain. The pain may last three days; the hives may last as long as three weeks. The reactions to these stings can be so rapid and serious that they are blamed for many drownings.

■ TREATMENT OF STINGS AND BITES

The first thing to do when you are stung or bitten is to get away fast. There may be other insects around, and some, such as bees and wasps, deposit a substance at the wound that attracts other insects.

If you are stung by a bee, knock the bee off immediately. Then scrape off the stinger and the venom sac as fast as you can with one swift scrape of the fingernail. Even after the bee leaves her stinger with the venom sac attached, the sac keeps contracting for two or three minutes and injecting more venom. Instant removal of the stinger and sac will prevent many of the harmful effects. Don't pick up the sac between your finger and thumb, because it only squeezes in more venom.

Hornets, wasps and yellow jackets can keep stinging you more than once, so after brushing them off, step on them to destroy them or get out of the area fast, because they will come back and attack you again.

The site of the sting or bite should be thoroughly washed with soap and water or an antiseptic solution.

Some of the pain and swelling will be reduced if you apply ice packs or hold an ice cube directly against the area. Do not use heat under any circumstances. If an arm or leg is involved, lie down and elevate the extremity. Letting the arm or leg hang down or exercising it will prolong the discomfort.

If hives form around the sting or bite or itching and swelling occur, take an antihistamine pill. Sometimes a steroid ointment on the bite will help alleviate pain as well. One effective treatment was described by a physician recently in the *Journal of the American Medical Association*. He wrote that he had steered his power mower over a nest of yellow jackets and received six very painful stings. He got immediate relief from the pain when he injected each sting with a drop of lidocaine (Xylocaine) in an epinephrine (Adrenalin) solution.

When there are multiple stings causing toxic reactions, then heroic medical measures are necessary with analgesic for pain, sedatives, intravenous fluids, antibiotics, antihistamines, steroids and other drugs.

If you have any symptoms other than a simple local one within the first twenty minutes after being stung, have someone get you to a doctor as fast as possible. You will probably need an injection of epinephrine quickly and other emergency treatment, such as oxygen.

If you have only mild symptoms and they don't start until about half an hour after the stinging, then the urgency is not so great, although you should be seen within a few hours, and should receive a small dose of epinephrine.

The shorter the interval between sting and development of symptoms of a systemic reaction, the greater the risk, even if you only begin to have generalized itching, redness of the skin or hives, or a feeling of heat throughout the body. It doesn't take long for these symptoms to develop to weakness, dizziness, nausea, vomiting, cramps, difficulty in swallowing and breathing and loss of consciousness or death.

If you tend to have more than a mild reaction from insect stings, you should wear an identification tag alerting others to your allergy and giving your physician's suggestions for first aid measures.

And persons who know they are allergic to insects and who have had general reactions previously should carry an emergency kit with them. It is inexpensive, compact and easy to carry, will slip into a pocket or purse. Each kit contains a preloaded sterile syringe containing epinephrine, two antihistamine tablets, two phenobarbital-ephedrine tablets, a tourniquet and alcohol pads. The epinephrine is injected and a tourniquet placed on the arm or leg to keep the venom from going to the rest of the body.

It is also a good idea to carry a bronchodilator aerosol spray with you in case you have difficulty in breathing after a stinging.

■ WHAT TO DO ON A LONG-TERM BASIS?

If you have shown sensitivity to insect stings or bites, you should consult with an allergist to decide your specific sensitivity and to determine whether you should have injections for immunization.

Whenever there is any doubt about what the exact species was that caused the reaction, it is generally suggested that a combination of several insect antigens be used for the desensitization program.

Desensitization does take time, but it's worth the time and energy because it is very often a lifesaving procedure. In the study by the American Academy of Allergy, investigators found clear evidence that preventive injection therapy is most helpful to persons allergic to insect stings. Progression to more serious reactions was halted for some 97 percent of treated persons, and usually their responses were reduced to those of normal people.

One man who had never had any reactions to stings before was stung by a wasp. He lost consciousness, had a convulsion, turned blue. His son gave him mouth-to-mouth resuscitation, then he was rushed to the hospital. He was treated by oxygen, cortisone, antihistamines, epinephrine and other drugs, and recovered. Desensitization was started. After he had received only about nine injections, he was again stung by a wasp. Terrified, he rushed to the doctor's office, but no reaction occurred. So desensitization does help.

Some people maintain their protection for many years, but a few lose their protection in less than a year; it is imperative that you keep in touch with your allergist so he can keep track of how the immunity is working in your particular case and how well protected you are at any time.

In most cases allergists feel that the hyposensitization therapy should be continued for the rest of the patient's life when he is allergic to insects. It is one thing to stop injections to ragweed and have the patient start sneezing or wheezing again. It's something else again to stop injections to insect venom and have the person get stung with the possibility of death.

Usually hyposensitizing injections are given subcutaneously at five- to seven-day intervals, starting with the equivalent of 1/100,000,000 of a sting and then using higher and higher concentrations until the highest tolerated dose is reached. After the maximum tolerated dose has been reached, usually injections of the same dilution are repeated at regular intervals during the insect season and every two weeks during the winter.

■ CONTACT DERMATITIS FROM INSECTS

Insects can also cause allergy just from a person touching them.

Allergists have reported that simple physical contact with cockroaches, for example, can cause asthma in sensitive people. One entomologist who worked with cockroaches had hayfever symptoms and skin reactions. Another entomologist says he has to wear a gas mask and rubber gloves when dissecting cockroaches in order to avoid terrible fits of asthma and itching eruptions of his hands. Cockroaches are one of the major causers of allergy in Puerto Rico where they routinely grow some two inches long.

Moths, whether full grown or in the caterpillar stage, are also notorious in certain areas for causing contact allergies.

Recently New York has been invaded by billions of caterpillars that have denuded trees and caused rashes and hives in thousands of people, especially children. In some neighborhoods they covered the doors, windows and steps and dropped out of trees like rain on children playing in the parks. Some entomologists say the infestation of caterpillars is occurring now because most birds in the city have been killed off by DDT and other pesticides.

In the United States the most irritating moth is the brown-tailed moth, found mostly in the northeastern part of the country, and the puss caterpillar or woolly slug living in the southern states. The ugly puss caterpillar when touched can inflict severe injury and can produce long-lasting pain and even paralysis in highly sensitive victims. Other less irritating caterpillars are the saddleback and io moth.

About the only thing that has been reported that helps a person with a dermatitis from moths is intravenous injection of magnesium thiosulfate and the rubbing on of camphor-menthol, calamine lotion, or menthol oil.

One corn moth is quite feared in South America. It forms swarms and is especially attracted by lights at night, so that people don't even light their houses at night for fear of an attack. One story is told of an oil tanker with a crew of fifty-five aboard that docked in Venezuela to take on oil. During the evening the ship's decklights were swarmed by flying insects, which then invaded every inch of the ship, covering everything including the crew. Bombs of insecticides were used against the insects, and in the morning carcasses of thousands of moths were washed overboard. The crewmen had inflamed eyes and itching skin and soon were covered with hives and eruptions that later became scaly and infected. The rash lasted for one week.

■ ALLERGIES FROM EATING INSECTS OR BREATHING INSECT DUST

Insects can also cause allergies when they are eaten or if bits of them floating in the air are breathed. We talked in the chapter on hayfever about how bits of insect dust breathed in by sensitive people often were the cause of hayfever symptoms. Many people who think they are sensitive to ragweed or grasses are actually allergic to insects.

Now other research has turned up the fact that these same bits of dust when in food can cause allergies when you eat the food. Dr. Harry S. Bernton, of Howard University, and Dr. Halla Brown, of George Washington University, have found allergic reactions to rice or black weevil, the fruit fly, Indian meal moth, saw-toothed grain beetle, red flower beetle, the lesser grain borer, and cockroaches. The Indian meal moth was found to be the most frequently involved in food contamination.

Many of the insect remains can cause allergy even after cooking, Dr. Bernton says. He believes that many supposed food allergies are really caused by allergies to insects contaminating the food. He points out that allergists frequently encounter patients who appear to be allergic to certain foods, but have negative results when tested for the food. Oftentimes, he says, these patients show positive tests to insects found in food, so possibly insects may play an even larger role in allergy than we realize.

Chapter 12

ALLERGIES TO DRUGS

It was a hot summer July afternoon when John Reynolds walked into his doctor's office for a penicillin injection to fight off an infection that was troubling him. Three minutes after he was given the injection he keeled over on the floor. In the next minute while the nurse ran for a bottle of epinephrine and a syringe, John Reynolds was dead.

A severe reaction like this to penicillin does not happen very often, but it does happen, and happens often enough now that physicians have been warned that whenever an injection of antibiotics is given to a patient, a syringe filled with epinephrine should be right there—not in the next room, but within arm's reach—just in case a reaction does occur.

Drugs are now among our most common causes of allergy. Fifty or sixty years ago we had very few drugs that would cause allergies; in fact we had very few drugs. But now with modern progress in medical treatment there are hundreds of drugs available to fight disease, and any one of them, if you are sensitive, can also cause an allergic reaction.

New drugs have made possible many of the advances of modern medicine. They have relieved much suffering, lengthened lives and prevented many deaths. They are indispensable. But as their number has grown, the incidence of allergic reactions to them has grown also. And in our overmedicated society, as the use of drugs increases, the incidence of allergic reactions will be even greater.

According to the Allergy Foundation of America, there has been a dramatic increase in recent years of the number of allergic reactions to drugs, especially to antibiotics. Thousands of reactions to penicillin alone have been reported, many serious, some fatal, the Foundation says.

"Drug reactions now comprise an amazingly large percentage of medical practice," says one physician.

Dr. John A. Benson, Jr., of the University of Oregon Medical School, reported at a medical symposium on adverse reactions that at one university clinic 5 percent of all patients admitted suffered from drug reactions, and at a hospital about 14 percent of all patients studied developed a drug reaction while in the hospital. "Since the average patient receives ten to fourteen drugs during a hospitalization, and since only about 10 percent of significant adverse reactions are voluntarily reported, the potential scope of this hazard is enormous," says Dr. Benson.

Not all of these reactions are allergic, but a good number of them are.

A disease that is caused by a treatment or procedure designed to cure another disease is called an iatrogenic disease. The physician must always be on the lookout for these side effects and allergic reactions, but he cannot let the danger keep him from using medications when they are clearly indicated.

■ TYPES OF DRUG REACTIONS

Whether sniffed, sprayed, rubbed on the skin, taken by mouth or injected, a medication can cause reactions. The effects can be as mild as a skin eruption or as serious as asthma, blood disturbances or even death.

Sometimes the reactions occur within a few minutes or several hours; or as in other allergies, they may be delayed, with the reaction not occurring until seven to fourteen days after the drug has been taken. Occasionally drug delayed reactions may not be evident for several weeks.

The amount of reaction to drugs increases as the dose of the drug increases; however, the smallest of doses is capable of causing a reaction in the person who is sensitive. The incidence of sensitization increases as treatment is prolonged with any drug or as courses of treatment are repeated. The fact that a person has tolerated a drug on a number of previous occasions is no guarantee that he will not get allergic symptoms with the next dose.

Certain underlying diseases may influence the incidence of symptoms because the drug may be broken down by the body in different ways or excreted more slowly. In patients with severe eruptions, for example, local applications of medications are more likely to sensitize the skin.

Some of the most serious allergic reactions can result from injected drugs. Antitoxin made from horse serum is particularly dangerous to those allergic to horses. Other injectable materials especially capable of giving allergic reactions are penicillin, insulin, vitamins, hormones, arsenicals and gold solutions. However, these drugs are often essential to treat certain conditions, so don't be afraid of them. It's just that you and your doctor need to have respect for their use and should always be aware of possible sensitivity.

Typical reactions include rashes, hives, asthma, hayfever, hemorrhages in the skin (purpura), gastrointestinal inflammations, circulatory disturbances and blood changes such as various types of anemia.

Sometimes blood vessels and connective tissues are affected. Sometimes there is also fever, enlargement of lymph nodes, changes in the blood, kidney disturbance or inflammation of the heart muscle.

There can also be reactions to drugs that are not allergic reactions, but are simply side effects caused by a distorted or exaggerated response to the drug. Some drugs, for example, are known to often cause a decrease in the number of white blood cells, so the resistance to infection is lowered. Several antibiotics are known to sometimes cause aplastic anemia. Liver damage can occur as a result of prolonged use of certain tranquilizers, sulfa drugs, tuberculosis drugs, thyroid drugs and gold salts. Sometimes we don't know whether a reaction is an allergic one or not.

Probably the three most common allergic drug reactions are as follows:

Anaphylaxis. The kind of severe total body reaction like that which sometimes occurs in insect stings. There is rapid onset, shock and occasionally death.

Serum Sickness. A delayed reaction to foreign animal serum. It is usually marked by hivelike skin eruptions, swelling of various parts of the body, enlargement of lymph nodes, joint pains, fever and weakness.

Contact Dermatitis. An inflammation of the skin from the application of medicines on the skin such as ointments or lotions.

■ DIAGNOSIS OF DRUG ALLERGY

Drug allergy must first of all be suspected by the physician or the patient. Any time a person is having strange symptoms, he should think about what medicines he is taking.

In most instances the physician who prescribed the drug sees the reaction, recognizes it and either treats it or discontinues the drug immediately. However, it becomes more difficult when physicians are called upon to diagnose reactions that may have been produced by drugs prescribed by others or that may have been produced by nonprescription substances, so it is important for you to tell your physician about any drug that you have gotten from others or any other new substances that may be causing the trouble.

Usually if there is a suspicion that a drug is causing symptoms, the drug is discontinued unless no substitute can be found. If the symptoms begin to improve within twenty-four to forty-eight hours after the drug has been stopped, it strongly suggests the possibility of drug allergy. Then if giving the drug again produces the symptoms again, this proves that it was the drug that caused the problem.

Sometimes, however, there are exceptions. Sometimes even though the drug was the cause, symptoms will continue after the drug is stopped. Particularly when the allergic reaction to the drug has been severe and produced tissue damage, recovery may be slow and incomplete. Sometimes the drug is long-acting, so that even if it is discontinued there is still a significant residual amount in the body that continues to produce symptoms.

Some people are sensitive to more than one drug or drug ingredient and tracing down the guilty factors in these cases can become a baffling task. One woman at age forty-two began developing chronic nasal blockage and lost her sense of taste and smell and within a few months began wheezing with asthma. The usual treatments did not help her symptoms, and the asthma was so severe that her doctor felt that it was necessary to give her daily treatment with corticosteroids. She had to be hospitalized six times in two years because of severe attacks of asthma, and in-between-times her symptoms were never really controlled. She had a severe attack of swelling of her tongue and multiple hives one day after taking two aspirin tablets for a headache. Her doctor told her she was sensitive to aspirin, but she would not accept the diagnosis and took some aspirin on two other occasions, each time developing a severe swelling of lips and tongue and asthma. Finally she stopped taking it, but then she used another product that contained a salicylate for headache and she had the same reaction of asthma and coughing. Then the patient and her physician became aware that a particularly tight cough and wheezing seemed to occur when she took drugs for the relief of asthma. Antibiotics did the same thing. Finally she was hospitalized, and all medications were stopped. In a week she was discharged symptom-free. But in two weeks the severe asthma had returned again. Within the next month she had to be hospitalized twice further with severe attacks of asthma. During this hospitalization she complained that she was having hot flashes because the usual hormone pills that she takes had not been brought to the hospital with her. She was given these pills, and her coughing and sneezing returned within three hours. Subsequently, it was established that this in addition to the aspirin had been the major troublemaker. When a different brand of the hormone was substituted, her asthma symptoms disappeared. She continued to do well for two months after discharge, but then shortly the cough returned. This time investigation revealed that it was due to a vitamin tablet coated with a yellow dye. A colorless vitamin not coated with the dye substance solved the problem that time. She now is free from asthma and is living a normal full life.

Sometimes it is difficult to decide whether a drug is causing a reaction or whether it is the disease itself causing symptoms. Infections alone can often cause skin rashes. Many people after an upper respiratory infection have pimples even when no drugs are given. Because of this, many times drugs are blamed for causing reactions when they are not at fault. Only by rechallenging the patient with that specific drug can accurate information be obtained.

Drugs can sometimes have a synergistic action with other substances—that is, the two of them together will produce some effect. For example, one woman who had always had normal blood pressure suddenly developed high blood pressure. She was given a drug containing chlorothiazide and cryptenamine, and in one week was completely paralyzed. It was learned she had been eating one whole package of licorice candy every night. When she stopped eating licorice, her paralysis cleared in three days and the high blood pressure disappeared in two weeks.

One drug when added to another can change the first drug concentration or can alter the patient's response to it. Some drugs will reverse the effects of other drugs. Some will limit the absorption of others. One of the few studies on interactions showed that the rate of adverse reactions rose from 4 percent when five or less drugs were given to an astounding 45 percent when twenty or more drugs were prescribed.

The best rule for both physicians and patients to follow—don't use three drugs if you can use two, and don't use two if one will be adequate. Treatment should always be simplified as much as possible.

Skin tests generally are of dubious value in revealing possible sensitivities to drugs. According to the Allergy Foundation of America, attempts to diagnose sensitivity to drugs through skin testing methods are rarely successful and may involve severe risks for the highly sensitive patient. "If testing is to be performed, the initial procedure should be a scratch test with very low concentrations of the suspect drug," the Foundation says.

However, there are some new tests that look encouraging. One is a blood test developed recently in Paris at the French National Institute of Immunobiology that promises to be useful in confirming cases of allergy to penicillin, aspirin and various other medicines. Others are being developed and tested.

Another new skin test to determine a person's sensitivity to penicillin uses penicilloyl polylysine (PPL). The new test, when it is used as a screening device, so far appears to pinpoint about 50 percent of the patients who are allergic to penicillin.

■ PENICILLIN ALLERGY

At least 5 or 10 out of every 100 Americans have an allergic reaction at one time or another from penicillin, according to the American Academy of General Practice. They can get the reactions from injections of penicillin, from penicillin tablets or from using a penicillin ointment. Some people can even get a reaction from milk and cheese that contain traces of penicillin because the cows producing the milk have been previously treated with penicillin for infection.

The reactions can vary. Some people develop hives and swelling; others develop fever or extreme exhaustion; and some people given an injection of penicillin will keel over and be dead before they hit the floor.

The problem of penicillin ointments causing contact dermatitis has become so bad that physicians simply do not use it for external application anymore.

There are two basic types of reactions to penicillin. One is a severe life-threatening shock reaction that occurs immediately. The other is a "serum sickness" reaction that occurs one to four days later.

The serum sickness reaction consists of hives, swelling, pain in the joints, fever, and sometimes it can also affect the kidneys and the circulatory system. The delayed reaction occurs one to four days after the injection and usually lasts about two to three weeks, but may vary from several hours to a year or more. Other delayed types of reaction from penicillin are peeling of the skin or diffuse body rash.

The most hazardous type of reaction to penicillin is that which occurs immediately after the injection, the life-threatening plummet into anaphylactic shock. Some physicians say this is the greatest single cause of death due to allergy today.

"It is difficult to estimate how often such reactions occur, but these immediate reactions are by no means rare," says Dr. Samuel M. Feinberg of Chicago. "On the basis of projection of statistics from surveys," he says, "it is reasonable to assume that 100 to 300 fatalities from such reactions occur annually in the United States."

"Nearly all of us know of one or two cases where an injection has been given and the patient hits the floor dead," says Dr. John P. McGovern of Houston, Texas.

The problem is especially drastic in Mexico, where anyone may go into a pharmacy and get an injection of an antibiotic of his own choosing without a prescription. The medications are administered by a pharmacist or sometimes are even given by well-meaning friends.

Penicillin is so widely self-administered that Mexican physicians are loath to ever prescribe it because of the high incidence of fatal reaction now occurring. At least one death a day due to penicillin reaction occurs in Mexico City, according to Dr. P. Mario Salazar Mallén, chief allergist of the General Hospital there.

When such a reaction does occur, immediate therapy is necessary. Antihistamine drugs aren't fast enough; neither are steroids or ACTH or any of the other usual methods. What the doctor needs to do is inject a large dose of epinephrine directly into a vein so that it may stimulate and support the body; then he puts a tourniquet around the site where the penicillin was administered, and makes sure the airway is open so that the patient can breathe. Sometimes a tracheotomy is necessary, with an incision made in the throat and an air tube put down into the trachea.

Sometimes a false allergic reaction will occur when penicillin is injected. Patients have been reported to have sensations of intense anxiety or even feelings of impending death and may also have visual or auditory hallucinations, feelings of lightheadedness or numbness. Usually the symptoms disappear within an hour although mild feelings of apprehension sometimes last for weeks. These reactions are not allergic ones, but apparently are due to inadvertent administration of the drug into a small vein. In these cases the person may continue to receive penicillin therapy if it is given with extreme caution.

The penicillin reactions are much less of a problem in children than in adults. In fact, one study shows that many reactions in children attributed to penicillin are really misdiagnosed and are due to other causes. The latest statistics are that only about one reaction occurs per year for every 100,000 children. Drs. C. Warren Bierman and Paul T. VanArsdel, Jr., from the University of Washington, reviewed several hundred case histories of children who were hospitalized with a diagnosis of penicillin allergy and found that many of them who developed rashes and hives during penicillin treatment actually did not have the reactions from the penicillin, but from something else.

Usually those who experience the serious systemic reactions have had previous milder reactions which they have ignored. If you ever have the slightest reaction after a penicillin injection or other medication, inform your doctor at once so that it may be added to your record. And be sure to tell any other doctors that you go to in the future.

It is extremely hazardous to try to desensitize persons allergic to penicillin, and the desensitization quite often is not effective. The only way really to deal with the problem is to scrupulously avoid the use of penicillin in any form if you are sensitive, and for the physician to use other therapy instead.

In some illnesses which do not respond to any other antibiotics, it can sometimes become necessary to give penicillin despite an allergy. For example, in meningitis which does not respond to other antibiotics, the effects of the disease are more dangerous than the penicillin. The same is true of subacute bacterial endocarditis, where penicillin can be lifesaving. Obviously in such cases the physician must proceed with infinite caution.

You must be careful of hidden penicillin also. The Food and Drug Administration prohibits the sale of milk from cows treated with penicillin. However, despite this regulation, there have been reports of allergic reactions to penicillin in milk.

■ OTHER ANTIBIOTICS

Streptomycin and sulfa drugs produce frequent allergic reactions. The newer sulfonamides are less prone to produce reactions than the older forms were, but the problem is still prevalent enough that few physicians will use them when there is any other choice of drugs.

Neomycin is rapidly approaching the same category. Present estimates are that 5 to 10 percent of patients react to neomycin.

Cephalothin was once thought to be an alternative antibiotic to penicillin in persons known to be allergic to penicillin; however, it has been found to be dangerous too. The antibiotic has an affinity for blood cells and does much of its damage to them.

The broad-spectrum antibiotics, such as the cyclines, rarely produce allergic reactions, although occasional cases occur. In a small percentage of patients tetracycline will produce skin rashes and other minor reactions, but this is considered one of the relatively safe drugs. Declomycin, however, does produce a photosensitivity reaction in a fair number of people, so that anyone taking this should avoid the sun while on therapy.

Novobiocin has a 9 or 10 percent incidence of skin rashes, but they are usually minor ones and most of them clear readily with antiallergic treatment.

Chloromycetin has been incriminated as the drug responsible for a number of deaths and is no longer used, unless under very exceptional circumstances. It causes a number of eruptions and drug fever.

Erythromycin is probably one of the safest antibiotics from a standpoint of sensitization. Very few allergic reactions to it have ever been reported, and those reported are usually mild skin rashes.

Lincomycin has also been reported to be a safe drug and is sometimes used in penicillin-sensitive patients.

Antibiotics can produce non-allergic side effects too. They can cause constipation or diarrhea, or because they destroy many of the bacteria in the intestinal tract, molds may develop and produce a black hairy tongue or mold infections in the vagina. Some women have a vaginal discharge that needs treatment every time they have antibiotic therapy for some other reason. Other people get an itch about the anal opening when they take antibiotics. These effects are not allergic ones, but are still effects to be on the alert for.

■ SENSITIVITY TO ASPIRIN

More than two hundred compounds that contain aspirin are sold on prescription or over the counter. It is a part of nearly every cold cure, headache remedy or pain-killer. A large number of people are allergic to it, though many are not aware of it. And even people who realize they are sensitive to aspirin still often get into trouble because aspirin and its related substances are encountered in so many different forms.

One fifty-two-year-old woman had a history of asthma and had had several episodes of severe anaphylactic shock following the ingestion of aspirin. She became very adept at avoiding aspirin; and knowing that her life was at stake, she learned to read labels carefully and in great detail. She went for years without any reaction because she was so careful. But one day she developed an abscessed tooth and went to a dentist. After taking her tooth out he put a tiny wick with just a touch of aspirin on it into the tooth socket. Within thirty minutes she went into severe anaphylactic shock and her life was saved only because a nearby physician rushed in and gave her repeated injections of epinephrine (Adrenalin). She had hives for most of the following week, and they did not disappear until the tooth socket was washed out with saltwater solution to remove the last traces of the aspirin.

People take aspirin so routinely and it seems so innocuous that sometimes it is difficult to convince them that aspirin, like all other drugs, can have inherent dangers. And the record of its havoc is long.

The first astronaut to wash out of the space program did so because of aspirin sensitivity. Navy Lieutenant Commander John S. Bull passed every rigorous test of physical stamina and instrument mastery and emotional coolness under pressure, but was disqualified because of the fact that he had aspirin-induced asthma.

The symptoms usually produced by aspirin sensitivity are hives or asthma.

Asthma that is induced by aspirin is usually violent in nature and is frequently accompanied by cyanosis. It can be fatal. Quite often the type of intractable asthma that develops rapidly in patients and which has no other obvious explanation is caused by aspirin sensitivity.

Dr. Max Samter, of the University of Illinois, warns that this peculiar sensitivity to aspirin could account for 2 to 8 percent of the known asthmatics, and he feels that aspirin asthma is on the increase.

It is not so surprising that there are so many reactions to aspirin when you consider that there are more than 9,000 tons of aspirin produced every year in the United States. One allergist says that whenever a patient comes in with massive hives of the face and neck, he always suspects aspirin until it is proven otherwise.

Aspirin can also cause ulcers and gastrointestinal bleeding, so that no one with ulcers or stomach problems should ever take them.

One gastrointestinal specialist reported that two out of every five patients who had had massive gastrointestinal hemorrhage had had aspirin within forty-eight hours of the bleeding.

Aspirin makes blood platelets less sticky, so that just one aspirin could have a serious effect on any blood condition for several days.

Aspirin is an ingredient in many patent medicines and cold preparations so that it may be taken unknowingly. If you are sensitive to aspirin, never take any cold pill without checking with your physician, because the chances are that there is aspirin in it.

Aspirin is acetyl salicylic acid. Some people who are sensitive to aspirin are allergic to other salicylate-related compounds also. Others are sensitive solely to aspirin and nothing else. For those who are allergic to only aspirin, there are some safe and reliable substitutes such as acetaminophen, available commercially under such trade names as Tempra, Tylenol and Nebbs.

For those who are also allergic to other salicylates, foods containing salicylates must be avoided also. The following list summarizes the foods, plants and other substances that should be avoided.

DRUGS

Acetidine
Alka-Seltzer
Anacin
Anahist
APC
Aspirin
BC
Bromo-Quinine
Bromo-Seltzer
Bufferin
Coricidin
Darvon
Dristan
Ecotrin
Empirin
Excedrin
4-Way Cold Tablets
Inhiston
Liquiprin
Midol
Pepto-Bismol
Persistin
Sal-Sayne
Stanback
Theracin
Trigesic

FLAVORING

Antiseptics
Gum
Lozenges
Beverages
Mouthwash
Oil of Wintergreen
Candles
Perfumes
Cosmetics
Toothpaste

Foods that contain salicylates in flavoring: ice cream, bakery goods (except bread), candy, chewing gum, soft drinks, Jello, jams.

FOODS

Almonds
Apples
Apricots
Blackberries
Cherries
Currants
Gooseberries
Grapes
Nectarines
Oranges
Peaches
Plums
Prunes
Raisins
Raspberries
Strawberries
Birch beer
Teaberry tea
Wines
Wine vinegar

PLANTS

Aspens
Birches
Poplars
Willows
Acacia
Spiraea
Teaberry
Calvanthus
Camellia
Hyacinth
Marigold
Milkwort
Tulips
Violets

MISCELLANEOUS

Acetyl salicylic acid
Aluminum acetyl salicylate
Ammonium salicylate
Arthropan
Calcium acetyl salicylate
Choline salicylate
Ethyl salicylate
Lithium salicylate
Methylene disalicylic acid (in lubricating oils)
Methyl salicylate
Para amino salicylic acid
Phenyl salicylate
Procaine salicylate
Sal ethyl carbonate
Salicylamide
Salicylanilide (anti-mildew)
Salicylsalicylic acid
Santyl (santyl salicylate)
Soap (green, wintergreen fragrance)
Sodium salicylate
Stroncylate
Strontium salicylate
Sulfosalicylic acid (chemical)
Suntan lotions

Patients who are allergic to aspirin are often allergic to pine pollen also, which is very closely related chemically.

People with aspirin sensitivity do not have a positive skin test to it, so it must be tested by trial and error to see whether a person is sensitive.

■ ALLERGY TO ANESTHETICS

The incidence of allergic reactions to local anesthetics is low; however, anesthetists, dentists and nurses do occasionally meet patients who have these sensitivities either of the immediate type or of the delayed reaction type. The reaction is often missed as an allergic reaction and is falsely considered to be a result of tissue injury or dental procedure.

Two of the most frequent causes of allergy among the anesthetic agents are benzocaine and Nupercaine. Xylocaine (lidocaine) is much less likely to cause a reaction, and patients who do not tolerate some other anesthetic agents can often tolerate it as a substitute.

Drugs to kill pain are basically divided into two groups. The first group includes tetracaine, chlorprocaine, monocaine and benzocaine. The second group is composed of drugs such as lidocaine, mepivacaine, prilocaine, dibucaine, and phenacaine. Drugs in the first group are somewhat related chemically, so that frequently there is cross reaction; that is, the patient who is allergic to one of the drugs may often be allergic to the others as well. However, they would probably not be allergic to one of the anesthetics in the second group.

Some people are also allergic to nitrous oxide.

Many of these substances are used both by injection, as when a tooth is extracted or local surgery is performed, and in ointments for the relief of itching or smarting from burns. The person allergic to them must be alert no matter what the form of its use and must warn any physician or dentist of his drug sensitivity.

■ ALLERGIES TO VACCINES AND TRANSFUSIONS

Many people have reactions from tetanus antitoxin, diphtheria antitoxin and other medicines made from animal serums. Again there can be either immediate reaction or delayed serum sickness syndrome. Purification of these antiserums in recent years has diminished the number of reactions considerably; however, some significant reactions do still occur.

People allergic to horse dander should beware of any injection that includes horse serum. If you suspect that you have such an allergy, a scratch test with horse serum will demonstrate the sensitivity, so that you can avoid medicines that would give you trouble. Sometimes when a person is sensitive to horse serum, medicines can be prepared from cow serum instead.

In order to avoid the necessity for using tetanus antitoxin after an injury, everyone should have routine immunization with tetanus toxoid. Then if the person is accidentally injured, a booster dose may be safely administered with little or no resultant reaction.

Another well-recognized type of allergy is the reaction to vaccines that have been grown on eggs or chick embryos. A person who is sensitive to eggs will quite often have a severe reaction when given such an injection of flu vaccine or other vaccine. If you have any trouble eating eggs, be sure to tell your physician about it and check before you get any injections, to find out what medium the vaccines have been prepared on.

Some people have allergic reactions to blood transfusions. Sometimes this is a reaction to a food or drug in the donor's blood to which the recipient of the blood is sensitive—as when, for example, the person has been receiving insulin, ACTH, heparin or hormone extracts. There can also be reactions from incompatible blood, but these generally are different in nature.

Gamma globulin infrequently has been reported to cause allergic reactions. It has many important and valuable uses, but it should not be used unnecessarily. It was formerly thought that gamma globulin was nonallergic, but repeated reports in the medical literature indicate that it can trigger anaphylactic shock in some patients.

It is reasonable and logical to use this drug to treat patients who have inadequate amounts of gamma globulin in their bodies; it is also of proved value for the prevention of measles and hepatitis, but it certainly should not be used indiscriminately to treat children for recurrent colds or infectious asthma, as is sometimes done. Actually there is no proof that such treatment is of value anyway.

■ OTHER MEDICALLY CAUSED ALLERGIES

Nearly any drug can cause a reaction in the person who is sensitive, but fortunately not all drugs are as likely to cause reactions as others. Coal tar derivatives are particularly notorious for causing reactions.

Following are facts about some of the drugs that have been reported to cause reactions in sensitive persons.

MERCURIALS

Ointments and antiseptics that contain mercury can cause a great deal of trouble, as can a substance named phenyl mercuric nitrate that is often used in ear and eye drops and other medicines as a preservative.

Mercury is present in many organic and inorganic compounds. A person may be sensitive to mercuric chloride, the mercury amalgam fillings in teeth, mercurial diuretics and to Merthiolate and Metaphen.

One man allergic to Merthiolate had a severe reaction when he used a Band-aid impregnated with it. His temperature rose to 103, he had headache, nausea, pain in the joints, and severe itching. Three days later the skin peeled off from about 70 per cent of his body.

A woman had a skin rash for years that never cleared completely until the mercury fillings in her teeth were removed.

SULFONES

This group of drugs is used mostly for the treatment of leprosy, but also for other purposes. It includes Diasone, Avlosulphone and Promacetin.

PHENOLPHTHALEIN

This drug is the basis of several laxatives. It is found in many medicines sold without prescription and also in preparations of petrolatum. Some of the medications containing phenolphthalein are Phenolax, Alophan, Ex-Lax, Phospho-Quinine, Evac-U-Gen, Taurophyllin, Carica-Bile tablets, Oxiphen, Lilatone, Nuchol, Veracolate, Caroid and Bile Salts. It is also a component of the laxative chewing gum Feen-A-Mint.

IODINE

There are at least 150 preparations that contain iodine which are available on prescription and over the counter. Iodine compounds are used for their expectorant value as well as their thinning ability, particularly in the treatment of asthma and also in contrast media for x-rays and fluoroscopy. They can produce a diffuse red pimply rash, hives, asthma or even anaphylactic shock.

FLUORIDES

A few patients have been reported sensitive to fluorides. They had some allergic symptoms from using toothpaste or vitamin preparations containing fluoride.

QUININE PRODUCTS

Reaction to quinine can take strange forms. Some people who are sensitive to it have ringing of the ears, impaired hearing, visual disturbances, shakiness, dizziness or gastrointestinal symptoms.

The main offenders are medicines used in treating malaria and heart disorders, but people can also have reactions after drinking tonic water alone or when quinine water is mixed with vodka or gin.

It may cause bleeding in some people. One woman developed blood blisters and black and blue spots all over her lips and mouth and had bleeding from her bowels and bladder after she drank cocktails with quinine water on three consecutive nights.

Even an infinitesimally small amount of quinine can cause reactions in the sensitive person, so persons who are sensitive to this specific drug must be very careful.

SEDATIVE DRUGS

About 3 to 5 percent of people who use barbiturates develop skin eruptions, hives, fever or other allergic reactions. More than 500 mixtures that contain barbiturates are on the market, and often the trade name of the preparation gives no indication of the fact that it contains a barbiturate. Assume that if it is a sedative, it probably contains barbiturate or a relative compound unless your physician says otherwise.

It is the barbiturates among other drugs that are likely to produce the "fixed drug reaction" in which an eruption or rash breaks out in one particular spot each time the drug is used.

NONDRUG MEDICAL ALLERGIES

Other substances besides drugs can produce allergy in medicine.

One fifty-nine-year-old woman came to her physician with headaches, lack of energy, blurring of vision, burning of the inside of her mouth, lack of appetite, and excessive salivation. She had been to five other physicians who had examined her but were not able to solve her problems, and she had been labeled as a severe neurotic. The sixth doctor that she saw was more attuned to the problems that allergies can cause, and he found that she was allergic to a prosthetic appliance that she was wearing that was made from Luxene. She discarded the appliance, had one made of metal, and all her strange symptoms disappeared.

Allergy to silk has frequently been troublesome in medicine. Many biological preparations are strained through silk, and when these are injected into silk-sensitive patients, serious reactions can occur. This manufacturing procedure is no longer used in the United States; however, silk sutures are still used in surgery as well as chromic catgut. Both of these can cause reactions in people sensitive to them.

Sometimes injection of preparations used for contrast in taking x-rays or performing fluoroscopy can produce hives or other reactions. It is not known whether these are allergic reactions or not.

■ PHOTOSENSITIVITY

In 1900 a Dr. Prine of Paris first noted a red reaction in twenty-six epileptic patients treated with eosin. Over the following years a number of other photosensitizing drugs were described, and now in today's drug-saturated society a remarkable number of drugs have been shown to be potential photosensitizers.

The incidence of photosensitivity reactions has increased drastically in recent times, basically due to two factors: the general public's current obsession with sunbathing and the ever-expanding quantity of photosensitizers in our cosmetics and drug environment.

Photosensitivity reactions can be caused either by a drug taken internally or by a cosmetic or chemical on the skin.

Probably the biggest causer of photosensitivity reaction is Declomycin. Somehow the drug sensitizes the skin in such a way that it overreacts to even small amounts of ultraviolet light, and the skin becomes red, swollen, blistered or scaly when exposed to sunlight. Sometimes the reaction is a transient one, but in other cases scaly or rough dark pigmented patches may remain for years. There also may be hives, eruptions or tiny hemorrhages.

Not much sunlight is necessary to cause a response; in fact patients can have the reaction on the exposed hands and face when outdoors in the middle of winter.

The hallmark of a photosensitivity reaction is the pattern of the eruption. The prominent areas involved are usually the exposed areas of the face, neck and arms and, in people wearing shorts, the front of the legs and the top of the feet. The left side of the face and the left arm often have a stronger reaction than the right side because of the exposure to the sun while driving. Usually there is no reaction on the upper eyelids, under the nose or on the inside of the wrists or elbows.

Clothing generally provides some protection, but reactions can be produced by the sun's rays penetrating right through fabrics.

Sometimes photosensitivity responses are used purposely in treatment. For example, coal tar and coal tar derivatives are often used in dermatology combined with light exposure to enhance their therapeutic effect. The drugs furacoumarin and Psoralen are used to stimulate pigmentation in a condition called vitiligo, in which the person has white splotches on the skin because of lack of pigmentation.

Both drugs and cosmetics can contain the photosensitizers. Substances in cosmetics that can produce the reaction include bergamot, lime oil, oil of cedar, vanillin oils, oil of lavender, oil of citron, sandalwood oil, coal tar and fluorescein in lipsticks.

In the past decade several antibacterial agents were incorporated in soaps to combat infection and reduce body odor, but some of them were noted to be photosensitizers. Between 1960 and 1962 one of these chemicals called tetrachlorosalicylanilide (TCSA) produced an estimated 10,000 cases of photosensitivity in England. TCSA was removed from general use, but a number of related compounds such as bithionol and another salicylanilide were also proved to be photosensitizers. Bithionol has been eliminated from incorporation into new preparations, but it is still in some creams and acne lotions. Other antibacterial and preservative substances including hexachlorophene, dichlorophene and carbanilides also will produce light sensitivity reactions on occasion, but not often.

A number of antiseptics found in soaps, cosmetics, detergents, shampoos and first aid creams are also significant causes of allergic reactions to sunlight.

Some of the common troublemakers in medicines are fluorescent dyes, coal tar derivatives, sulfonamides, antifungal agents, such as griseofulvin, diuretic agents such as the thiazides, some antibiotics and even some antihistamines. Others are the diabetic drugs, such as chlorpropamide and tolbutamide, some tranquilizers such as chlorpromazine, and other phenothiazines, Psoralen and hexachlorobenzene. Antibiotics showing the reactions include Aureomycin, Terramycin, Vibramycin. The photosensitizing antihistamines include Phenergan and Benadryl.

Plant-induced sun sensitivity can also create a number of problems. The pattern of the rash produced depends on the sites exposed and may assume a number of peculiar patterns. For example, if one develops a reaction from squeezing Persian limes, the rash will localize on the backs of the hands and in the webs of the fingers. Stripes on the back are common in Europe where the people tend to sunbathe in fields which contain a number of plants that cause photosensitivity. A violent reaction sometimes occurs among celery harvesters when they encounter a substance in celery infected with a pink rot disease.

Other causes: optical bleaches added to detergents, the yellow and red dye used in tattoos, and the artificial sweeteners cyclamate and saccharin.

And some people simply react to sunlight itself, being sensitive to the sun's ultraviolet rays. Sunlight energy itself cannot act as an antigen, but allergists think it might act as a triggering agent to convert something in the skin that becomes an antigen. These people, when they are exposed to excessive sunlight, may get eczema, red patches, hives or other reactions.

Photosensitivity is prevented by elimination of the drug or ointment that is causing the trouble. Or if it is necessary to use that drug, then stay out of the sunlight completely.

Treatment for the reaction includes cool water soaks and the application of corticosteroid preparations. Even after the drug is discontinued, sunlight must be avoided as much as possible until the sensitivity disappears.

Generally, stopping the drug causing the problem will prevent further reaction. However, some patients may become persistent light reactors, with the trouble continuing even though the drug is stopped. These patients must then limit even the mildest exposure to the sun to control their severe skin reactions. They should wear long sleeves and long pants, stay in the shade when possible or wear a sunscreening lotion. One lotion that has just been reported as especially effective is a combination of para-aminobenzoic acid and alcohol. But none of the current products will give absolute protection. Therefore, the hypersensitive individual must carefully determine the extent of protection any one product can provide him.

One must also be careful of sunscreens, because sometimes they themselves can produce a photoallergic reaction.

■ HIDDEN ADDITIVES

Many times there can be allergic reactions not to the drug itself, but to additives in the drug such as preservatives, coloring in the coating, or fillers. Just as hidden chemicals and dyes in food can cause allergic reactions, so can hidden chemicals and dyes in drugs. And often the very same allergens are involved in both food and drugs.

One man who was violently sensitive to peanuts had his first episode of anaphylactic shock after he ate a doughnut that had been deep-fried in vegetable fat that contained peanut oil. The second attack occurred after he received a drug suspended in peanut oil.

The Food and Drug Administration checks drugs for ingredients that might cause cancer or birth defects, but it does not check drugs for potential producers of serious allergy reactions.

During the past several years numerous reports have occurred concerning reactions from dyes and other additives in vitamins, drugs and other pharmaceutical materials. They can produce catastrophic effects.

Almost never are the sensitizing substances listed with the ingredients of the medicine so that the task of the physician in trying to determine a diagnosis is doubly difficult. Many allergists recommend that the laws be changed to require listing of dyes on both food and drug packages. For the sensitive person the labeling could be lifesaving.

It is a sad fact that many of the coloring and flavoring agents in medicines are made of coal tar derivatives and other chemicals that frequently produce allergy, so that over and over again the medicines given to people to cure them end up causing them more trouble. Many of the same additive agents that cause trouble in foods are used in medicines: vanillin, chocolatin, strawberrin, raspberrin, brilliant blue, amaranth, naphthol yellow and orange.

They are even used to flavor and identify antihistamines, steroids, and other drugs that are used in the treatment of allergic reactions. One allergist reports that one yellow dye, tartrazine, has caused at least nineteen allergic reactions that he knows of when it was given as part of hayfever medicines.

One sixty-year-old man was given an antibiotic tablet for an infection. About forty minutes after he took the first tablet he developed severe itching all over his body. Then he got hives that were so severe that they joined together in huge swellings. Later testing showed he was sensitive to the yellow coloring in the tablets. When he changed to the type of tablet that did not contain the yellow dye, he experienced no further untoward reactions.

It is because of the additives in drugs that one brand of drug is different from another brand. Practically every preparation has a filler, a dye or an additive substance of some type that can make it react differently in different people. This is why so many physicians feel that it is important to prescribe drugs by their brand names rather than by the generic names alone allowing pharmacists to provide the cheapest or most available drug.

One allergist says, "Since the physician has the responsibility for the outcome of the case, he certainly should have the authority to give the patient the medication he considers the choice one and not to subject the patient to the perils of any substitution."

■ PREVENTION AND TREATMENT

The best way to prevent having allergic reactions to drugs is to avoid drugs as much as possible. Physicians like to avoid prescribing a drug unless it is strictly indicated. Make sure you don't pressure your physician into giving you antibiotics for a simple cold or other drugs that you don't really need.

The second preventive measure your physician can take is to give preference, whenever there is a choice, to the drug that is least toxic and least likely to produce sensitivity. For example, newer forms of ACTH and new synthetic penicillin are less likely to produce sensitivity reactions than the forms that first came out.

Before treatment is ever given with any drug, a complete personal and medical history should be taken in the doctor's office or in the hospital to help reveal any sensitivity to drugs or other substances. Always cooperate with the physician or nurse when they take this history, and be sure to tell of any reactions you have had in the past.

Also any time you are taking medicines and you get any strange symptoms, no matter how mild, you should report them to your physician because sometimes they herald the onset of more severe reactions or they can mirror changes in the blood that your physician can check up on with laboratory tests.

Drug-sensitive patients should always be avid label readers. Read the label of any medicine you buy, whether it is by prescription or over the counter, and do not take it if it contains the drug you are sensitive to.

Sometimes reactions occur because people take pills without a doctor's advice. One young woman had been taking a drug—she didn't know what—under a doctor's directions for years. She knew that the doctor suggested that she take the pills at the onset of a cold or a viral infection. A friend was visiting her, apparently in the beginning phase of a severe cold. The woman gave her several of her pills. In half an hour her friend was wheezing and having difficulty breathing. Before an ambulance could even be called, she died. The drug she was given was penicillin. The only previous indication that the girl had had penicillin allergy was a mild case of hives that she had as a child.

A seemingly harmless pill that causes no side effects in one person can cause serious side effects, even death, in another. Don't pass pills around. Only use those that have been specifically prescribed for you by a physician.

There is one other major way to make certain that in an emergency you are not accidentally given something you are sensitive to. Patients who know they have sensitivity to a drug or a combination of drugs should carry this information with them in the form of a medical tag or an identification card.

The following lists have been prepared to show what pharmaceutical products contain penicillin, sulfonamides, tetracycline, iodine and mercury, all of which sometimes produce allergic reactions. If you are sensitive to any of these substances, you should avoid all medicines listed under that category. (Lists adapted from those of Dr. Stephen D. Lockey.)

PREPARATIONS CONTAINING PENICILLIN

ABBOCILLIN (Abbott Laboratories)
ALBA-PENICILLIN CAPSULES (The Upjohn Company)
ALUMINUM PENICILLIN TABLETS (Hynson, Westcott & Dunning, Inc.)
BICILLIMYCIN (Wyeth Laboratories)
BIOSULFA (The Upjohn Company)
CER-O-STREPS (The Upjohn Company)
CER-O-CILLIN (The Upjohn Company)
CILLIMYCIN (Wyeth Laboratories)
CILLORAL (Bristol Laboratories)
COMPOCILLIN (Abbott Laboratories)
CORICIDIN w/PENICILLIN TABLETS (Schering Corporation)
CRYSTICILLIN (E. R. Squibb & Sons)
CRYSTIFOR (E. R. Squibb & Sons)
DEPO-CER-O-CILLIN (The Upjohn Company)
DEPO-PENICILLIN (The Upjohn Company)
DIURNAL (The Upjohn Company)
DRAMCILLIN (White Laboratories, Inc.)
DROPCILLIN (White Laboratories, Inc.)
DURACILLIN (Eli Lilly & Company)
DURYCIN (Eli Lilly & Company)
FLAVOCILLIN (Philadelphia Laboratories, Inc.)
GANTROCILLIN (Roche Laboratories)
HYASORB PENICILLIN (Key Pharmaceuticals, Inc.)
K-CILLIN (Mayrand, Inc.)
K-PEN (Carrtone)
K-P.G. (Physician's Products Co., Inc.)
LEDERCILLIN (Lederle Laboratories)
LENTOPEN (Wyeth Laboratories)
NEOPENZINE (Eli Lilly & Company)
NOVAHISTINE w/PENICILLIN CAPSULES (Pitman-Moore Company)
PALOCILLIN (Palmedico, Inc.)
PENALEV (Merck Sharpe & Dohme)
PEN-G-CAPSULES (The Upjohn Company)
PENICILLIN G POTASSIUM (Abbott Laboratories) (Eli Lilly & Company)
PENICILLIN, RAPID (Wyeth Laboratories)
PENICILLIN-STREPTOMYCIN READIMIXED (The Upjohn Company)
PENICILLIN & STREPTOMYCIN (Parke, Davis & Company)
PENICILLIN S-R (Parke, Davis & Company)
PENICILLIN S-R-S (Parke, Davis & Company)
PENICILLIN OPHTHALMIC OINTMENT (Rexall Drug Company)
PENICILLIN TOPICAL OINTMENT (Rexall Drug Company)
PENICILLIN TRIPLE SULFONAMIDE TABLETS (Rexall Drug Company)
PENIORAL TABLETS (Wyeth Laboratories)

PEN-TABS (Rexall Drug Company)
PENTID (E. R. Squibb & Sons)
PENTRESAMIDE (Merck Sharp & Dohme)
PEN-VEE-CIDIN CAPSULES (Wyeth Laboratories)
PLASMACILLIN (Rexall Drug Company)
PROCAINE PENICILLIN G (Breon Laboratories, Inc.)
PRONAPEN (Pfizer Laboratories)
REMANDEN (Merck Sharp & Dohme)
STREP-COMBIOTIC (Pfizer Laboratories)
STREP-CRYSDIMYCIN (E. R. Squibb & Sons)
STREP-DICRYSTICIN FORTIS (E. R. Squibb & Sons)
STREP-DISTRYCILLIN (E. R. Squibbs & Sons)
SUGRACILLIN (The Upjohn Company)
SULFA-SUGRACILLIN (The Upjohn Company)
TRISEM-PEN (The S. E. Massengill Company)
TRUO-CILLIN (Abbott Laboratories)
V-CILLIN (Eli Lilly & Company)

SYNTHETIC PENICILLIN

CHEMIPEN (E. R. Squibb & Sons)
DARCIL (Wyeth Laboratories)
MAXIPEN (J. B. Roerig & Company)
PENBRITIN (Ayerst Laboratories)
POLYCILLIN (Bristol Laboratories)
PROSTAPHLIN (Bristol Laboratories)
RESISTOPEN (E. R. Squibb & Sons)
RO-CILLIN (Rowell Laboratories, Inc.)
SEMOPEN (The S. E. Massengill Co.)
SYNCILLIN (Bristol Laboratories)
SYNDECON (Bristol Laboratories)
TEGO-PEN (Bristol Laboratories)
UNIPEN (Wyeth Laboratories)
V-CILLIN SULFA (Eli Lilly & Company)
V-KOR DISKETS (Eli Lilly & Company)
WYCILLIN (Wyeth Laboratories)

PREPARATIONS CONTAINING SULFONAMIDES

ACR ALLANTOMIDE OINTMENT (The National Drug Company)
ACUSUL (Philips Roxane Laboratories)
AFLUHIST (Palmedico, Inc.)
AFLUS-P (Palmedico, Inc.)
ALDIAZOL (The S. E. Massengill Company)
ALLANTOMIDE OINTMENT (The National Drug Company)
ALMOCETAMIDE (Ayerst Laboratories)
ALULOTION SULFATHIAZOLE (Wyeth Laboratories)
AUREOMYCIN TRIPLE SULFAS (Lederle Laboratories)
AVC CREAM (The National Drug Company)
AVC SUPPOSITORIES (The National Drug Company)
AZO-ENTUSUL (U. S. Vitamin & Pharmaceutical Corp.)

AZO-GANTANOL (Roche Laboratories)
AZO-GANTRISIN (Roche Laboratories)
AZO-KYNEX (Lederle Laboratories)
AZO-SULFSTAT (Saron Pharmacal Corp.)
AZO-SULFURINE (Table Rock Laboratories, Inc.)
AZULFIDINE (Pharmacia Laboratories, Inc.)
AZOTREX (Bristol Laboratories)
BICILLIN SULFAS (Wyeth Laboratories)
BIOSULFA (The Upjohn Company)
BLEFCON OPHTHALMIC OINTMENT (Madland Laboratories, Inc.)
BLEPH SOLUTION (Allergan Pharmaceuticals)
BLEPHAMIDE OPHTHALMIC LIQUIFILM (Allergan Pharmaceuticals)
CETAPRED OPHTHALMIC OINTMENT (Alcon Laboratories, Inc.)
CETAZINE (Bowman, Inc.)
CITRASULFAS (The Upjohn Company)
COCO-DIAZINE (Eli Lilly & Company)
COCO-SULFONAMIDES (Eli Lilly & Company)
COMPOCILLIN-VK w/SULFAS (Abbott Laboratories)
CREMODIAZINE (Merck Sharp & Dohme)
CREMOMYCIN (Merck Sharp & Dohme)
CREMOSUXIDINE (Merck Sharp & Dohme)
CREMOTHALIDINE (Merck Sharp & Dohme)
CREMOTRES (Merck Sharp & Dohme)
CRIONIL LOZENGES (Research Products Corp.)
DELOMETS (S. F. Durst & Co., Inc.)
DELTAMIDE (Armour Pharmaceutical Co.)
DUOZINE (Abbott Laboratories)
ELKOSIN (Ciba Pharmaceutical Co.)
ENTEROSULFON (G. M. Campbell Products Co.)
ENTUSUL (U. S. Vitamin & Pharmaceutical Corp.)
ERYTHROCIN-SULFAS (Abbott Laboratories)
ERYTHROMID (Abbott Laboratories)
ERYTHROSULFAS (The Upjohn Co.)
ESKADIAZINE (Smith Kline & French Laboratories)
GANTANOL (Roche Laboratories)
GANTRICILLIN (Roche Laboratories)
GANTRISIN EAR SOLUTION (Roche Laboratories)
GANTRISIN (Roche Laboratories)
GLUCO-FEDRIN w/SULFATHIAZOLE NASAL SOLUTION (Parke, Davis & Company)
ILOSONESULFA (Eli Lilly & Company)
ILOTYCIN-SULFA (Eli Lilly & Company)
INCORPOSUL (The Blue Line Chemical Co.)
INTESTOL (First Texas Pharmaceuticals, Inc.)
ISOPTO CETAPRED OPHTHALMIC SOLUTION (Alcon Laboratories, Inc.)
K-CILLIN SULFA (Mayrand, Inc.)
KECTIL (Bristol Laboratories)
KYNEX (Lederle Laboratories)
LIPO-GANTRISIN (Roche Laboratories)
LIPO-SULFALOID (Westerfield Laboratories, Inc.)

MADRIBON (Roche Laboratories)
MAGMOID SULCO (Pitman-Moore Co.)
MESULFIN (Ayerst Laboratories)
METIMYD (Schering Corporation)
MIDICEL (Parke, Davis & Company)
MUCAMIDE (Warren-Teed Pharmaceuticals, Inc.)
NEOPENZINE (Eli Lilly & Company)
NEO-SYNEPHRINE SULFATHIAZOLATE (Winthrop Laboratories)
NEOTHALIDINE (Merck Sharp & Dohme)
NEOTRESAMIDE (Merck Sharp & Dohme)
NEOTRIZINE (Eli Lilly & Company)
NISULFAZOLE (Breon Laboratories)
OTOMIDE EAR SOLUTION (White Laboratories, Inc.)
OTOS-MOSAN EAR SOLUTION (Ayerst Laboratories)
PAMOLIN (Winthrop Laboratories)
PANSULFA (The William S. Merrell Co.)
PAOGUAN (The S. E. Massengill Co.)
PAREDRINE SULFATHIAZOLE (Smith Kline & French Laboratories)
PECTOGUANIDINE (Carrtone Laboratories, Inc.)
PENSUL (Savage Laboratories, Inc.)
PENTID-SULFAS (E. R. Squibb & Sons)
PEN-VEE SULFAS (Wyeth Laboratories)
PENTRESAMIDE (Merck Sharp & Dohme)
PHTHALYLSULFACETAMIDE (Various)
PHTHALYLSULFATHIAZOLE (Various)
POMALIN (Winthrop Laboratories)
PROKLAR (Westerfield Laboratories, Inc.)
PYRIDIUM TRI-SULFA (Warner-Chilcott Laboratories)
QUADSUL JUNIOR WAFERS (The Vale Chemical Company)
RENASUL (Carrtone Laboratories, Inc.)
RESION P M S (The National Drug Company)
RHINAZINE NASAL SOLUTION (Lederle Laboratories)
ROSOXOL-AZO (Robinson Manufacturing Co.)
RO-SULFA (Rowell Laboratories)
SEBIZON (Schering Corporation)
SECOMAT (Texas Pharmacal Co.)
SODIUM SULAMYD (Schering Corporation)
SONILYN (Mallinckrodt Chemical Works)
SUCCINYLSULFATHIAZOLE (Various)
SULADYNE (The Stuart Company)
SULAMYD TABLETS (Schering Corporation)
SULF-30 (Smith, Miller & Patch, Inc.)
SULFABED (The Purdue Frederick Co.)
SULFA CEEPRYN (The William S. Merrell Co.)
SULFACETAMIDE (Various)
SULFADIAZINE (Various)
SULFAGUANIDINE (Various)
SULFAMERAZINE (Various)
SULFAMYLON (Winthrop Laboratories)
SULFA-PLEX VAGINAL CREAM (Rowell Laboratories)

SULFAPYRIDINE (Various)
SULFA STATIN (Crookes Barnes Laboratories, Inc.)
SULFA SUGRACILLIN (The Upjohn Company)
SULFASUXIDINE (Merck Sharp & Dohme)
SULFATHALIDINE (Merck Sharp & Dohme)
SULFATHIAZOLE (Various)
SULFATRIAD (Smith, Miller & Patch, Inc.)
SULFA-TRIO (Rexall Drug Company)
SULFEDEX (Abbott Laboratories)
SULFEDEXAN (Abbott Laboratories)
SULFID (Philips Roxane Laboratories)
SULFONAMETS (The National Drug Company)
SULFONAMIDES (Eli Lilly & Company)
SULFONOSOL (The National Drug Company)
SULFOSE (Wyeth Laboratories)
SULFSTAT (Saron Pharmacal Corp.)
SULFURINE (Table Rock Laboratories, Inc.)
SUL-PONDETS (Wyeth Laboratories)
SUL-SPANSION (Smith Kline & French Laboratories)
SUL-SPANTAB (Smith Kline & French Laboratories)
SULTACOF (Table Rock Laboratories, Inc.)
SULTRIN (Ortho Pharmaceutical Corp.)
SYRASULFAS (The Upjohn Company)
TAOMID (J. B. Roerig & Company)
TAO SULFA (J. B. Roerig & Company)
TERFONYL (E. R. Squibb & Sons)
TETREX (Bristol Laboratories)
THALMYD (Schering Corporation)
THIOSULFIL (Ayerst Laboratories)
THIZODRIN (Eli Lilly & Co.)
TOUR-AID (First Texas Pharmaceuticals, Inc.)
TRIAMIDE JR. (Haberle Drug Company)
TRI-AZO-MUL (First Texas Pharmaceuticals, Inc.)
TRIFONAMEDE (Mallinckrodt Chemical Works)
TRICOMBISUL (Schering Corp.)
TRIONAMIDE (Tilden-Yates Laboratories, Inc.)
TRIPLESULFAPYRAMIDINES (Lederle Laboratories)
TRIPSUL (Carrtone Laboratories, Inc.)
TRISEM (The S. E. Massengill Co.)
TRISEM-PEN (The S. E. Massengill Co.)
TRISULFAMINIC (Dorsey Laboratories)
TRI-SULFANYL (U. S. Vitamin & Pharmaceutical Corp.)
TRISULFAPYRAMIDINES (Various)
TRISULFAZINE (The Central Pharmacal Co.)
TRISUREID (Reid-Provident Laboratories, Inc.)
TRUOZINE (Abbott Laboratories)
TYMPANIDE (Warren-Teed Pharmaceuticals, Inc.)
URIPLEX (Westerfield Laboratories, Inc.)
UROBIOTIC (Pfizer Laboratories)
URONAMIDE (Flint Laboratories)
UROSULFIN (Warner-Chilcott Laboratories)

UROSULFON (CWC)
UTRASUL (Conal Pharmaceuticals, Inc.)
VAGIPLEX (Rowell Laboratories, Inc.)
VASOCIDIN (Smith, Miller & Patch, Inc.)
VASOSULF (Smith, Miller & Patch, Inc.)
V-CILLIN K SULFA (Eli Lilly & Co.)
WESTHIAZOLE VAGINAL JELLY (Westwood Pharmaceuticals)

PREPARATIONS CONTAINING TETRACYCLINE

ACHROCIDIN (Lederle Laboratories)
ACHROMYCIN (Lederle Laboratories)
ACHROSTATIN (Lederle Laboratories)
AUREOMYCIN (Lederle Laboratories)
AZOTREX (Bristol Laboratories)
BRISTACYCLINE (Bristol Laboratories)
CANCYCLINE (Canfield)
COMYCIN (The Upjohn Company)
DECLOMYCIN (Lederle Laboratories)
DECLOSTATIN (Lederle Laboratories)
KESSO-TETRA (McKesson Laboratories)
MAYTREX (Mayrand, Inc.)
MYSTECLIN-F (E. R. Squibb & Sons)
OXYTETRACYCLINE (Various)
PALTET (Palmedico, Inc.)
PANALBA (The Upjohn Company)
PANMYCIN (The Upjohn Company)
RETET (Reid-Provident Lab., Inc.)
RONDOMYCIN (Pfizer Laboratories)
SAROCYCLINE (Saron Pharmacal Corp.)
SIGNEMYCIN (J. B. Roerig & Company)
STECLIN (E. R. Squibb & Sons)
SUMYCIN (E. R. Squibb & Sons)
SYNTETRIN (Bristol Laboratories)
TERRA-CORTRIL (Pfizer Laboratories)
TERRACYDIN (Pfizer Laboratories)
TERRAMYCIN (Pfizer Laboratories)
TERRASTATIN (Pfizer Laboratories)
TETRACHOL (Rachelle Laboratories)
TETRACYCLINE (Various)
TETRACYDIN (J. B. Roerig & Company)
TETRACYN (J. B. Roerig & Company)
TETRAMAX (J. B. Roerig & Company)
TETRASTATIN (J. B. Roerig & Company)
TETREX (Bristol Laboratories)
UROBIOTIC CAPSULES (Pfizer Laboratories)
VELACYCLINE (E. R. Squibb & Sons)

PREPARATIONS CONTAINING IODINE

AMEND'S SOLUTION (The Leeming & Co.)
AMMONIUM CHLORIDE (Haberle Drug Company)

ANAMEBA (Campbell)
BETADINE (Physicians Products Co., Inc.)
BEXCEMINS (Haberle Drug Company)
BIVAM (U. S. Vitamin & Pharmaceutical Corp.)
BRACODIN (McNeil Laboratories, Inc.)
CALCIDIN (Abbott Laboratories)
CALCIDRINE (Abbott Laboratories)
CALCIHAB (Haberle Drug Co.)
CALCINATAL (Nion Corporation)
CAL-OB (Warren-Teed Pharmaceuticals, Inc.)
CAL-RON (Rowell Laboratories, Inc.)
CONTRAST MEDIA FOR X-RAY EXAMINATIONS (Various)
DI-ODINE (The Brown Pharmaceutical Co.)
DIODOQUIN (G. D. Searle & Co.)
DOMEFORM-HC (Dome Chemicals, Inc.)
EN-CEBRIN (Eli Lilly & Company)
ENDOLAC (Endo Laboratories, Inc.)
ENFAMIL (Mead Johnson Laboratories)
ENGRAN (E. R. Squibb & Sons)
EPHED-ORGANDIN (Wampole Laboratories)
FELSO (American Felsol Company)
FERRONORD PROGRAVA (Nordson)
FILIBON (Lederle Laboratories)
FLURA-PREN (Kirkman)
FORMTONE (Dermik Pharmacal Inc.)
HEB-CORT V CREAM (Barnes-Hind Pharmaceuticals, Inc.)
HESPERO-C PRENATAL (The National Drug Co.)
HYQUIN CREAM (Texas Pharmacal Company)
IODACREST (Nutrition Control Products)
IODASEPT (Guardian Chemical Corp.)
IOD-ETHAMINE (Pitman-Moore)
IODETINA (Italian Drugs Importing Co., Inc.)
IODIZED LIME (The Upjohn Company)
IODIZED TABLE SALT (Various)
IODOGENOL (E. Fougera & Co., Inc.)
IODO-ICTHOL (Ulmer Pharmacal Co.)
IODOLAKE (Lakeside Laboratories, Inc.)
IODO-LIPALONE (Spirt & Company, Inc.)
IODO-NIACIN (Cole Pharmacal Co., Inc.)
ISUPREL (Winthrop Laboratories)
ITRAMIL (Ciba Pharmaceutical Company)
K-I-N TABLETS (Irwin Neisler)
LIDAFORM-HC (Dome Chemicals Inc.)
LIDA-MANTLE CREME (Dome Chemicals Inc.)
LIPIDOL (E. Fougera & Co., Inc.)
LIPOLODINE (Ciba Pharmaceutical Company)
LUGOL'S SOLUTION (Various)
MEVANIN-C (Beutilich, Inc.)
MOEBIQUIN (C.M.C.)
NEO-DOMEFORM-HC (Dome Chemicals Inc.)
NEO-LIDA MANTLE (Dome Chemicals Inc.)

NIODOLIN (Lincold Laboratories, Inc.)
NUATELS (Abbott Laboratories)
NYSTAFORM (Dome Chemicals Inc.)
OBNATAL (Boyle & Company)
OMINAL (Kenwood Laboratories, Inc.)
ORGANIDIN (Wampole Laboratories)
OS-CAL FORTE (Marion Laboratories, Inc.)
OS-VIM (Marion Laboratories, Inc.)
PALAFLOR (Parke, Davis & Company)
PANVITEX PRENATAL (Fellows-Testagar)
PEDIACOF (Winthrop Laboratories)
PENTACORT (Dalin Pharmaceuticals, Inc.)
PHORM (B. F. Ascher & Co., Inc.)
POTASSIUM IODIDE (Various)
POTASSIUM IODIDE THEOCALCIN (Knoll Pharmaceutical Co.)
PRAMET (Abbott Laboratories)
PRAMILETS (Abbott Laboratories)
PRECALCIN (Walker Laboratories)
PRE-FLUR (S. J. Tutag & Company)
PREFORT (Amfre-Frant, Inc.)
PREVAM (U. S. Vitamin & Pharm. Co.)
RADIOACTIVE IODINE (Abbott Laboratories)
SEDORZL (Wampole Laboratories)
SODIUM IODIDE (Various)
SOSAL COMPOUND (Haberle Drug Co.)
SYRUP HYDRIODIC ACID (Eli Lilly & Company)
THEOBROMINE-PHENOBARBITAL COMPOUND (The Upjohn Company)
THEONATAL-E (The Central Pharmacal Co.)
THEO-ORGANIDIN (Wampole Laboratories)
THESODATE w/PHENOBARBITAL & POTASSIUM IODIDE (Brewer & Company, Inc.)
THYROID STRONG EMPLETS (Parke, Davis & Company)
TINCTURE OF IODINE (Various)
TOPIGEL (Reed & Carnick)
TUSSI-ORGANIDIN (Wampole Laboratories)
VI-AQUAMIN (U. S. Vitamin & Pharm. Corp.)
VICALMIN (Smith, Miller & Patch)
VIOFORM-HYDROCORTISONE (Ciba Pharmaceutical Co.)
VIO-HYDROSONE (North American Pharmacal, Inc.)
VIO-PRENATE (Rowell Laboratories, Inc.)
VIRAC (Ruson Laboratories, Inc.)
VI-SYNERAL (U. S. Vitamin & Pharm. Co.)
X-RAY CONTRAST MEDIA (Various)
YODOXIN (Glenwood Laboratories, Inc.)

PREPARATIONS CONTAINING MERCURY

AMMONIATED MERCURY OINTMENT (Various)
AR-EX SORSIS (Ar-Ex Products Company)
BLUE OINTMENT (Norwich Pharmacal Company)

CUMERTILIN (Endo Laboratories, Inc.)
DERMA ZERMA (Standard Laboratories, Inc.)
DICURIN PROCAINE (Eli Lilly & Company, Inc.)
EUDICAINE (Rexall Drug Company)
HERMESOL (Kahlenberg Laboratories)
HYDROPHEN (Amfre-Grant, Inc.)
KAY-SAN OINTMENT (Commerce Drug Company, Inc.)
MAZON OINTMENT (Thayer Laboratories)
MERCIREX OINTMENT (The Mercirex Company)
MERCUHYDRIN (Lakeside Laboratories, Inc.)
MERCUPROCYL (Barrows Biochem. Prod. Corp.)
MERCUROCHROME (Various)
MERCUROPHYLLIN (Various)
MECUZANTHIN (Campbell)
MERSALYN & THEOPHYLLIN (Various)
MERTHIOLATE (Eli Lilly & Company, Inc.)
MYCOZOL (Parke, Davis & Company)
NEOHYDRIN (Lakeside Laboratories, Inc.)
NEOMERSYL (The Central Pharmacal Co.)
PALMER'S "SKIN SUCCESS" (E. T. Browne Drug Co., Inc.)
PREPARATION H (Whitehall Laboratories, Inc.)
PRIVINE HYDROCHLORIDE (Ciba Pharmaceutical Company)
RIASOL (Shield Laboratories)
SALCRESIN (The Upjohn Company)
SALYRGAN & THEOPHYLLIN (Winthrop Laboratories)
SORIDEX (Kahlenberg Laboratories)
SPERTI OINTMENT (Whitehall Laboratories, Inc.)
THANTIS LOZENGES (Hynson, Wescott & Dunning, Inc.)
THIOMERIN (Wyeth Laboratories)

■ SOME TYPES OF DRUG REACTIONS AND THEIR CAUSES

Table 1.

SYSTEMIC DISEASES CAUSED BY DRUGS

Causative Agents	*Disease or Syndrome*	*System*
Anesthetics, mercurials, penicillin procaine, penicillin, sulfonamides, sera, acetylsalicylic acid, insulin	Anaphylactic shock Polyarteritis nodosa	Vascular
Penicillin, chlortetracycline HCl, meperidine HCl, mercurials, para-aminosalicylic acid, arsenic, acetylsalicylic acid, belladonna	Asthma	Pulmonary

From *Medical Science,* June 1967. Original from the Fenton-Rom Clinic, Detroit, Michigan, Revised by Stephen D. Lockey, M.D.

Table 1. *(cont.)*

Hydralazine HCl	Lupus erythematosus-like	Collagen
Oxygen in premature infants	Retrolental fibroplasia	Metabolic
Chlorpromazine, HCl, thiouracils, methimazole	Jaundice-intrahepatic obstruction	Hepatic
Phenacemide, phenylbutazone, isonicotinic acid hydrazides	Hepatitis	
	Hepatic coma	
Sulfonamides, trimethadione, chelating agents, autonomic blocking agents	Nephrosis Acute urinary retention	Renal
Tranquilizers, particularly trifluoperazine, perphenazine, prochlorperazine, reserpine, rauwolfia, steroids, streptomycin sulfate, dihydrostreptomycin sulfate	Convulsive disorders and parkinsonism Psychoses Eighth nerve	Neurologic
Antithyroid drugs, phenylbutazone chloramphenicol, amphetamines, trimethadione, methylphenylethydantoin, diphenylhydantoin, tolbutamide, chlorpromazine, HCl aminopyrine	Hemotoxic drug reactions	Hematologic

Table 2.

DERMATOLOGIC MANIFESTATIONS OF DRUG REACTIONS

Type	*Most Common Offenders*
Hives	Organ extracts, penicillin, streptomycin, salicylates, sera, foods with artificial coloring, flavoring and preservative agents of coal-tar origin
Allergic eczema	Sulfonamides, penicillin, mercurials, arsenicals, local anesthetics, quinacrine HCl, quinine, aniline dyes, arsphenamine
Fixed eruptions	Barbiturates, phenolphthalein, quinacrine HCl, sulfonamides, gold, phenacetin, antipyrine
Erythema multiforme and nodosum-like lesions	Bromides, iodides, salicylates, phenacetin, sulfonamides, penicillin, phenolphthalein
Purpura	Barbiturates, gold salts, iodides, sulfonamides, arsphenamines, acetylsalicylic acid

Table 2. (*cont.*)

Exanthematous	Barbiturates, sulfonamides, heavy metals, arsenic, salicylates, foods with artificial coloring, flavoring and preservative agents of coal-tar origin, penicillin
Bullous eruptions	Iodides, gold salicylates, sulfonamides, phenolphthalein
Exfoliative dermatitis	Arsenicals, barbiturates, gold salts, mercurials, quinacrine HCl, belladonna

Chapter 13

ALLERGIC HEADACHE, EARACHE, SINUS TROUBLE AND OTHER ALLERGIC SYMPTOMS

An astounding number of maladies can be caused by allergy, some of which you might not have considered possible.

We have talked about how an allergy can cause eye problems, respiratory symptoms, gastrointestinal upsets, skin disturbances, anaphylactic shock and even emotional and personality disturbances, but the list of strange symptoms that allergy can initiate is even longer than this. An allergy can upset any system of the body and can mimic almost any disease or condition known to man. Allergy has been called the great masquerader.

An allergy can cause earache, headaches, sinus trouble, certain types of pneumonia, cough, dizziness, deafness, a form of epilepsy, disturbances of the heart and circulatory systems, and malfunctioning of the bladder.

■ HEADACHES

The causal relationship between specific allergies and certain types of headache has been known for many years, yet today allergy is frequently overlooked as a factor when headache is treated.

Many times the wrong factors get blamed for causing a headache. One middle-aged man went to several doctors with a complaint that he had recurrent severe headaches, but only on Thanksgiving, Christmas and New Year's Day. Finally he visited an allergist who found three factors commonly involved on the headache days: he always ate and drank a lot, his mother-in-law always came for dinner and the main dish was always turkey.

There were many hurt feelings and unkind words, especially from his mother-in-law, until after much study his allergist found he was sensitive to penicillin. His holiday turkeys came from a state where they were fed on a mash containing penicillin.

Dr. Leon Unger of Chicago studied 55 patients who had had severe attacks of headache and found that 80 percent were either completely or almost completely relieved of their headaches when allergies to food were detected and the involved foods eliminated.

Particular allergic factors that should be considered when trying to learn the cause of headache are inhalants such as animal dander, dust, mold spores and pollen, foods such as milk, wheat and chocolate, drugs that contain aspirin, sulfonamides or phenolphthalein and drugs used in the treatment of high blood pressure.

Allergic reactions can involve the arteries leading to the brain. Often pain can be caused by stretching of these arteries, and the alternate stretching and relaxing of the vessels can produce the throbbing pain so often associated with headaches.

Allergically caused headaches can also be caused by swelling and congestion of the nose or sinuses. These are often more severe in the early morning hours when the patient wakes. Sinus headaches are usually frontal ones and are often associated with a sensation of pressure and pain around the sinuses, the nose and the eyeballs. The headache that occurs when allergy causes swelling of the inner structures of the nose can also, by referred pain, produce headache in other parts of the head as well as into the neck, back, shoulders and upper arms.

How can you tell if particular headaches are due to allergy? A headache attributable to allergic causes should generally satisfy one or more of the following criteria:

There are other allergy conditions in the patient or his relatives.

Attacks occur after the person eats certain foods or after exposure to other specific substances.

Positive skin tests indicate specific hypersensitivity.

Results are obtained by eliminating the food or other causal factor or factors.

Allergic headaches may occur immediately after exposure to a substance, or in a delayed reaction may occur sometime later, often as late as twelve to twenty-four hours.

Frontal headache is the most common type of head pain due to allergic factors. It occurs in about 75 percent of headaches. It usually occurs on both sides and often is accompanied by a stuffed-up or runny nose. Skin tests are usually positive, showing sensitivity to food or inhalant allergens. Also in some instances the headache can be reproduced by injection of the antigen into the patient.

There is probably a vascular basis for frontal headaches because there are often warning symptoms such as visual changes, nausea, vomiting and driving pain.

Sometimes the attack is also preceded by swelling of the hands, feet and face, and the patient gains weight just before getting the headache, and urinates a great deal and loses weight at the end of the headache.

Migraine headaches can also be caused by allergies. A migraine headache is defined as one that begins suddenly with intense, throbbing pain and is caused by changes in size and degree of pulsation of certain blood vessels in the head.

It is estimated that about 8 to 12 percent of the population of the United States suffer attacks of migraine. For some reason it seems to affect city dwellers and white-collar workers more than country people and manual workers. More than half the cases of migraine start between the ages of twenty and thirty years, although cases do occur in childhood and in late life. When parents have migraine headaches, about half the children also develop migraine.

The migraine attack passes through three stages: The prodromal symptoms may be very disturbing and may include feelings of euphoria or depression, body disassociation, feelings of alteration of body size, and the patient may see flashes of light or hear things. This is usually followed by the major throbbing head pain usually on one side, often followed by nausea or vomiting. There is also usually an after-pain due to swelling of the walls of the arteries and muscle spasms.

Numerous factors can cause migraine headache—allergy, emotional or physical stress, premenstrual tension, hypothyroidism, gastrointestinal upset, infections, precipitous weather changes, overexertion or menopause. One or several of these factors may exist in the same person at the same time, or each may exist separately at different times.

One of the major contributors to migraine is allergy to food. When offending foods are eliminated from the diet, many migraine patients are quickly relieved of their attacks.

One allergist believes that a good number of people who suffer from migraine may be allergic to sodium propionate, which is found in some forms of Swiss cheese and is used as a preservative in tobacco and many foods, including bread.

Another kind of common headache is the tension headache, which bears a very close relationship to the migraine. In fact, if effective medication is not taken early enough, migraine headaches may follow tension headaches.

Tension headache is variable in character and can be burning, pressing or throbbing. Once it begins, it may persist for hours or sometimes days. Usually along with it there are muscle contractions and tender spots in the neck and the scalp. This type of headache is not allergic. There is usually a large emotional factor involved that causes the tension and contraction of the neck and scalp muscles that in turn leads to the pain of the headache.

Another type of headache is called histamine cephalalgia. It is uncommon and occurs mostly in men over age forty. When it does occur, the pain becomes so intense that many times patients wake up in the middle of the night screaming, or may even contemplate suicide to obtain relief. This kind of headache is often caused by food allergies, and many reports have been made of patients who have been completely relieved of pain when the foods precipitating this type of headache were removed from their diet.

Headache, of course, can be caused by many other things in addition to allergy. The cause can be as simple as poor ventilation in the room resulting in an imbalance in the air you breathe, or you may get a headache if you skip a meal, if you have a fever, or if you concentrate on one task too long, straining your muscles. It can be caused by an infected tooth, eye strain, ill-fitting dentures or out-of-line teeth that have an imperfect bite.

Sometimes they can be caused by serious underlying disorders such as high blood pressure, brain tumor or hemorrhage in the brain.

Danger signals to look out for are: if frequent headaches begin in someone not previously headache-prone, if headaches of a long duration have a sudden change in pattern, if headaches begin increasing in severity and frequency, if headaches are aggravated by coughing, straining or stooping, or if headaches are associated with other symptoms such as high fever or paralysis or increasing sleepiness.

See your physician if you have frequent headaches. Before you can assume headaches are due to food sensitivity or other allergy, your physician must rule out all other potential causes.

Successful treatment of the allergic headache must begin with an accurate diagnosis; then complete avoidance of the offending allergens should be sought. Your physician can give you several medicines to help cope with the acute attack of headache. Antihistamines are sometimes helpful. Tranquilizers will help with the muscle spasms and raise the pain threshold. Ergot preparations are helpful, as are anti-serotonin agents such as Sansert and Periactin which have proved helpful in many patients to both treat and prevent headaches.

In some patients anticonvulsant drugs such as phenobarbital and Dilantin are useful in preventing migraine headaches. A new drug called only BC-105 is still experimental, but appears to have an even better effect in preventing migraine headaches.

■ SINUS TROUBLE

Chronic sinusitis is a problem for nearly ten million people in the United States, and of these only about one out of three are under a doctor's care.

People use the term "sinus trouble" to mean many things. What it is really is an infection or an allergy that stuffs up the sinus cavities that are in the forehead and the upper part of the cheeks.

Leonardo da Vinci is credited with the first description of the sinus cavities in 1489. Their function appears to be threefold: they aid in warming and moistening the inspired air; being filled with air they lessen the weight of the skull and give it better balance; they contribute to the resonance of the voice. Some people believe that earlier in evolution they were used for smelling; then when man's need for an acute sense of smell decreased, they gradually became closed off. Infections occur readily because there is little ventilation and drainage.

Some of the sinuses are present at birth; some of them appear later.

Any infection or allergy that involves the mucous membrane of the nose can quickly affect the sinuses, and a case of acute sinusitis often begins in the late stages of a cold or hayfever attack, although sometimes something like an abscessed tooth can be the cause. It is estimated that up to 70 percent of cases of chronic sinusitis have an allergy as an underlying cause, with infection as a complication.

Neglecting an acute sinus attack that occurs after an infection or hayfever attack is one of the major causes of long-term chronic sinusitis. With each attack there is injury and swelling to the membranes, and permanent changes occur to make the condition a chronic complaint.

Other factors that can favor the development of sinus trouble are mechanical obstructions such as septal deformities, swollen membranes in the nose, malformation in the nose, polyps or other obstructions or impaired activity of the cilia. Other contributing factors include diet and vitamin deficiencies, anemia, blood disorders, psychosomatic factors, hormone upsets, changes in the weather, and excessively dry air. Swimming and diving can bring on sinus trouble also, probably because bacteria are driven into the sinus cavities under pressure. Similarly it can be caused by the pressure that occurs during air travel. People who are bothered by sinus trouble should not fly when they have an upper respiratory infection. Many people find it helpful to use a vasoconstrictor just before take-off and again before descending.

Headaches that seem to recur every morning can be caused by sinus infection or nasal allergy. Nasal discharge that has accumulated during the night is prevented from draining into the nose by the swollen sinus openings, and the pressure from the accumulated discharge causes the headache.

The kind of headache or pain one has depends upon which of the four sinuses is infected. If the frontal sinuses are involved, the headache can be very painful, sometimes with a throbbing feeling over the eyebrows. If it is the cheek sinuses, the pain may be over the cheekbones or around the eyes.

The pain of sinusitis tends to be unilateral or at least worse on one side. It is often increased in severity by leaning forward or when you jar your body by a sudden movement. If you press your finger over the sinus or under the roof of the eye and press upward, it often produces tenderness or pain.

Sometimes during a sinus attack people lose their sense of smell. You may or may not have other symptoms such as nasal congestion, fever, malaise and muscular aches. Sometimes there is swelling of the skin over the involved sinus. Sometimes what seems like a toothache is caused by sinus trouble.

Treatment of sinus trouble is aimed at eliminating the infection or allergy, restoring ventilation and adequate drainage, and providing symptomatic relief.

Antibiotic agents are often used to control the infection. Drainage and ventilation are obtained with vasoconstrictive drugs, often administered in a flushing-out procedure by the doctor. Other times a nasal spray is used. Antihistamines are helpful. Analgesic drugs are helpful in controlling pain.

It also helps to drink a large amount of liquid, to apply heat and to use steam from a vaporizer. During the acute phase, bed rest is usually recommended. After the acute stage passes, your doctor may continue treatment until he feels the infection is under control, irrigating the sinus cavities with a warm salt solution, sometimes with a vasoconstrictive drug, an antihistamine or an antibiotic.

Sometimes surgery is needed, but not very often. It is a relatively minor procedure when used. Sometimes the doctor may have to puncture an opening in the floor of the sinus. Sometimes he needs to remove polyps or to remove some structural impediment that is interfering with good drainage.

Whenever a diagnosis of sinusitis is made and the patient is subject to frequent episodes, allergic factors must be seriously considered as a cause, and careful and intensive study by a competent allergist of the patient should be a *must*. To proceed otherwise on a makeshift basis is a gross error and an injustice to the patient.

If the disease is allergic, a search needs to be made for the offending substance or substances, so that the basic cause of the sinus trouble can be removed.

■ SEROUS OTITIS MEDIA

An achy ear or one that is congested or seeping with infection can often be caused by allergy. This condition is common in infants and children (see page 28), but it also frequently occurs in adults. The attacks can be acute or chronic or intermittent.

It quite frequently happens that the ear problem coexists with an upper respiratory tract allergy, so that the patient will have hay-fever symptoms at the same time he has his ear problem. Any time a person has frequent ear problems and any other signs or symptoms of allergy, the allergy should also be suspected as the basis of the ear problems.

Symptoms usually appear suddenly. One day the patient hears well, and the next day he doesn't. There is also usually a history of recurrent earaches or diminished hearing following colds. The voices may echo in the ear or sound as though you were talking into a well or a barrel, or your ears may feel as they do when you get off an airplane or have been swimming. Sometimes you may even hear or feel fluid moving in the ear when you change your position, or your ear or head may feel full, heavy, blocked or congested.

Because the hearing is often affected, people, especially young children, are often labeled as inattentive, stubborn, or disobedient when actually they are having difficulty hearing and understanding. Hearing tests should always be performed when there is a suspicion that this might be true.

When patients fail to respond to treatment initially, or they respond for only a short time to antibiotics, then soon after have other flare-ups of the condition, chances are an allergy is the underlying cause.

In one large study of more than 500 patients with secretory otitis media, Dr. John McGovern found that 96 percent of those who had a flare-up of otitis also had nasal symptoms such as nasal itching, sneezing, stuffiness or a runny nose. "Allergic mechanisms are frequently overlooked in otitis media," says Dr. McGovern. "Allergy is often the major cause in chronic cases."

It is believed that what happens in allergic-based ear problems is that the tissues become swollen as an allergic reaction, only in this case the tissue swelling leads to obstruction of the eustachian tube (a canal connecting the ear to the nose), which prevents drainage of secretions from the middle ear and prevents air from passing through the tube and thus equalizing pressures. Another factor is that in allergy-prone children or adults who have many upper respiratory infections there is an extension of the infection from the nose and throat to the eustachian tube and thus into the middle ear.

If you have this problem, it is often helpful to chew gum frequently to stretch the eustachian tube. This lets in a little air and often helps reduce the pain and permits fluid to drain out.

If the ear problem is being caused by allergy, then treatment consists of avoiding the cause, whatever it is in the environment, and having a complete allergic diagnostic survey. Medication and hyposensitization will produce excellent results in about one out of four people, almost eliminating attacks, and in nearly all others will produce good results, with a considerable reduction of the attacks.

There can be other causes of the condition also. And for these, some beneficial effect has been reported with tonsillectomy and adenoidectomy, with radiation treatments, and with drainage of the fluid through a catheter. But many times these techniques fail, and in these cases it might be wise to again think in terms of hidden allergies that might not have been detected previously.

■ CHRONIC PNEUMONIA

There are several types of pneumonitis or pneumonia that can be due to allergy. One physician reported on five patients at a medical meeting, all of whom had pneumonia with shortness of breath, high fever, weight loss, pockets of fluid in the lung and the typical x-ray appearance of inflammation. All five were severely ill, and some appeared close to death when hospitalized. Treatment with antibiotics brought no response; x-ray findings became increasingly severe. Finally the pneumonia was treated as an allergy, and the patients were given corticosteroids. Within forty-eight hours there was improvement, and within a week the x-rays were clear and the patients were well.

Occasionally the patients had recurrences with x-ray patterns of the exact size, shape and location as in the initial episode of pneumonia, suggesting that parts of the lungs may become particularly sensitized.

Diagnosis of allergic pneumonia may be made by lung biopsy. It should be suspected any time a patient has asthmalike symptoms at the same time he has pneumonia symptoms, and if the disease becomes progressively worse despite antimicrobial treatment. In these cases steroid therapy should be tried.

One type of pneumonialike lung disease caused by allergy is pigeon breeders' disease. Persons who have this illness suffer from fever, chills, coughs, pain in the joints and general malaise, as well as inflammation of the lungs, whenever they go near pigeons or their lofts.

It is an occupational problem similar to other allergic lung diseases caused by inhaled organic dust. Others include farmers' lung, bagassosis (resulting from inhaled dry sugarcane fibers), mushroom pickers' disease, maple bark strippers' disease, and snuff takers' disease.

One case has been reported of a six-year-old city boy who lived near a market where live chickens were sold. He had recurrent pneumonitis and was admitted to the hospital with fever, cough, dizziness and sinus infection. While he was in the hospital, his symptoms cleared. But within a few hours after he returned home, his temperature rose and his respiratory difficulty began again, so he had to be hospitalized a second time. Despite a severe pneumonitis, again no bacteria were recovered from his nose or throat or lungs. He was treated for two and a half weeks in the hospital and returned home again. The very next day the problem started all over again. Despite the fact that the child lived in the city, the doctor thought his disease seemed similar to pigeon breeders' disease. Upon investigation he discovered the boy's home was only 200 yards from the live-chicken market. When he told the family to keep the child away from the chicken market, all symptoms disappeared and he remained well.

Another case has been reported where a person living in the city had the same pneumonialike symptoms from parakeet droppings.

■ DIZZINESS

Dizziness or ringing of the ears is fairly frequently due to allergies. This can occur when the labyrinths of the inner ear are affected causing dizziness, difficulty in hearing or sometimes even nausea. Many doctors have reported cases such as this due to various food allergies.

Dr. William H. Wilson, of Denver, says that upper respiratory allergic symptoms do not always occur at the same time as the allergy-caused dizziness. However, flatulence and abdominal bloating do often occur. Wheat ranks high on the list of common food offenders in people suffering from labyrinthine dysfunction, he says, as do coffee and milk. In fact, Wilson says, any frequently used food requires investigation, especially if the history suggests a craving for that food.

There is a disease called Mènière's syndrome, characterized by severe dizziness and nausea, that may occur in frequent completely debilitating attacks. Sometimes surgery helps, sometimes nothing does. A doctor suffering from the condition himself, Dr. Fred W. Wittich, of Minneapolis, Minnesota, found he could treat the condition successfully by giving himself repeated injections of histamine during an attack. The histamine reduces the increased volume of fluid in the inner ear which causes the dizziness.

■ ALLERGIC COUGH

There is nothing rare about a cough caused by allergy.

The allergic cough is often unproductive and is very intense, with chains of paroxysms that may last for minutes or for days. There is often scratching or itching deep in the throat also, as well as some degrees of hoarseness. The cough is usually a noisy hoarse barking one, in some instances almost doglike, and it often occurs in sudden spurts of increasingly severe attacks. Some patients have wheezing with the cough, some do not. Patients usually have a general appearance of good health despite the severe cough, but it can lead to more serious troubles, so should be treated.

There can be other causes for a cough, too, of course, as we discussed in the chapter on emphysema.

Nighttime coughing is often due to allergy. Try dust-proofing the bedroom or using a humidifier at bedtime.

When a cough is established as being due to allergy, one can expect to obtain an excellent response by the institution of competent allergic management. Results are the most dramatic when the allergen can be avoided. Sometimes it's as simple as getting rid of the family cat, or dog and the cough clears up.

However, usually there are several causes, and not so easily gotten rid of. In these cases, injection treatment should be tried for two to three years for best results.

Menthol preparations for rubbing in the chest or vaporizing not only don't help much, but sometimes may cause a worsening of the cough. Even treatment with antihistamines has been disappointing. Sometimes the only palliative medication that seems helpful is administration of steroids, despite their side effects.

Patients with an allergic cough, of course, would do well not to smoke.

■ ALLERGIC CONVULSIONS

It was not too long ago that the occurrence of convulsive seizures in allergic disease was considered coincidental. Now allergists have learned that allergic reactions can occur in the brain just as they can in other parts of the body, and one symptom that can be produced is a seizure.

Over the years physicians who have been suspicious of allergy as a possible cause of convulsions have reported cases of epilepsy connected with milk allergy, other food allergies, pollen allergy and allergy to cat dander.

Further definitive work was done by studying the brain-wave patterns of allergic children. It was found that there was an abnormally high percentage of irregular brain waves in allergic children, and sometimes marked changes in the brain-wave patterns appeared during acute attacks of asthma. Then other researchers studying epileptic children found that some of the children were allergic. When they kept them away from what they were allergic to, they no longer had convulsions.

There are many factors that can cause epilepsy, but allergy as a causative factor is one that is often ignored and should be considered and thoroughly investigated in any patient.

One doctor reported on a housewife who had epilepsylike attacks. She was sick nearly all her life with wheezing, headaches, blackouts, staggering gait and depression, and she had muscle and joint pain so bad that she had to be helped from chairs. She frequently spent months confined to her bed. The only time she seemed well was when she was outside, which her friends and relatives attributed to the beneficial effects of sunshine and air. She had several attacks in her kitchen that her family doctor diagnosed as epilepsy, but after years of suffering it was determined that she was allergic to the gas in gas stoves and gas furnaces.

Drs. Bernard T. Fein and Peter B. Kamin, of San Antonio, Texas, studied eighteen patients who had both allergies and convulsive disorders. Of these, nine had either petit mal or grand mal seizures, five had convulsions from fever, and others had convulsions from some unknown cause. When skin tests for allergy were performed, the patients were shown to be allergic to such things as ragweed, tree pollen, grass pollen, weed pollen, milk, chocolate, eggs, citrus fruits, pecan, house dust and molds. Treating the allergies helped some of the patients, but not all of them.

■ HEART ATTACKS

Attacks of upset in heart rhythm can often be due to allergy. Dr. Joseph Harkavy, of Mount Sinai and Montefiore Hospitals, New York, studied and reported on several patients who had irregular heartbeats caused by hypersensitivity to various foods, inhaled matter or bacterial substances.

The arrhythmias included extra heartbeats, excessively rapid heartbeats and an uncontrolled writhing of the heart muscle called fibrillation. All of the patients had had several attacks, and sometimes they were associated with other symptoms such as asthma, diarrhea, hives or skin rash. Some had the attacks during hayfever or after eating specific foods.

Repetitive exposure to the offending agents would induce an attack, Dr. Harkavy said, and the attacks were controlled by having the patients avoid what they were allergic to and also by giving them desensitization injections. Treatment of specific attacks was effective with the use of antiallergic medication in combination with other drugs.

"In view of these findings," Dr. Harkavy said, "it would seem advisable that patients with normal hearts who manifest arrhythmia of unknown origin be investigated from the point of view of hypersensitivity."

Allergies can also cause an allergic reaction of the blood vessels. Usually the changes produced are temporary and easily reversible, but sometimes they are more persistent, and permanent damage is done to the veins and arteries and capillaries. If the condition persists without treatment, then further damage is done—for example, to the kidneys, as the blood vessels deteriorate.

Often associated with allergic reactions of the circulatory system are such things as asthma, involvement of the joints, kidney problems and skin rashes, especially with purple patches.

This condition is very serious, and treatment should be tended to without procrastination. Most patients require fairly large doses of corticosteroid drugs, and, of course, the primary cause should be found and eliminated.

■ CATARACTS

Cataracts are usually due to some different causes than allergy, but research indicates that when cataracts occur during early adulthood, especially in the thirties, they are often closely associated with allergies, especially with dermatitis. The reason for the relationship is not known.

Other allergies of the eyes can occur also. There are, of course, the usual redness and itching of hayfever that every allergic person is familiar with, but there can also be reactions of the eyelids, of the outer scleral coverings of the eyes, of the inner pigmented areas of the eyes and even of the lens itself and the optic nerves.

■ DROWSINESS

Allergy, by affecting the central nervous system, can also cause extreme drowsiness and sleepiness. One man walked around in a daze, constantly falling asleep in the middle of the day during the two months of ragweed hayfever season. This went on every year for eleven years. He had no usual symptoms of hayfever, but when tested for allergy to ragweed, he was strongly positive. When he was treated with injections of ragweed pollen extract, his symptoms promptly disappeared.

■ CANKER SORES

Many strange reactions can occur in the mouth. Dental plates can cause an allergic reaction from contact sensitization as well as irritation from simple mechanical pressure. There can be swelling of the lips from sunlight or inflammation due to allergy. Some of the most common and recurrent troublesome things are fever blisters and canker sores. These sores are due to infections with a virus called herpes simplex, that causes the sores when the general resistance is low, when there is systemic infection, when the membrane of the mouth is injured, or when patients eat something they are allergic to. Some patients get them because viruses and fungi grow in the mouth when normal bacteria have been killed by an antibiotic taken for one reason or another.

Chapter **14**

PHYSICAL ALLERGIES: COLD, HEAT AND LIGHT

Strange as it may seem, there can be allergic reactions to purely physical things such as heat, cold, light, injury and mechanical irritation. Despite the fact that the first case of hives due to cold was described a hundred years ago, we still do not understand how these physical things can really cause allergy, but they do.

It is not yet known whether the physical agents themselves act as specific exciting factors or whether they work through some other secondary system to set up an antigen-antibody reaction to precipitate the allergic attack. One theory is that the physical agents act on the skin, altering tissue proteins in such a way that the proteins then act as antigens to cause the allergic reaction. Another theory is that there is some substance present in all human tissues that is liberated with exposure to the physical agent, but which produces allergic reaction only in susceptible persons who are hypersensitive to this substance.

Allergic reactions to physical agents can be contact reactions where the allergic response occurs directly in the tissue exposed to the physical agent. Or they can be reflex reactions where the response is not in the tissue exposed to the physical agent, but in other tissues in another part of the body. Or the reaction may be generalized with symptoms occurring over the entire body.

The most common responses in physical allergy are diffuse itching or hives, but there also may be eczema, hayfever, asthma, purpura, gastrointestinal symptoms, dizziness or blood in the urine. Some people will develop hayfever or asthma symptoms in a very hot room or very cold room or with a sudden change in temperature.

■ HYPERSENSITIVITY TO COLD

The most common form of cold allergy is hives. In some people the tendency to get hives when exposed to cold temperatures runs in families and is transmitted by heredity from one generation to another. The other form of cold allergy is acquired and has no relationship to heredity.

In one family studied, 23 out of 47 of the relatives were affected with allergy to cold. The inherited type reactions are often noticed in the newborn infants right in the delivery room and almost always occur within the first four months of life.

There is some controversy over whether the inherited type of hives due to cold are allergic. But the later acquired type is definitely allergic. Signs and symptoms differ somewhat. The hives produced from the inherited type of cold reaction have a burning or smarting sensation, while the hives produced by the acquired disease are itchy. People with the inherited kind of reaction also usually have chills, fever, aching joints and headaches with their reaction. Usually the onset of noninherited cold allergy is sudden and unexplained. It can appear at any age and without any apparent reason.

Reactions vary a great deal even within the same person. Sometimes extreme cold is not necessary to bring about the reaction, only a slight chilling, and the length of exposure needed can vary from a few seconds to several minutes.

The hives generally occur in the area that is exposed to the cold where there are no protecting clothes, but if a person is very sensitive there can be a generalized reaction of the body. Sometimes if the person swims in cold water or takes a cold shower, his body becomes completely covered with hives and he may even show signs of going into shock. There is great danger in these people of death from drowning because they can have this generalized reaction when swimming in cold water.

In one study, patients who had hypersensitivity to cold were told to immerse their hands in very cold water for three to six minutes. Their hands became pale in the water, then when they took them out, they became red, swollen and hot. In a few minutes blood pressure dropped, their pulse skyrocketed rapidly, and they became very dizzy. It took about ten to fifteen minutes for them to recover.

Allergy to cold may be treated rather successfully in three or four weeks by gradually exposing the body to cold by immersion in cold water. This gradually builds up resistance to the cold.

Antihistamines can also help in controlling and treating the condition.

■ HYPERSENSITIVITY TO HEAT

Allergic responses to heat, just like allergic responses to cold, can be local with hives appearing only on the exposed areas of the skin, or they can be general with hives appearing all over the body.

In addition to hives there may be asthma, migraine headache, dizziness, irregular heartbeat or rapid pulse produced by the reaction to heat. Sometimes there are also systemic reactions at the same time, such as abdominal cramps, diarrhea, faintness, sweating, flushing and salivation. Sometimes the person collapses.

The reaction can be brought on by external heat or by body heat from physical exertion, effort and stress. It can be brought on by being in a warm room, eating hot foods on a hot day, wearing hot clothes, developing a fever, taking a hot bath, or it can be brought on by emotional stress. In very susceptible individuals, the hives can be precipitated by an increase of body temperature of less than one degree Fahrenheit.

A person can be tested for heat allergy by immersion of a hand in hot water, as in the experiment with cold water previously discussed.

It is believed that the heat reaction takes place because the warm blood stimulates the heat-regulating center of the brain of the sensitive person, and this in turn stimulates the parasympathetic nervous system (the one that controls your automatic body function). Then a chemical is released and reacts with the skin of the hypersensitive person to produce the hives.

Antihistamines are helpful to relieve the symptoms, and the attacks can also be diminished by applying cold water or ice water to the hands and arms as soon as possible during the attack.

The heat-allergic person can be desensitized much as the cold-allergic person by careful, gradual exposure to increasing amounts of heat with hot baths.

■ HYPERSENSITIVITY TO LIGHT

Some people are sensitive to light. Their skin becomes intensely inflamed from sunlight even at low exposure levels that would produce no reaction at all on a normal skin. Even slight exposure in them may cause hives and other skin disorders. Sometimes there are the little reddish purple hemorrhages in the skin called purpura and other lesions that simulate more serious diseases.

There can also be eruptions of eczema, as well as redness or itching pimples and papules. Eruptions usually appear on the face, ears, neck, hands or upper surfaces of the arms. There also may be mild or severe swelling.

When there is eczema, there is often oozing and crusting and thickening, and then a flaking off of skin. Sometimes there are red pimples all over the nose, cheeks and other parts of the face and neck. This form of reaction occurs most often in men. Sometimes there are plaquelike lesions that are pink and scaly. A person may have any one of these symptoms or a combination of them at the same time.

In severe allergy to sunlight, the typical reaction is that after brief exposure to intense sunlight, large red wheals appear on the exposed areas. Then if the exposure is prolonged, hives appear all over the body and there is swelling. The patient becomes dizzy, and shock often occurs. The attacks may last from several hours to two days.

Sometimes the allergy may appear suddenly, may last for several years and then disappear. At other times the allergy persists throughout life. There is very rarely any improvement in sensitivity in those who are allergic to visible light only, but spontaneous improvement does sometimes occur in those sensitive to ultraviolet light. The attacks occur three times more often in women than in men.

Most allergic light sensitivity is in the ultraviolet range of light rays—that is, between 2,900 and 3,900 angstroms.

Some patients who are very sensitive are also sensitive to the ultraviolet light coming from fluorescent light fixtures. The radiation does not usually escape because of the fluorescent coating in the glass wall of the tube, but the blue light itself may cause a reaction.

Hypersensitivity to light also occurs when a light-absorbing substance causes a specific photochemical reaction. This can result from various dyes, cosmetics and drugs, as discussed in previous chapters. It can occur whether the photosensitivity-producing substance is applied to the skin or taken in pill form.

Skin lesions due to the sun are often misdiagnosed, and sun and light allergy is probably much more common than is generally reported.

One important point to remember is that the sun's rays that produce the photosensitivity are not filtered out by glass; therefore you can develop a reaction while sitting in the window light of your home or office.

The best way to treat allergy to sunlight is to avoid exposure to it. If it is a photosensitizing drug that is causing the problem, extra precautions must be taken to stay out of the sun, and if necessary the photosensitizing substance can be eliminated.

The use of chemical sunscreens helps in prevention. Dermatologists have found that two preparations are much better than others and longer lasting. They are PABA (para-aminobenzoic acid) and Escalol. But they must be in an alcohol solution. These preparations have been on the market for years, but not in alcohol solution. The researchers found after studying commercial preparations over three years that the PABA in a 5 percent ethyl alcohol solution and the Escalol in a 2.5 percent alcohol solution protected even fair-skinned people, offered protection after sweating, and remained on the skin after bathing or swimming.

Antihistamines, antimalarial drugs and hormones have also been reported of some value. Desensitization by gradual increases in the amount of ultraviolet light has on several occasions worked.

■ HYPERSENSITIVITY TO MECHANICAL IRRITATION

Probably the most common physical allergy is dermographia. If you stroke the skin with a fingernail or other mechanical stimulus in people who have this condition, you will get a raised line. It isn't the usual white line that most people get, but it raises in typical allergic-type wheals surrounded by red flares on the skin. Generally the response is immediate; sometimes a delayed response occurs three to six hours after the original trauma and disappears slowly.

This is different from the normal red, raised, inflamed site a person gets when lashed with a stick or other violent injury. The hypersensitive person has redness and itching (rather than pain) from a mild stimulus, a stimulus that to the rest of us would be a normal mild sensation, nothing unusual.

Pressure urticaria is similar; in fact, it is probably a type of dermographia. It occurs in areas that receive constant pressure, such as the buttocks, which are sat upon, or the soles of the feet, which are walked upon, and in other areas where clothing might constrict the skin. It develops usually after a latent period of several hours or even a day.

Aside from hives, mechanical stimulation can cause an irritation of the skin similar to a contact dermatitis; or it may cause eczema, scaling or other skin reactions.

If the person rubs or scratches at the area it may, of course, compound the trouble.

Antihistamines have been successful in suppressing some symptoms of allergy from mechanical irritation. Some people need to have continuing antihistamine therapy; others simply take the tablets when occasion demands. Local areas may be temporarily desensitized by continued mechanical irritation, such as stroking of the skin with a stiff hairbrush several times a day to diminish the intensity of reactions.

Chapter **15**

GOING TO THE DOCTOR

First, how do you go about finding a competent allergist?

If you have faith in a physician that you are at present going to and you feel you need an allergist, discuss it with him. He will be happy to recommend one in your area to you. If you have moved into a city recently and have not yet made contact with a family physician, you may call your local county medical society to find an allergist with offices near you. Simply look in the telephone book under "Blank" County Medical Society.

Some doctors are full-time allergists specializing in allergy and treating only allergy patients. Other doctors specialize in internal medicine with a subspecialty of allergy, and so devote only part of their time to allergy. In either event the men who really know something of allergy will be members of either the American College of Allergists or the American Academy of Allergy—these are the two national allergy societies of standing. You can check this out with any physician simply by asking him, or you can call or write the American Medical Association at 535 North Dearborn St., Chicago, Illinois.

They will give information on any physician concerning his education, specialty, academic appointments and membership in professional societies.

You may be going to a doctor for the first time for your allergy, or you may have had a series of frustrating encounters with many physicians and with many bewildering suggestions and remedies and may be beginning to doubt the effectiveness of modern medical science.

Whatever your experience, keep in mind that the allergist is not God, but neither is allergy an uncontrollable or mysterious disease. It can be checked. You can be helped.

The road leading to successful treatment of an allergic patient is not always straight, smooth or even clearly marked, but if you go to a competent allergist, he has a variety of tools at his disposal that can usually guide you along the best route to a successful result.

When you visit the allergist on your first trip, go with as much specific and objective information as you can. Be ready to tell him exactly what your symptoms are, precisely where they occur and when, what time of day or what time of year, whether they seem to occur after any special event, or are worse at any particular times.

If your allergy just began, try to figure out if the beginning coincided with anything specific, such as starting a new job or using new materials on the job. Determine whether the reaction occurs on a day off or on a working day. The day of the week is important. Monday usually means you've been handling soap for washing. On Fridays you may be eating fish or preparing it.

The season is important too. For example, a dermatitis in the summer might have something to do with plants, gardening, handling of certain foods or flowers in season, summer sports activities, special summer clothes. You might have a rash on your hands from a golf club, or you might have a shoe leather dermatitis in the summer because your socks are thinner then.

If you think foods might be part of your trouble, make a list of the foods you suspect and another list of the foods you dislike. It sometimes helps to run through a list of foods and check those you eat often and those you eat occasionally. Refer to our lists in the back of the book and in the chapter on food.

If your doctor is not sure whether you have allergy or not, but he is suspicious that you do, he may use a diagnostic aid called an Allergic Index. It is a simple list of the major symptoms and contributory factors of allergy, with each of the symptoms and factors being given a numerical value reflecting its relative importance in the total picture. By checking through it, your doctor can determine whether a complete diagnostic allergy work-up is in order.

ALLERGIC INDEX

Symptoms	*Unit Weight*
Heredity	
Bilateral inheritance	2
Unilateral inheritance	1
Bronchial asthma	5
Colic	1
Chronic gastroenteritis of allergic cause	1
Infantile allergic dermatitis	3
Tonsillectomy and adenoidectomy twice or more	3
Pollinosis	
One season	2
Two or more seasons	3
Recurrent upper respiratory infections	1
If associated with perennial allergic rhinitis or seasonal repetition	2
Perennial allergic rhinitis	2
Chronic allergic cough	2
Intermittent hearing loss	1
Allergic eye irritation	1
Recurrent croup	1
Bronchiolitis, two or more episodes	1
Paroxysmal sneezing	1
Hives	1
Chronic clearing of throat	½
Visceral pain, including spasms of intestines	½
Drug allergy	½
Migraine	½
Recurrent nosebleeds	½
Canker sores	½

When the "unit weight" of symptoms totals 5 or more units, experience has indicated that the patient should undergo an allergic investigation. Any of these symptoms, even though given a relatively low unit value in the Allergic Index, may indicate a significant allergy requiring treatment if it manifests itself to a severe degree or if it tends to recur frequently.

Your physician must have a thorough clinical history of your past illnesses and problems. Your allergy has been writing its own story, but it is up to the examining physician to read, translate and interpret it. Besides a complete and detailed picture of your environment and daily routine, the doctor will want the full story of any symptoms that you have, whether they seem to relate to the allergy or not.

If you have a notebook with your medical history in it, take this with you.

Tell your doctor on the first visit whether any other doctors have done allergy tests on you, or whether you have received any previous treatment. Tell him if you are receiving any medications for other disorders.

Also in the interview the doctor will want to do some psychological evaluation to determine any emotional factors that may be affecting your allergy.

Don't be offended by the number of questions the doctor asks you or the time it takes. Remember tracking down the cause of an allergy is a matter of sifting many bits of evidence to uncover the triggering factor, and the success in your particular case may depend on just how skillful your doctor is in questioning you and interpreting your answers. Tell him everything, even the smallest, remotest details, and do not hesitate to offer your own observations no matter how silly you think them to be or how embarrassed you are in mentioning them. It's amazing how often these seemingly silly or irrelevant questions and statements contain information that gives the key to a vital aspect of the case.

A rectal itch may be a clue that a food may be causing the allergy. If a child continually stuffs objects in his nose he could be suffering from an airborne allergy that attacks his nasal passages.

In no other branch of medicine is the painstaking search for clues more important. You never know what clue is going to bring the whole picture together.

Dr. Constantine Falliers, Denver allergist, writes in *Hospital Practice* of the importance of these first interviews between the allergist and the patient. He recommends that a patient list what he thinks brings on attacks, emphasizing what he has noticed, as well as what he has heard from others. Details should be brought out, such as the time interval between events and the attack, and specific examples should be discussed, such as damp weather or an argument. Then the doctor can present an additional list of possible precipitating factors, and the patient can indicate which, if any, apply. The list might include such things as chest colds, overexertion, weather, excitement, emotional reactions, worry, anger, sadness, laughing, crying, hard breathing, coughing, pollens, dust, animals, foods and drugs. After the list is obtained of what factors might be affecting him, the patient is asked to rank the triggering factors in order of their importance in causing his symptoms. Then he tries to estimate the frequency with which a given triggering factor is tied to the onset of the attacks and the severity of attacks caused.

You have to learn to be an astute observer.

When you go to the doctor, besides asking you seemingly hundreds of questions, he'll also give you a physical examination, will do lung function studies if indicated and will do several laboratory tests. Sometimes the examination is relatively simple; other times there may have to be extensive tests including electrocardiograms, thyroid tests, blood tests, x-rays, breathing tests and other things.

The examination, of course, will partly depend on your case and your symptoms. If you have respiratory symptoms, the doctor is going to be looking into your nose and throat and listening to your lungs. If you have a contact dermatitis of the big toe, he's going to spend more time looking at your big toe.

Sometimes the doctor's job is harder than it should be—patients withhold information. One allergist tells the story of a bride who used an allergy to asparagus as a way to avoid entertaining her mother-in-law. She hated her, and so each time the mother-in-law was due for a visit the bride secretly ate some asparagus and brought on an asthma attack. For years her mother-in-law was blamed for the attacks until the girl finally confessed.

Another case is told of a patient purposefully using an allergy. One of the actors in *Oh, Calcutta!* found a way to upstage the other actors in the nude scenes. Before the performance each night he ate a food he was allergic to so his would be the only body on stage with a rash.

Your doctor must do a thorough physical examination because there may be things causing your symptoms other than allergy. Wheezing can be caused by lung cancer or heart trouble, as well as by asthma. Severe abdominal distention can be due to eating certain foods, but it could also be due to an intestinal obstruction. Itching could be due to allergy, but it could also be due to diabetes, leukemia, liver disease, scabies or fungal infection. A decrease in the red cell count could mean an anemia due to allergy or another cause.

Say you go to the doctor for a cough and you suspect it's an allergic one. You'll tell him why you're there, what your problem is. You'll answer whatever questions he asks, and you'll offer any thought you have about possible related circumstances and causes. He'll ask you some obvious questions like how many cigarettes you smoke, and he'll check more subtle causes like possible allergy to pollens, grasses, animal dander, etc.

He'll check to see if you are exposed to dust or gases from air pollution or chemicals on your job that might be causing the cough. He'll ask you about wheezing or feeling of a heavy chest or whether you get short-winded easily. He will do some skin tests. He'll look in your ears to find if there's any excess wax or other odd things like beans or bugs that could be setting up a cough reflex. He'll look in your nose and throat to see if any allergies or sinus trouble or infections might be causing a dripping down the back of your throat.

He'll look at the mucous membrane inside the nose to see if it is swollen and pale and boggy, which strongly suggests that you have nasal allergy. He'll look in your throat to see if any little bumps of tissue might be causing irritation. He'll look at your larynx (the voice box in your throat), where he might find a cyst or other growth causing the problem. He'll look for irritation along your windpipe that might cause a dry hacking cough. He'll check for inflammation due to influenza or a cold and will take your temperature for a sign of low-grade fever. He may have your chest x-rayed for telltale signs of tuberculosis, cancer, pneumonia, sacs of infection or swallowed objects. One woman had lost a pin into her lungs after holding pins in her mouth while sewing. He'll listen for fluid accumulation. As another check for lung cancer he'll look at a sample of your saliva under the microscope for malignant cells and will look into your lungs with a bronchoscope.

He'll check your heart, since some types of heart failure or abnormal heart rhythm can cause coughing. He'll investigate the possibility of its being a psychogenic cough, since some people start coughing because of excitement, fright, embarrassment or self-consciousness or apparently for no reason at all.

There are also many little signs that the alert physician will notice as he is examining you. He may see a rash, or evidence of scratching, or the allergic salute, or the nasal fold or wrinkle across the bridge of the nose that often is evidence of your having allergically "saluted" for years. Or he may notice that you breathe through your mouth or repeatedly clear your throat or have dry lips or have red eyes or are short-winded.

He may notice that you have some particular nervous habit. One woman used to run her hand through her hair all the time. A rash she had between the third and fourth fingers of her right hand proved to be a reaction to her hairsetting fluid.

If you have a skin allergy, he will study the appearance of the rash to give him clues to the cause. If a rash is dry and hard, it usually means it is a chronic reaction and would indicate some constant occupational contact or some item of clothing that is worn repeatedly. A very irritated and swollen rash, on the other hand, suggests a single contact rather than a repeated one. Clear-cut stripes suggest a reaction to adhesive tape; widely separated bumps suggest a reaction to pollen or bits of chemicals. If the rash does not go into the folds of the skin, the lesions are probably due to a solid agent. If the rash is in the folds, then it is probably caused by a liquid.

He may after this first visit tell you to try something straightforward like giving up cigarette smoking or installing a humidifier in your house to correct dry winter air that often causes coughing. Or he may want you to come back for more diagnostic tests or for treatment with desensitization injections.

■ SKIN TESTS

There are several skin tests the doctor can use to find what you are sensitive to. The scratch test is the one most often used and the safest.

Usually many tests are done at one time, with the doctor making the scratches in the skin by pressing a scalpel lightly onto the skin; then extracts—dry powders of solution—of suspected substances are rubbed into the scratches. Sometimes as many as twenty-five or fifty substances are tested, with the scratches an inch apart.

The extracts to be tested are taken from tiny tubes and gently rubbed in the scratches, usually with a sterile toothpick. A separate test substance is used for each site.

The reactions usually appear in sensitive individuals within about ten minutes with redness, itching and hives. The reactions increase for about fifteen to thirty minutes and then slowly subside. Two scratches are made and no allergen is rubbed in, so that they can be used as controls to compare the other reactions with.

It is considered a positive reaction if a mosquito-bitelike hive is produced that is at least one-fourth inch in diameter or larger, or if it is surrounded by a large area of redness. The doctor scores each reaction if positive as one to four plus, according to the size of the positive reaction.

Sometimes delayed reactions take place, and a red itchy area or wheal develops twenty-four hours or so later, but usually it appears within ten to fifteen minutes.

A similar test based on the same principle is the intradermal test in which a diluted extract of the allergen is actually injected into the middle layers of the skin. This test is used if the scratch test with the same substance is negative, but it is still suspected.

A third method is the eye test, used if the scratch tests are negative. A small amount of dry pollen or other allergen or a solution of it is dropped into one eye. If the eye reddens and waters, the test is positive. However, this test is not nearly as accurate, and only one allergen can be tested at a time, while with the skin tests a whole series can be done at one visit.

Another method that is used even less frequently is the passive transfer test. This is indirect testing. The serum from a blood sample of the allergic person is injected into several areas of the skin of a volunteer. Then forty-eight hours later the volunteer is given an intradermal test at the same site. This test is used as a double check when the doctor suspects that a patient is allergic to something, but it doesn't test positively using a standard skin test. It can also be used when there is a skin disorder or other illness that would make the skin test inconclusive or when other special conditions prevent direct testing.

Patch tests are done when one is trying to find out what is causing a contact dermatitis. The suspected material—either in its natural form, in a diluted form or in a laboratory-prepared extract—is placed on a small patch of gauze and is fastened to the skin with adhesive tape. This is examined one to three days later. If redness, swelling or blistering occurs, it indicates a positive reaction.

Skin testing may be performed successfully at any age. The skin reactions of younger children tend to be a little smaller than those of older children and adults, and they tend to become red when the test is positive with not so much of the large hive being formed. But the reaction is strong enough so that a competent allergist can tell whether the test is positive or negative.

Most pediatric allergists feel that children should be tested by both the scratch and intradermal techniques. Since scratch tests are the simplest and safest, they should be used first. Then the child can be

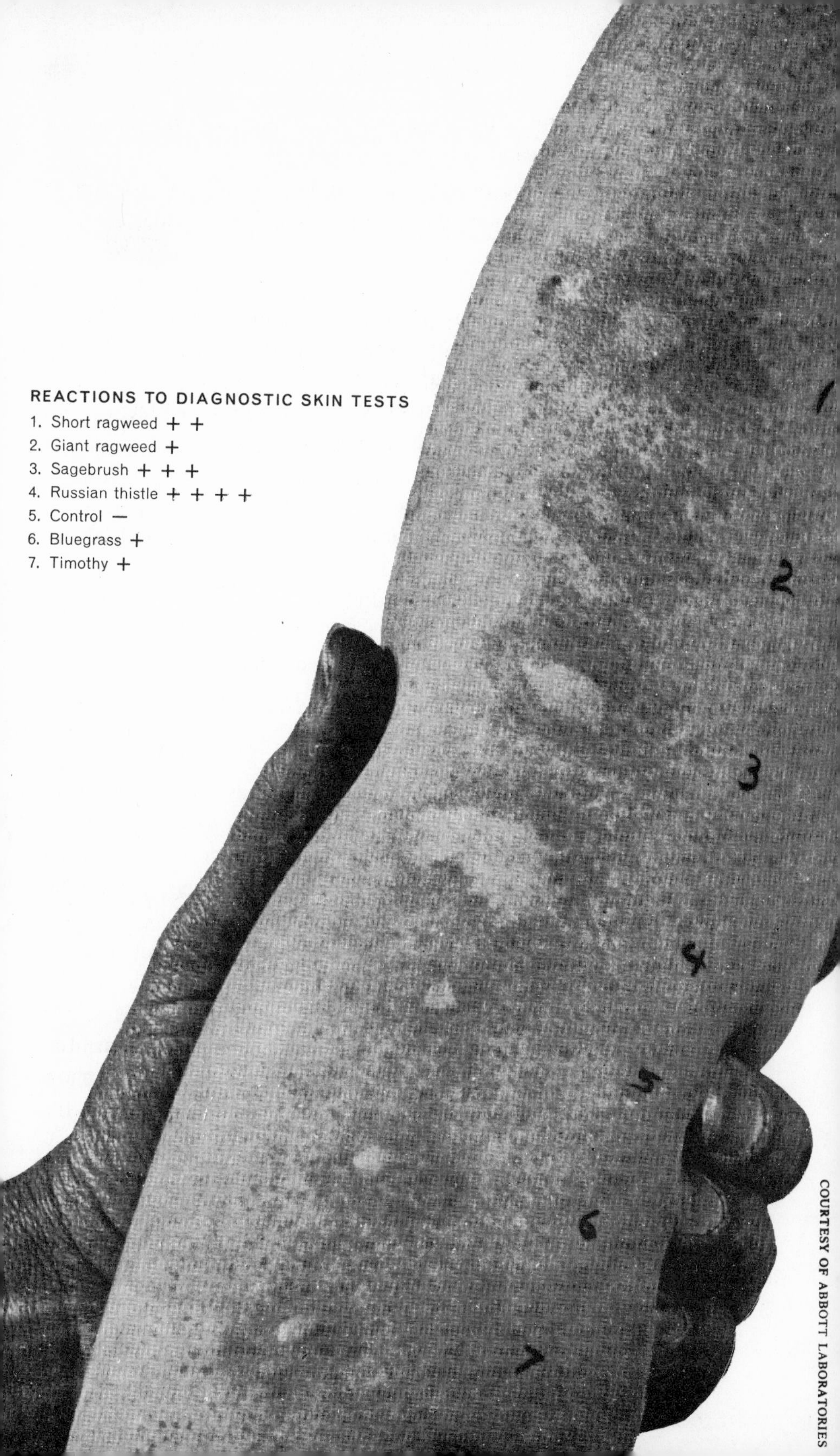

REACTIONS TO DIAGNOSTIC SKIN TESTS

1. Short ragweed + +
2. Giant ragweed +
3. Sagebrush + + +
4. Russian thistle + + + +
5. Control —
6. Bluegrass +
7. Timothy +

COURTESY OF ABBOTT LABORATORIES

checked again with intradermal tests for those substances which showed a negative reaction with the scratch test.

When neither of the two skin tests shows any allergy reaction to pollens or other substances, the eye test can be used in older children or adults.

In Negroes it is sometimes difficult to see the skin test reaction because of the dark skin. Dr. Herbert Kaufman of the University of California, and Dr. Marion Sulzberger, of Letterman Hospital, have used a special instrument that detects the heat rays given off by a positive reaction. Test sites that show no visible positive reaction will still show a higher reading on the heat detector.

What do the skin tests mean and how important are they? They are not infallible. They sometimes give misleading results, but in most cases they are very helpful. They don't give the entire answer in themselves, but when correlated with the other facts from the patient's physical examination and from the history interviews, they provide invaluable evidence.

The skin tests are the most valuable and reliable in detecting airborne allergens such as pollens, dust, molds and animal danders. They are much less reliable for food and drug allergies and contact allergies.

One major problem arises when there is a positive skin test, but the patient does not have the clinical symptoms to this particular substance. Actually such positives may indicate past or future sensitivities and may prove important, especially in children, in the total management of their allergy.

Sometimes a person was allergic to a substance when he was younger and still gives a positive reaction to the test although the substance no longer bothers him. Sometimes a material that is new to a person's environment may test positively without being harmful.

Young children between about ages two and five commonly show positive tests to pollens, but do not have any symptoms during the pollen season. The majority of such children shortly develop symptoms to that particular pollen, generally within two years.

The National Jewish Hospital and Research Center in Denver reports a particularly high incidence of such "illogical" positive reactions to skin tests for house dust, strawberries, spinach and chocolate. A harmless substance may be labeled responsible for being the cause of an allergy a surprisingly great number of times, they say, and if the results are not confirmed by additional diagnostic study, patients can be given unnecessary desensitization shots or told to avoid a long list of substances, unnecessarily making their lives complicated and difficult. Some patients have come to them, they said, having been told that they were sensitive to over 400 different materials. One woman was told that she was allergic to everything but water. Obviously these patients had not consulted competent allergists.

Fortunately these cases are rare. But they do make the point that a suspected material may not be judged innocent or guilty on the basis of skin testing alone. This is why the doctor needs to learn from you as much as he can about your symptoms and the details of your attacks.

The doctor could do hundreds of skin tests to possible allergens, but this is unnecessary because of the other facts gathered. Because of the information you give him about when and where your sneezing or hives or other symptoms occur, he can narrow down the possible allergens to a smaller number. For example, if you develop hayfever symptoms at the same time each year, it is likely that they are caused by pollens or mold spores, and he will test for these. If your symptoms develop irregularly or are continuous all through the year, then a complete allergic study must be done.

■ OTHER TESTS

The doctor may need to do other tests also to study your problem. Bits of evidence can be gathered through laboratory examination of nasal smears, stool samples and blood samples. There is often an increase in the blood, for example, in the number of white cells called eosinophils when an allergy is present.

Sputum studies may show special crystals in cells present in the sputum of patients with allergic asthma that are not present in other people. In contrast, special large cells containing granules of pigment called "heart failure cells" are found in patients with congestion of the lungs due to heart failure.

X-rays can be helpful in the differential diagnosis of upper respiratory conditions. In allergic rhinitis, for example, the sinuses are usually clear or only slightly clouded. When the sinus areas are fuzzy or clouded on the x-ray it means an infection or perhaps a growth or thickened membranes.

When food allergies are suspected, elimination diets may prove useful. The patient is maintained on a diet that has been stripped of nearly anything that might cause allergy. Then slowly, one by one, the physician reintroduces suspected foods until the guilty one is discovered.

Another diagnostic technique is the provocative test. Natural full-strength substances are used to try to provoke an attack. If it is suspected that a patient is allergic to a certain food, he is fed this food to see if he reacts to it. If this test is used, the doctor must be extremely careful to avoid causing a severe reaction during the test.

Frequently tests will be made of pulmonary function—the efficiency of your breathing. The doctor may want to check if there is any interference with breathing function so he can estimate any impairment in your lung function and gauge the possibility of improvement.

He may want to test whether the amount of air you breathe increases during exercise. He may want to measure the volume of air breathed, the rate of breathing, whether you breathe deeply or shallowly.

He may have you blow out a lighted match or candle or use a special test whistle, or he may test you with fancier instruments called spirometers, pneumotachographs, body plethysmographs—all these designed to measure air flow rate, airway resistance or other factors in lung function.

Measuring the various blood gases in the arteries and veins can tell how well your lungs are working to get oxygen into the blood and carbon dioxide out.

The different kinds of records made on these tests can help him decide whether your lungs are healthy or whether you have emphysema or asthma or a tumor.

Sometimes despite thorough questioning and exhaustive testing, the elusive allergen causing the trouble cannot be found. In these cases it is sometimes necessary to hospitalize the patient to minimize the outside influences and to permit even more complete study within the controlled environment of the hospital where no strange foods or pollens or other factors can sneak in unnoticed.

■ TREATMENT

Once an accurate diagnosis is made, specific treatment to eliminate or reduce attacks can be undertaken with remarkable success. Many of the treatment failures of the past were actually due to wrong diagnoses. The real troublemaker was not being treated.

Allergic management consists of two major approaches: removing or avoiding the specific cause of the allergy, or increasing your immunity or tolerance to it. Avoiding the allergen is the best procedure whenever it's possible. This may mean getting rid of a cat or a feather pillow or a particular food, air-conditioning your home or office to filter out pollens or molds, changing occupations or changing locations. The way to increase your immunity is to have desensitization injections against what you are allergic to.

Your doctor will suggest two other things to you also: lighten your allergic burden by trying to control some of the factors that add to your allergic problem, and with various medications treat symptoms as they occur.

To lighten your allergic burden, your doctor will probably advise you to do such things as dust-proof your house, avoid exposure to pungent odors or fumes and stay out of drafts.

RELIEVING THE SYMPTOMS

Many medications are available for reducing or controlling symptoms: pills, tablets, capsules, nose drops, cough medicines, eyedrops, ointments and lotions.

They can all be helpful. But they do not cure allergy. They only control symptoms. But if your allergy is mild, this may be enough.

ANTIHISTAMINES

The most widely used allergy medicines are the antihistamines. They can be a most effective weapon, working by counteracting the histamine of the allergic reaction.

The antihistamines are most valuable in treating mild seasonal hayfever. They are helpful at putting an end to itching eyes, dripping nose and sneezing. They are particularly good also in treating skin rashes, hives, swelling and itching. But they have limitations. They are less effective in relieving nasal blockage that often occurs during and at the end of the pollen season. They occasionally produce relief in allergic bronchitis, but are of no value in preventing or treating asthma attacks. Their drying-up effect only intensifies the asthma and makes it more difficult to cough up the troublesome thickened and tenacious sputum of asthma.

In general it is safe to take antihistamine drugs. However, the drugs do have some side effects. Drugs show different side effects in different people, so you and your physician must work out the most effective drug with the least side effects in your particular situation.

The most common side effect is sedation. On the pills, you may have difficulty in concentrating or may feel extremely sleepy or dizzy. Because of the drowsiness and slowed reaction time, you should not take any antihistamine pills if you are going to drive a car or if you have a job that requires mental alertness and motor coordination. such as being a punch press operator.

Sometimes the drowsiness disappears after the antihistamine has been used for two or three days. But if it persists, try reducing the dose. If that doesn't work, try another antihistamine. Consult your allergist. It takes a bit of trial-and-error experimenting to find the best one for you.

Because of the depressive action of the drugs, if you are taking them, you should not drink alcoholic beverages or use other drugs that depress the central nervous system, since the effects would be additive. If a simple overdose of, say, two tablets instead of one is taken, the person will become extremely sleepy, unable to hold his eyes open, and usually will simply sleep off the effects for four hours. However, if a great number are taken, death can occur, so every precaution should be made to keep the medicines away from children.

Some physicians as a last resort to counteract drowsiness add a stimulant such as ephedrine or amphetamine. Beware of these mixed preparations, however. They can be dangerous to patients who have high blood pressure, heart disease, arteriosclerosis, enlarged prostate gland, glaucoma or thyroid disease.

Antihistamines have also, but not commonly, been known to produce symptoms of excitation such as insomnia, tremors, nervousness, irritability and convulsions. And the same action that produces dryness of the nose can make your mouth dry, can produce blurred vision, urinary retention, low blood pressure, fast heartbeat and impotence. In other people certain of the antihistamines may produce lack of appetite, abdominal pain, nausea, vomiting, diarrhea or constipation. If antihistamines are taken over a very long time, some blood reactions can take place. But these side effects are all rare.

Sometimes antihistamines are combined with pain-killers, corticosteroids or antibacterial agents, as well as stimulants. Many physicians do not like any of these combination pills. They prefer to carefully adjust the dosage of the individual ingredients, and they also want to make sure that sensitivity to any of the agents has not developed.

In general antihistamines should be taken orally rather than being applied as creams or ointments, even if they are for skin rashes. They tend to produce rashes when applied directly to the skin, and frequently will also produce photosensitivity.

OTHER METHODS OF TREATMENT

We have discussed most of the other methods of treatment in previous chapters. Breathing exercises, moving to a new climate, bacterial vaccines, diet, psychotherapy, can all be helpful in the right circumstances.

Cortisone drugs and ACTH are used by physicians only under special conditions such as in a prolonged attack of asthma or to tide the patient over a critical period in a severe allergy. Because serious side effects can occur, these drugs should be used only temporarily until more suitable allergic management can be begun.

The major thing to do at any time that you hear of some treatment that you have not heard of before or is not covered in this book is to consult with your allergist and to be guided by what he has to say.

HYPOSENSITIZATION INJECTIONS

It was in 1911 that two English doctors named Noon and Freeman first reported successful inoculation against hayfever. Although it has been improved upon a bit, their technique is still basically the same one used now as the most effective weapon against allergy.

The principle is the injection of increasingly larger amounts of extracts of the substance the patient is sensitive to, thus stimulating the production of increasing quantities of blocking antibody and building up resistance. In time, with the increasing buildup of antibody, the body becomes competent to cope with the person's trouble-making substance.

The technique, when used properly, can now be expected to provide good to excellent results in most patients with allergies. Untoward reactions in the hands of competent physicians are rare, and for the most part not a serious problem.

Usually the immunity is built up by injections of the substance into tissue under the skin in the person's upper arm. However, in food allergy sometimes it is possible to achieve a tolerance by oral desensitization. The food is eaten in very small amounts daily, gradually increasing the amount until you are able to eat the food without any problem. This technique, however, has been largely abandoned during the past twenty years.

Hyposensitization—also called desensitization or immunization—is the only immunologically sound means of treating allergy. It is the only technique aimed specifically at achieving control over the substances that are really responsible for the symptoms.

These injections aren't miracle workers, although some patients claim that for them they have been. But they do yield good results, and they do prevent the allergic person from being a helpless cripple bowing to his ruthless allergy.

The injections are not an overnight cure. The process of building up immunity is slow and tedious and many visits are required over several years.

There are several ways of carrying out the hyposensitization treatment. Treatment can be preseasonal, perennial or coseasonal.

Optimally the preseasonal injections are begun about fifteen to twenty weeks before your symptoms usually appear. Injections are given at four- to seven-day intervals, with the dosage carefully increased until it reaches a maximum just before the seasonal symptoms usually begin. Then the injections are continued usually at the same or a reduced dosage through the pollinating season at five- to seven-day intervals.

In the perennial type of treatment the preseasonal schedule is used to start the treatment, but instead of stopping the injections at the end of the pollinating season, the maximum dose is continued at two- or three-week intervals through the winter months. Then shortly before the seasonal symptoms are due to begin again, the schedule is stepped up to weekly injections and increased in concentration, and these are maintained throughout the season. The schedule drops back to twice a month again during the winter.

In coseasonal treatment, used after the season starts, the size of the dose of allergen used for the injections is smaller and the strength is weaker. The dosage starts at very low concentrations of about 1:500,000 and then is gradually increased with daily injections until the point of tolerance is reached and the symptoms are controlled. Then the optimum dose is maintained with a gradually increasing interval between doses.

Treatment schedule for the preseasonal or perennial injections should be arranged so that the strongest dose of the graduated series is given about ten days before the height of the pollen season in the patient's locality. For a patient with ragweed hayfever in the north, central and eastern states, for example, the highest dose of ragweed pollen extract should be given prior to August 10. In the West the highest dose would be given as early as August 5; in the South as late as July 20. In Florida the ragweed season may begin as early as June.

For the patient with allergy to grass pollen in the North, the top dose should be given on or about May 20. In the South and Southwest, where the grass season is considerably longer, year-round treatment is required.

Most allergists find that the perennial injections schedule yields results far superior to either the preseason or coseasonal treatment schedules.

The time interval between injections should be as regular as possible. If you have discontinued treatment for more than a week, then at the next visit the dosage will be reduced. If you wait too long between injections, then your doctor may consider it necessary to return to the starting dosage level for safety's sake. Also for safety, some physicians suggest you wait in the office for fifteen to twenty minutes after an injection.

The materials used for desensitization shots (as well as for testing materials) are gathered by field crews of eleven major companies who scour the country in search of pollens and other allergens ranging from cat dander to special molds. Some of the more rare substances sell for as much as ten dollars per gram, much more costly than gold.

Pollen from ragweed is fairly easy to gather. It is vacuumed right off the plant. Other pollens have to be cut early and kept in incubation rooms to ripen. All materials have to be sifted or washed to remove foreign matter. Some of the substances are sold directly to doctors to be used in powder form. Others are sent to pharmaceutical houses for extraction; that is, solvents are used to draw out the parts of the allergens used for injection.

Sometimes if stock solutions off the shelf do not help with your particular problem, your physician may want you to collect the dust in your own home or your office to make a vaccine that is specific to your needs. A regular vacuum cleaner can be used. It should be cleaned out first; then dust should be collected from the furniture, bed slats, mattresses, drapes, pillows and rugs. Always be sure to collect the dust from shelves in your home or office and from rafters and high ledges of barns or factories. These often harbor the air-borne particles that are causing the most trouble. Do not vacuum entrance halls where outside dust collects and do not collect dust from rugs that have been treated with moth crystals or other poisonous chemicals. Also avoid any floor collection if the surface has been treated by oil, solvent or chemical substances.

If your physician suspects that a pet is causing the trouble, he may want you to collect some of the pet fur and dander. This is best done by placing the animal on a newspaper and giving him a brisk brushing and clipping, or vacuum his sleeping blanket for hair and dander. At least a cupful of the sample is needed. If birds are suspected, feathers may be collected at molting time.

The collected samples are taken to the doctor or shipped to the laboratory he indicates. The laboratory will test the sample for any bacteria and any poisonous substances and then will prepare the extract and send it to your physician.

Should you get injections or shouldn't you? Are they worth the trouble and bother of the repeated trips to the doctor's office? It is a long-term procedure. Physicians and patients who expect to see a cure within a few months will be severely disappointed. Progress in controlling allergy is measured in years, not days. But it is largely effective.

Hyposensitization gives the best results against inhalant allergies. In fact, in patients with simple uncomplicated hayfever, nine out of ten have good results; that is, there are either minimal symptoms or they disappear completely. In those with asthma complicating their hayfever, about 75 percent have good results, and of those who have complicating sinus infections or other allergies, about 80 percent have good results.

The larger the doses of pollen extract that the patient can tolerate, the more effective they are in combating the allergy. Dosage is tailored to the patient's tolerance level.

Once the patient has had two successive years marked by significant improvement, treatment may be discontinued. But the patient should still report every six months so that his status may be reviewed.

There have been assertions that for some patients receiving treatment for respiratory tract allergy, treatment goes on year after year without a "cure." But the fact is that adequate management usually yields some relief in a matter of weeks or months, depending on the individual circumstances, and that control can generally be achieved within two or three seasons. The patient whose illness has not been controlled within a reasonable length of time is not getting the proper treatment, or else he let it go untreated so long that it progressed beyond the reach of therapy.

There have been assertions that medications available in any drugstore are perfectly adequate to relieve the symptoms of allergy, and that nothing further is required. But the fact is that a good percentage of the case load of virtually every practicing allergist consists of patients who were dosed for years with nose drops or expectorants or cough medicines or sedatives, before somebody finally realized that something more effective was indicated.

There have been assertions that skin-testing is nothing but "mumbo-jumbo," or a subtle form of torture, and that the results are accepted only if they agree with what the allergist knew all along. But the fact is that skin tests are an essential part of a complex diagnostic process that is designed to reveal every detail of the patient's history—medical and personal—that will help develop a clearer picture of the total illness and aid the physician in decisions as to how to set up a treatment program.

There have been assertions that hyposensitization with specific antigens offers no greater benefit than treatment with a placebo. The fact is that recent scientifically controlled studies in many allergy centers demonstrate conclusively that such treatment has *great* value.

Hyposensitization is still the sole means available to combat the causative factors of this difficult chronic illness. And it is the best means of preventing the development of serious complications, such as the pollen asthma that is frequently seen subsequent to untreated pollinosis.

To mix a few architectural metaphors, hyposensitization with the correct antigens is the foundation, the cornerstone and the keystone to today's treatment of allergic disease.

REPOSITORY IMMUNIZATION

For the uncomplicated hayfever sufferer, a single large injection has been used by some allergists to replace the thirty or so separate shots usually necessary in the long tedious treatment to build up immunity against ragweed pollen. The single-shot treatment is still controversial, but it has been of help in many people.

At present the material used for the repository injections has not been given government approval and is not commercially available to physicians. It is available *only* on a research basis.

With the single-shot method the pollen extract is emulsified in a mineral solution and so is released very slowly over a long time. Sometimes it is given in two or three injections instead of just one.

First to develop the technique was Dr. Mary Hewitt Loveless, of Cornell University Medical College. She cautiously tried the new slow-release method for the first time on a human volunteer in 1947. Then in a ten-year study, she tried the method on 117 more volunteers who had hayfever, alternating the slow-release shots with conventional aqueous shots to compare results.

Results were promising and she then gave more than 1,500 treatments and reported it "an effective and safe method of annual immunization that has possibilities of benefitting thousands of hayfever sufferers." Unfortunately many severe reactions were encountered.

Field trials on the one-shot treatments were carried out a few years ago, with doctors giving the single-shot treatment to hayfever sufferers in clinics of twenty-five medical schools throughout the country. To make the field trials as uniform and valid as possible, all doctors gave the injections with the same kind of needles, with the same technique and with the identical extract made in one laboratory from one lot of ragweed. Patients kept daily charts of their symptoms, and the results of the single-shot immunizations were compared with those of regular multiple injections.

The findings showed that in patients getting the one-shot treatment, 74 percent had at least moderate or marked benefit. About 15 percent had fair relief, and 11 percent had none.

Where comparison with conventional shots was made, over half of the patients felt they got better results with the one-shot treatment than with the conventional series of shots they had had previously.

When you get a repository injection, first you have to be tested with skin scratch tests to make sure of what you are really allergic to. If you are not allergic to ragweed, giving you the repository shot for ragweed can make you allergic to it in the future.

The doctors have to decide how large a dose of the long-lasting extract you can tolerate, since the single shot contains 50 to 100 times more extract than normal injections. They can decide this by checking how large a dose of extract you received last year, or by giving you several small old-type injections first.

Sometimes the injection is given in three divided doses at fifteen-minute intervals.

You sit around for about an hour to see if any reactions occur of swelling, tenderness, redness, itching or sneezing. Some people have an itchy, swollen arm for several days; some do not. After the injection has been given, you usually take antihistamine tablets three times a day for the next two days as a safeguard against any delayed reactions.

There is still much controversy about the repository shot injection. Most allergists feel that we need to know more about how it is absorbed, how it actually works and how safe it is. Some doctors report that the patient's arm can sometimes become permanently swollen where the shots have been given. Some warn that an infection or an open ulcer might be created or a local tumor formed. Others are worried about long-term effects such as the mineral oil causing cancer. Also the dose is so much stronger than the usual injection dose that if the mixture is not properly prepared and given, there could be a serious shock reaction.

OTHER KINDS OF INJECTIONS

Because of the controversy over the use of mineral oil as the base for the repository shots, attempts have been made to find other substances that will produce the same slow-release effect.

For instance, allergists are trying a substance called alginate colloid, which is a kind of gel derived from seaweed.

Another approach is to prepare extracts with a substance called pyridine and then to precipitate them with alum. The resulting mixture is called Allpyral.

The Allpyral extracts are absorbed from the injection site more slowly than with the conventional aqueous material, but the effect is not as long-lasting as the mineral oil repository injections. The release occurs for one to three weeks. Fewer injections are required than with the conventional aqueous injections, and there is less risk of systemic reaction and other problems found with the mineral oil repository shots.

First clinical reports of these Allpyral shots seem favorable. Doctors reported that as few as six to eight injections per season were giving adequate protection and that dosage levels could be given safely that were many times higher than those that could be given with aqueous material.

The method seems a decided improvement over the other methods, especially for those extremely sensitive patients who could not tolerate high enough dosages of aqueous material to provide protection.

Several physicians say that they have used the Allpyral material for injection treatment in thousands of patients with low reaction rate and effective results. Lately, however, a number of investigators have raised questions about the Allpyral preparations. They feel that a closer examination is needed of the substance and its effectiveness.

Some investigators say that the Allpyral works in patients when the pollen count is under 200, but when the count is greater it does not seem to yield as good results as the aqueous injections. Others say that when patients are switched from Allpyral suspension to aqueous injections, they sometimes have reactions to the aqueous material even though it is in lower concentrations.

In fact, the manufacturer of Allpyral cautions, "never attempt to switch a patient directly from treatment with Allpyral suspensions to conventional aqueous solutions of allergens."

Doctors also are finding that some patients have a flu-like reaction three to six hours after the injection.

Allergy is a chronic illness requiring close supervision over many years. In this age of antibiotics and sophisticated medicine most physicians and most patients are not accustomed to dealing with long-term illnesses, and both can be easily discouraged when treatment does not have a prompt effect. Unfortunately quick cures are not part of the allergy picture.

On the other hand, allergy will not disappear if ignored, and it usually gets worse. So proper long-term management is needed.

The allergy patient can help himself by avoiding allergens where he can, by eliminating outside additive factors to lighten his allergic load, by seeing a competent allergist who understands allergic illness and its possible complications and by taking the medications and desensitization therapy that his doctor suggests.

Chapter **16**

RESEARCH AND THE FUTURE

Research isn't always glamorous. In fact, it seldom is. Research starts with filling out grant applications to raise money for your research work. Then it's spending day after day in a laboratory with test tubes or mice, maybe spending hours trying to find a way to make a guinea pig sneeze. It's spending months or years on a project and then perhaps finding you've run up a blind alley, all your efforts wasted, that your theory was wrong. It's spending months or years testing hundreds or thousands of drugs on animals to find one—perhaps—that may work on humans. It's poring over graphs and figures and analyzing results.

It's tedious trials and keeping track of millions of facts and carefully and slowly building up bits and pieces of evidence, hoping that someday they may lead to a new explanation or understanding of how a tiny bit of the universe works or may lead to a new way to treat a disease or to somehow make people happier, more comfortable or more useful.

Sometimes you come up with a beautiful theory or results but fail to convince other people that it's valid. But once in a while when you do find some new nugget of information or some new treatment to help a suffering human being, it's marvelous.

Research is people, and there are more people involved in allergy research than just allergists. The physiologist investigates how histamine works and what the other mediators in the immunology system are. The biochemist works on synthesizing new products which might be useful and studies chemical changes in the body caused by the disease. The immunologist works to identify the antigens and antibodies and study the allergic reactions. The pharmacologist searches for more effective drugs. The public health specialist surveys various populations to learn the scope, the incidence and age and inheritance factors of allergy. The specialist in preventive medicine studies environmental and occupational effects, air pollution and other factors, and analyzes what can be modified to prevent allergies.

Others in medical schools and pharmaceutical companies and hospitals across the nation are seeking new methods of diagnosis, new or improved treatments, new drugs with fewer side effects. Investigators are trying to find out how allergy develops and why some people develop allergy and other people don't. They are standardizing materials used for desensitization injections. They are studying the relationship of allergy to other diseases. They are studying the effect of emotional stress on allergy.

Finally when a new method or new product is developed and has been tested in animals, the allergist in clinical practice tries it on patients with their consent and determines whether it is effective, whether it is safe and whether it is an improvement over already known methods.

Research is also money. One large supplier of funds to allergy research is the National Institute of Allergy and Infectious Diseases, which is part of the U.S. Public Health Service. It is presently funding about twelve million dollars a year into several hundred allergy research projects.

Aside from government grants, money for research also comes from private donors, industry, pharmaceutical companies and various other organizations. One of the functions of the Allergy Foundation of America, for example, is to stimulate research on allergic diseases and to have qualified investigators commit themselves to study particular problems. Recently, however, government grants as well as private funds have been sharply reduced and because of the cutback, monies for allergy research can scarcely be found.

■ IN THE BEGINNING

The history of allergy goes back through the ages. One of the earliest records was an order written in 3000 B.C. from Shen Nung, the emperor of China, who ruled that pregnant woman should not eat fish, chicken or horse meat. It was said that these foods caused ulceration of the skin. Some scholars believe that many of the dietary restrictions mentioned in the Old Testament were formulated because it was noted that eating certain foods caused allergies.

In the first century B.C. Lucretius first stated the now well-known adage, "One man's meat is another man's poison." Galen in the second century A.D. described people who always sneezed in the presence of certain plants and flowers. Hippocrates wrote about asthma and stated, "It is a bad thing to give milk to persons having headache."

It was early in the nineteenth century that Dr. John Bostock of London described the symptoms of hayfever. He thought they were due to summer heat or sun, having suffered with them himself since childhood. Then Dr. William Gordon described similar symptoms and called them "hay asthma." Dr. John Elliotson linked hayfever to pollen of grass, and argument raged in medical circles as to whether heat or pollen caused hayfever. Another Englishman, Dr. Hyde Salter, then showed allergy could also be caused by animal fur and foods.

Then Dr. Charles Harrison Blackley, who had hayfever himself, accidentally bumped a vase of grass arranged by his children and went into a hayfever attack. He began some experiments and proved the case for pollen.

In America, doctors were beginning to talk about ragweed causing hayfever in the fall. But the theories were not accepted completely. Some still claimed bacteria or emotional problems for hayfever.

During the last half of the nineteenth century several investigators injected test animals with the serum of other animals. They observed that rabbits when injected repeatedly with dog serum sometimes showed strange and unaccountable reactions following the second injection. Other animals did the same.

Credit for understanding and explaining the strange phenomenon goes to Dr. Charles Richet and his associates of France. They took the poison from the Portuguese man-of-war, a jellyfish, and injected it into dogs, trying to make them immune. To their surprise, the poison gave no reaction on the first injection, but sometimes proved severely toxic, even deadly, when it was injected the second time several days after the first injection. It was a curious phenomenon—their scientific appetites were fired. Diphtheria was the critical illness at that time, and diphtheria antitoxin was being used intensively. Richet recognized that the dog reaction was the same as commonly seen in diphtheria patients. They named the reaction "anaphylaxis," which meant without protection, as opposed to "prophylaxis," which means protection. The chance discovery later won Richet a Nobel Prize and set up basic concepts which still have application. One was that a foreign substance which on first injection may be relatively harmless may on reinjection become severely toxic, even fatal, when given in the same or even smaller dosage. Second was that an interval of several days must elapse between the first and second injections.

In 1906 Professor Clemens Von Pirquet, a pediatrician, suggested the term "allergy" in place of "anaphylaxis." Von Pirquet is considered the father of modern-day allergy. He and his loyal friend and associate Professor Bela Schick collaborated on a monumental study on serum sickness that is the background for present-day allergy practice. In commenting on this first scientific paper and the term "allergy," however, one reviewer said that the paper was not important, that it was a superfluous publication introducing a new and useless term. It was a rather inauspicious and frustrating beginning for allergy and allergy research, but it survived the now unknown reviewer.

It was in these same years that Professor Von Pirquet and Professor Schick teamed up in Vienna, working with patients in the old scarlet fever pavilion of the St. Anna Kinderspital. They believed that some of the delayed complications of scarlet fever might be due to a form of allergy. They were correct. This is accepted today as one of the autoimmune diseases. Then, still thinking in terms of allergy, Bela Schick developed the Schick test for testing patients for diphtheria. The test showed whether people were immune to diphtheria already or required immunization against it. Von Pirquet developed the first test for tuberculosis—the tuberculin test.

Schick went on to become chief of the children's department at Mt. Sinai Hospital in New York and continued a considerable amount of clinical research.

He remained interested in allergy; because of his great personal influence as a teacher, he was greatly responsible for the acceptance of allergy in important medical circles both here and abroad. For many years he and his wife Catherine traveled to Europe each summer and lectured to physicians there. Many of the European physicians as well as Americans at first were skeptical of the report of the great frequency of allergic conditions in children. But Schick constantly cited work coming out of many clinics in the United States and began to convince physicians of the importance of allergy.

It was following this that allergy as a specialty in medicine became more accepted, and major research projects began. Allergy and allergy research advanced considerably in the next fifty years.

■ BASIC RESEARCH—LEARNING WHAT ALLERGY REALLY IS

In allergy, and in other fields of medicine as well, there are two different kinds of research. There is basic research—designed to learn fundamental facts of how and why things work as they do. There is applied research—designed to find practical applications for knowledge, such as new and better ways of diagnosis or treatment.

The allergic response is a complex process. We know it begins with the introduction of an antigen into the body by one means or another, and it ends with the production of antibodies and in many instances clinical symptoms of allergy. Many of the steps involved in between are still not established. Trying to learn these steps and determine the mechanisms comprise the greatest part of basic research in allergy.

One place these studies begin is with the beginning of life itself. Allergy and immune mechanisms are vitally important in pregnancy. For years medical researchers have puzzled over the question of why a woman's body tolerates the growing embryo, whose genetic and protein makeup is different from hers. Why doesn't her body reject it, as it does an organ transplant or skin graft?

Alterations of the immune responses during pregnancy have been observed for many years, but they haven't been fully understood. For example, skin grafts were observed to survive longer in pregnant animals and in some pregnant women.

Part of the answer may be a hormone manufactured during pregnancy that cuts down on the body's ability to produce antibodies.

It may be that an antigen from the fetus enters the mother's circulation in amounts just large enough to build up tolerance rather than immunity, and that this is the reason that pregnancies continue to term instead of being rejected.

No one knows what really causes a pregnancy to terminate. One theory is that allergy may well be the initiating spark that starts the chain reaction that finally results in the contraction of the uterus and the delivery of the baby.

Many investigators are also studying the newborn infant. It cannot form antibodies and cannot develop its own immuity, but it is afforded protection with gamma globulin and other substances transmitted from its mother until it's able to develop its own immunity. At about three months of age the human infant begins to show in its bone marrow a certain cell, called a plasma cell, which is believed to be a precursor of the later cells that produce antibodies. Then it can develop its own resistance to germs and other foreign bodies.

Allergy and immune mechanisms are particularly significant in relation to Rh babies. The problem arises when the mother has the negative blood cells and the fetus has Rh positive cells. Previously many of these infants were born dead or died shortly after birth. Sometimes they have been saved by total removal and replacement of the infant's blood. Now when blood tests show the mother has Rh negative blood, she can be immunized before she has her baby and all problems will be prevented for the future. This development of being able to immunize mothers against having Rh babies was a great step—the first practical application of completely preventing a dangerous and possibly fatal allergy.

The biggest question in basic research is why some people develop allergies and others don't. What is the allergic mechanism? What really happens? From infancy on, the body builds up a defense mechanism consisting of specific antibodies that fight against any invasion of a foreign biological substance. This principle is usually good, often lifesaving. It helps us build up immunity to bacteria. Jenner and Pasteur applied the principle and developed vaccinations (immunization). But when the mechanism works poorly, it produces allergies. Why?

Some scientists believe that a mixup in the body's metabolism is the reason. Their theory is that allergic conditions are caused by the malfunctioning of an enzyme that metabolizes epinephrine. The constitutional abnormality could be inherited or could be acquired later. They believe that the constitutional abnormality in metabolism—the enzyme disturbance—produces the susceptibility and tendency to be allergic, and the allergy-producing substances, whether food or ragweed or dust or mold, act as triggering mechanisms.

Other researchers are studying the thymus gland, thinking it may be the key to this enigma. This small gland in the chest seems to be at the very heart of immunological capability. If you remove the thymus in newborn mice, they develop normally for a few weeks, then die from symptoms resembling graft rejection. On the other hand, when the thymus gland is removed in people receiving kidney transplants, it seems to help prevent rejection of the transplanted kidney. There also appears to be a relationship between the thymus gland and the development of autoimmune diseases.

The white blood cells called eosinophils are being studied by other investigators, to learn just how they are related to allergic reactions. They use "skin windows." An area of the skin is abraded and a thin glass cover slip applied to the area. Various antigens are added, and what takes place at the cell level is examined microscopically. When ragweed extract is injected into the skin of an allergic person, eosinophil cells appear in about fifteen minutes in great numbers. They do not appear in nonallergic persons.

Indeed some researchers have found that allergic sensitization can be transmitted from one person to another by white blood cells. Because of this, they advise against the use of allergic persons as blood donors. One person, allergic to horses, donated blood to a friend. The friend visited a stable about two weeks later and had a severe attack of asthma.

Other investigators are studying antibodies to try to find clues. There are two forms of immunological reactions in the body, they find. One is due to antibodies found in blood plasma and other body fluids; the other is due to antibodies associated with certain white blood cells. The white cell antibodies produce allergies, cause the rejection that occurs with transplanted organs and provide immunity to diseases. The other newly discovered antibodies seem to control the development of the cellular antibodies, but little else is known.

It could well tie in with what other researchers say about a second separate immune system apparently localized in the mucous membranes and secretions of glands. They note, for example, that sniffing a vaccine or spraying it into the nose often achieves a more effective immunization against respiratory viruses than injection does. At the State University of New York at Buffalo a dentist doing research work says that some of the evidence of this second local immune system indicates that it may be possible to use it to immunize people against dental disease.

Also in the quest to learn what is different in allergic people, researchers have recently discovered a substance called gamma E. It is a gamma globulin found only in allergic people. Two Denver doctors, Teruko Ishizaka and Kimishige Ishizaka, found that this gamma E acted differently from any of the other known gamma globulins, having a special affinity for white blood cells. It may be that the gamma E induces the release of histamine from these cells to produce allergic symptoms.

Another special gamma globulin—globulin A—has been pinpointed as the probable cause of reactions from blood transfusions. Life-threatening anaphylactic reactions occur occasionally despite careful cross-matching procedures before transfusions. Dr. Herbert Perkins, of the University of California, made the discovery when he was treating a woman who required three or four units of blood at regular intervals. She had several reactions, so the next time she needed blood, Perkins and his team took special precautions, inserting a tube into her vein to be instantly ready if they had to inject medications quickly. They gave her some plasma from a donor she had previously reacted to and stood around for about thirty minutes watching carefully.

Said Dr. Perkins, "There was no particular reaction, so we went downstairs for lunch. We had hardly gotten off the elevator when there was a call for me. When I got back up to the woman's bedside she complained of shortness of breath and a feeling of acute discomfort. I gave her an antihistamine, but she did not respond. Then to my alarm she suddenly fell unconscious. I quickly gave her some epinephrine via the previously inserted cannula and she recovered immediately."

Later, trying to find out why the woman had reacted so severely, the research team found special antibodies to globulin A circulating in her blood, implicating that the donor's globulin A had caused the transfusion reaction.

Some scientists are trying to find other mediators of allergic reactions. They think a major substance may be some chemicals in the blood plasma called kinins. They are released by special enzymes. The kinins are known to increase capillary permeability, just as histamine does, and have been observed in large amounts in human plasma during allergic reactions.

Another theory being studied involves tiny receptors in the body called beta-adrenergic receptors. They are found in the glands, smooth muscles and blood vessels. Some scientists believe that it is a disturbance in these receptors that causes bronchial asthma. But most of the work on this theory has been performed on animals, and thus far no one has shown it in humans.

Other investigators are studying the role of hereditary factors. How large a role does heredity play? Does inheritance of allergy occasionally skip a generation or two and then reappear, or do some parents have allergies that they are not aware of that their children inherit? Some physicians think that heredity may give a person a predisposition to poor quality of skin or mucous membranes that makes them more permeable and lets antigens through that normal skin would block.

Laboratory animals are being studied to try to find out just how much of a heredity factor there is. One public health scientist has spent several years studying the genetic characteristics of three strains of guinea pigs. He finds that one strain is quite resistant to allergies, another is moderately susceptible, and a third is highly susceptible. He is now crossbreeding allergic and nonallergic animals to study the hereditary mechanisms.

But in contrast, another investigator studied fifty-nine identical twins and found only seven showed identical allergies, which he said sheds doubt on the influence of heredity.

Environmental factors play a significant role, too. Some areas have been called "hotbeds of asthma." In certain regions in northeastern France, for example, as many as 20 to 30 percent of the children are asthmatic. Investigators say that genetic factors can not be involved because the working population has changed in a series of waves of Italians, Poles and North Africans coming in one after another, with the number of asthmatic children remaining almost constant. In other villages epidemics of asthma have affected as much as 50 or 60 percent of the population.

One of the major problems in allergy research has been the difficulty in being able to produce symptoms artificially in animals, and until relatively recently no animals were known that had allergies naturally. So the researchers had no laboratory animals to work with.

This situation has improved somewhat. Dr. Ando Szentivanyi, pharmacologist at the University of Colorado School of Medicine, has devised a technique of artificially establishing an allergic reaction in guinea pigs.

Another scientist has succeeded in transferring human allergies to monkeys by injecting serum into them. So now guinea pigs and monkeys can be used for tests and for allergy studies under controlled conditions in the laboratory.

Dr. Roy Patterson, of Northwestern University, has found some dogs who have hayfever and pollen asthma and is trying to find other dogs in the country with allergies so that they can be bred. One of his first dogs, Pansy, a female terrier, had one of the most severe cases of hayfever even seen in man or beast. Dr. Patterson asks anyone who has an allergic dog to contact him at Northwestern University in Chicago. If he can borrow a few dogs for a short time, he can breed them, keep the puppies to start a colony of hayfever dogs, and return the original dogs to their owners.

As doctors are able to gain a better understanding of allergies in animals, they can try to relate the knowledge to humans. They can also test various drugs and other methods of treatment on the animals before trying them on humans.

■ INVESTIGATING THE TROUBLEMAKERS

Another area in allergy research is aimed at the things that cause the allergies—the pollens, molds and the other influencing factors that impinge upon these. For example, as the ragweed pollinates year after year, researchers intensify their efforts to dislodge the secrets of the weed, to find ways to counteract its effects or to discourage its growth.

Their research tools include indoor gardens to grow ragweed, wind tunnels, human test chambers and electronic probe counters for monitoring pollen clouds in the air.

They are studying just how ragweed and other plants pollinate and how the pollen is diffused into the atmosphere and how it reaches the mucous membranes of human beings.

At the University of Michigan researchers are studying how ragweed is dispersed over long distances. They measure the pollen as it is blown across Lake Michigan, since the lake itself is free of ragweed and provides a natural experimental setup to permit the evaluation of pollen transport.

Not all research yields medical breakthroughs. At the University of Michigan a team of investigators had high hopes of being able to make both short-range and long-range predictions about pollen concentrations. They figured if weather conditions in the spring or early summer indicated that there were going to be large stands of ragweeds, allergists could then treat their patients more intensively and very sensitive persons could perhaps plan to flee the area during the hayfever season. During the season, if on one day weather conditions suggested that the pollen count would be especially high the next day, sensitive person could take extra medication or plan to stay at home with air conditioners running. Meteorological records were collected for several years from the university meteorological laboratories, and records of local pollen counts were obtained for the same years. The scientists painstakingly analyzed the days of the highest pollen counts, noted whether curves of pollen count throughout the season skewed or peaked or sloped gently, compared the counts in various years, then correlated all this information with the Weather Bureau records. They said in a lengthy report they "so far have had no success at all in arriving at a method of long-range predictions." They're still working on it.

As part of the campaign to try to control ragweed, some investigators have discovered that certain molds will infect and destroy ragweed. This could open the door to the possibility of controlling the ragweed by natural means.

Others have found that some significant inroads can be made in controlling ragweed if destruction is concentrated in the perimeter zones around cities and in industrial and farming zones where new ground is broken. This is where ragweed usually grows—where nothing else grows on bare soil.

How do airborne pollens actually cause people to develop hayfever? A pathologist from the University of California at San Diego found in his research that some large protein molecules can pass unchanged right through the membranes of the lungs into the blood. This may be the way that ragweed molecules slip into the body.

In the same vein (if you will excuse the pun), a doctor at Louisiana State University reports that people with allergies have an important difference in the way protein antigens are handled as they come in contact with body membranes. He believes that allergic persons have a permeability defect in their membranes allowing the antigens through.

Other investigators have been trying to find out just what it is in pollen that causes allergic reactions. For example, at Rockefeller University and at Johns Hopkins Hospital doctors have isolated the two most active allergens in ragweed pollen. Then other doctors tried using this pure fraction of the ragweed pollen for hyposensitization treatment. The antigens were found to be one hundred times more active than an extract of the whole ragweed pollen. But so far results have not matched those achieved with the injections given with the whole ragweed extract. Apparently there are other antigens in the ragweed that are necessary, too. And the search for these goes on.

Similar studies are under way as to what the factors are in house dust that cause allergy. Evidence now points to the fact that mites of submicroscopic size may be the chief cause. If injections of mite extract prevent allergy to house dust, it will be a great boon to tens of thousands of persons. This is still being studied intensively.

Why do some patients have symptoms before the pollen season begins and some have symptoms long after the pollen season ends?

Dr. John T. Connell, of Roosevelt Hospital in New York, came up with interesting evidence that the initial or priming exposure to pollen at the beginning of hayfever season takes place only in the nose, not in the whole body, as previously supposed. In fact, he found that when one nostril of a patient was primed with pollen every day for five days while the other nostril was closed, hayfever symptoms usually developed in the primed side of the nose only. The procedure was also found to be reversible—that is, after two or more days without subsequent pollen exposure, even a large pollen dose is relatively innocuous, and very little reaction occurs. However, the longer the patient is exposed to ragweed during the priming period, the longer it takes to reverse the procedure, so that in patients who are exposed to ragweed pollen every day during the ragweed season the reversal of the priming effect requires three to six weeks. This may explain "hangover" effects.

The priming effect with the ragweed can also affect reactions to other pollens and molds. It was found that if a patient's nose is primed with one type of pollen, it becomes hyperactive to all other airborne allergens to which the patient is allergic. So a person who is allergic to two different pollens whose seasons overlap could have a much worse time than if he had a free interval in-between for his reactivity to pollen to decrease.

Several investigators are studying the effect of air pollution and other environmental factors on hayfever and asthma. At the Hospital for Sick Children in Washington, D.C., a submarine type unit called an environmental control center is being used to study the effect of air pollution on children with chronic asthma and other respiratory ailments. The two-room unit has air that is completely filtered, and it is entered through two submarine doors. The idea was conceived from the book *Under the North Pole,* by Captain William R. Anderson of the U.S. Navy, who wrote that in the *Nautilus* submarine there was no air pollution and crew members never felt better in their lives—no colds, coughs or respiratory symptoms. In the environmental control center physicians sit at a control panel and monitor barometric pressure, temperature and humidity inside the rooms. They are able to duplicate any environment in the United States, including dirty city air.

Three children can stay in the unit at a time, usually eating, sleeping, studying and undergoing various tests there for three weeks within the controlled environment. The present project is to determine whether there is any improvement in asthmatic children who are moved from dirty city air to clean air. If there is improvement, they want to find out whether it is due to any specific agents in the air.

Allergists from the University of Michigan studied allergic persons in a state prison in southern Michigan. Here men were living in a controlled environment, ate the same food, lived by the same schedule. Volunteers who had hayfever or asthma were kept under close medical observation, and their symptoms were correlated with observations of daily pollen count from a sampler set on a roof within the prison walls and by samplers in each subject's room. Lung function was measured daily; blood counts were taken. The allergists found, not surprisingly, that symptoms increased with pollen count, but less expectedly they found that although the drop in pollen count near the end of the ragweed season brought some relief to asthmatics, it did not bring much relief to hayfever sufferers. Another puzzling fact was that although the highest pollen count was recorded from 8:00 A.M. to noon, almost every patient reported that he had the least symptoms between six and nine in the morning.

Other people have been comparing the incidence of allergy of persons born and reared in the United States and persons coming from other countries. When university students were studied, few of the foreign students had hayfever or asthma in their own countries, but they frequently developed allergies in this country after being here three to five years. The allergies were almost always to ragweed at first. Some allergists feel that this indicates that allergies develop only on exposure to especially powerful allergens, such as ragweed, and that this exposure somehow triggers immunological imbalance. They found that persons initially allergic only to ragweed often developed other allergies later.

■ DIAGNOSTIC TESTS

The key to successful treatment of allergy is the correct diagnosis of the allergy. You've got to know exactly what you are allergic to before you can be successfully treated. So one of the areas in which concentrated research is focused is for better diagnostic tests.

Reports of several new tests have been appearing in the recent scientific literature. Some involve taking a sample of the patient's blood and testing for allergies with test tube methods, which might eliminate the need for skin tests. But a great deal of corroborative effort needs to be done yet before they are acceptable for routine clinical application.

One test uses red blood cells that have been coated with an antibiotic called cephalothin. It can detect persons who are allergic to penicillin.

Several other tests have been devised that may prove helpful in diagnosis of drug allergies. They use blood samples also. One causes a change in the white blood cells in the sample when a drug is added that the patient is sensitive to. Another measures the effect of serum on strips of monkey muscle. With another new test blood cells are placed under the microscope, and various antigens are tested on it. Those that cause certain blood cells to bud out and start to reproduce after five days of incubation are considered positive.

Another test is performed on the patient's skin. An area of skin is abraded. The drug in question is applied to it, and a cover slip placed over the area. In twenty-four hours the cover slip is studied under the microscope. The presence of certain white blood cells indicates whether the patient was sensitive to the drug or not.

Another doctor has devised an instrument to measure the amount of carbon dioxide in the blood of persons who come in with severe asthma attacks. He has found that when the carbon dioxide level goes up, it is a serious sign. If a small incision is made in the trachea immediately, the sticky mucus suffocating the person can be removed.

Several patients have been saved from death by being made able to breathe again.

A diagnostic test for asthma has been developed at the National Jewish Hospital at Denver. Called a quantitative inhalation challenge apparatus, the machine enables doctors to measure the degree of bronchial reaction to a known quantity of whatever substance is being tested. The patient inhales a mist containing the substance suspected of causing his trouble to see if he has a reaction, and if so, how much exposure is necessary to induce breathing difficulty. Later the same apparatus can be used to determine how well the patient is responding to treatment.

Another new diagnostic approach is being used at St. Vincent's Hospital and Medical Center in New York. There, in what they term "the cleanest room in the world," a controlled environment has been established with no contaminants. Measured amounts of a suspected allergen are released into the air to test the patient's reaction.

■ NEW METHODS OF TREATMENT

The eventual goal of nearly all the research is better treatment for the patient. Researchers across the nation are trying to find new drugs or new methods of treatment or modifications of old ones to try to better battle the many allergies and the frustrating symptoms that the allergic person suffers from. Several new drugs look promising.

At Johns Hopkins University on the East Coast and at California Institute of Technology on the West Coast, a new substance is being tested that promises to be useful in both the treatment and prevention of allergy. The substance is called an allergoid. It is produced from some substance that produces allergy, such as ragweed pollen, but in the process it is detoxified. This is similar to the way vaccines are produced. The result—the product can stimulate immunity to the allergy without causing serious allergy symptoms, just as vaccinations protect against a disease.

Allergoids have been developed on an experimental basis with grass and ragweed pollens, and tests are now under way to see how effective they will be. The allergoid is prepared by incubating the pollen in formaldehyde for thirty-two days. The resulting substance retains about 60 percent of the natural pollen's ability to stimulate the production of antibodies, but is hundreds or thousands of times less irritating than the natural pollen, so that large amounts of it theoretically could be injected without producing untoward symptoms. If these substances prove of value in clinical trial, it could be one of the greatest breakthroughs in the history of allergy.

Other treatment advances are being reported also. At the University of Utah, injections of heparin are producing interesting results in treating stubborn cases of allergy. Heparin, used mainly in medicine as an anticoagulant, seems to counteract the excess of histamine that is released from the cells during the allergic reactions.

At St. Joseph's Mercy Hospital in Madison, Wisconsin, a drug called glucagon is proving useful in asthma. Glucagon has been well known as an agent against diabetes, but just recently has been helpful for asthma patients, apparently acting as a bronchodilator. Only a few patients have been studied so far, but when they were given injections of glucagon, nine out of the ten showed prompt improvement.

At McGill University in Montreal, a substance taken from tomato stalks has been shown to have some effect on allergy. The substance, called tomatine, had previously been shown to counteract fungal infections, and now has been found to counteract the effects of histamine.

Another substance, called disodium cromoglycate, has been found capable of reducing the amount of steroids needed in asthma. Both in the United States and England, physicians found that if they gave the cromoglycate at the same time they gave steroids, a much smaller amount of steroids could be used to produce the same elimination of symptoms. A group of 56 patients, aged 12 to 78 years, received the added drug for 20 months. In some of them requirements dropped from almost three tablets of steroid needed daily to one tablet by the end of the study period.

Research at Johns Hopkins University indicates that perhaps the injections of allergens that have been used in desensitization therapy have not been strong enough. They found that when injections of ragweed extract were increased about eightfold to levels much higher than had ever been given to patients before, the symptoms decreased tremendously. Many of the patients had had the more conservative series of injections over several years, but their severe symptoms had not been helped.

At another university some of the same techniques that have been used to break down viruses into separate fractions are now being used to break ragweed pollen into different fractions. One fraction has been isolated that constitutes only 6 percent of the ragweed protein, but it is believed to contribute about 90 percent of effectiveness of the allergen. This could lead to more effective desensitization for ragweed hayfever and could eliminate many of the complications.

Meanwhile, as some researchers search for new drugs, other researchers investigate some old-fashioned remedies to see if there is any truth to them. Dr. William Peterson of Ada, Oklahoma, for example, has found raw honey a help to his hayfever patients. He says raw honey—and it must be raw—contains all the pollen, dust and molds that cause most hayfever and so builds up the person's immunity. He prescribes one teaspoonful of raw honey a day.

Research goes on, too, on the role of emotional factors in allergic disease. Anxiety or depression can precipitate or worsen allergic symptoms, and so investigators search for ways to ease emotional pressure and help relieve symptoms.

Other investigators are teaching their patients self-hypnosis and are finding this may be helpful in controlling the symptoms of asthma, hives and general swelling. In Houston, a psychiatrist and an allergist together treated twenty-four adult patients who had not responded to any other medical treatment. They found that 80 to 90 percent responded to self-hypnosis after two or three sessions. The best improvement is found, they said, if the patient continues the self-hypnosis exercises himself for two to three years.

Other doctors are studying the patients who use their allergies as emotional weapons, sometimes to the point of self-destruction. Because of trying to punish somebody, because of trying to be defiant, or because of trying to aggrandize their suffering self, they either refuse to accept treatment or deliberately expose themselves to whatever they're allergic to. When their willfulness or martyrdom is extreme, it can sometimes lead to accidental suicide. One twenty-one-year-old patient had a history of nine years of asthma, and a record of consistent defiance toward any medical recommendations. She was advised not to bear children, but she had a child anyway. She courted exposure to house dust unnecessarily, although she had been told to avoid it. She refused psychotherapy, and finally died in an asthmatic seizure a little more than two years after she was first seen.

Many patients seem to have a built-in inertia. They don't seek help when they should, and—this is the most baffling to physicians—when help is offered to them, they often do not carry out the directions the physician gives them. This is true not only with allergy patients but with other patients, too.

To combat this problem both individual doctors and pharmaceutical companies have designed special pill dispensers. These dispensers usually have a month's supply of dated pill-packs and record the day each pack is supposed to be removed. One even has a uranium plug so that when each pill is removed, the plug is lowered and the radioactivity makes a mark on a sensitive strip of film. A series of even marks indicates the pills were removed every day. When there are heavy marks followed by blanks, it means that the patient missed taking the medication and pulled out the extra pills to catch up to the current date.

Some researchers are finding that variations in biological rhythms in humans are a factor in how effective medications are. There are daily, weekly and monthly changes in biological rhythms, and medications at one point in a cycle will be more effective than at another point. In one city doctors are using computers to map out the person's patterns of body rhythms.

Studies of treatment are being made in special areas, too, such as allergies that occur in pregnant women. Women's allergic symptoms lessen in pregnancy, with the hormones of pregnancy apparently counteracting the allergy. Many women with eczema have better-looking skins during pregnancy than at any other time of their lives.

However, a few cases have been reported of women who have terrible symptoms of allergy during pregnancy. Dr. Donald Unger, of Chicago, describes the case of one woman who finally asked to be sterilized after six almost-fatal pregnancies because of the severity of her asthma when she was pregnant.

Pregnant women should not take any drugs that they do not absolutely need, and this pertains to allergy medications also. Iodides and steroids and excessive use of antihistamines should be avoided. It is acceptable to have hyposensitization injections during pregnancy.

Allergy research even gets involved with sex. Doctors are finding that many women who cannot become pregnant are allergic to their husbands' sperm. A doctor in Honolulu has devised a test with a radioisotope that determines how much a woman's antibodies oppose sperm. The woman's blood serum is mixed with sperm from her husband. A radiation counter is used to determine the degree to which his sperms have become coated with radioactivity that was in the woman's serum.

Experimental treatment of infertility has been for the husband to use a prophylactic for a time so that the woman is not repeatedly exposed to sperm. When the antibody level is reduced in the woman, then the prophylactic can be discontinued.

Sometimes the man can have antibodies to his own sperm also. And he can also be allergic to his wife's sexual secretions.

The researchers involved say that there is little doubt that allergy is the cause of many cases of unexplained infertility.

The reaction has possibilities for effective birth control. You can produce sterility consistently in male guinea pigs by injecting a vaccine derived from sperm. The sterility lasts for six to eight months; then the animals become fertile again.

Similarly when guinea pig sperms were injected into female guinea pigs, antibodies were formed and the females were sterile for a year or longer.

It would seem logical that with this system the female who is repeatedly in contact with sperm and ejaculation fluid would normally become sterile, but Dr. Seymour Katsh, pharmacologist at the University of Colorado, doing research in this field, explains that there are enzyme systems both in the testes and serum of men and in the uterus and serum of women that destroy these foreign antigens. The female who becomes allergic to male sperm probably has an inadequate enzyme system for inactivating the antigens.

One recent research report describes a woman who was allergic to her own sex hormone. She had such deep painful ulcers of the mouth before each menstrual period that she requested that her ovaries be removed. After the operation, she had no further problems.

Some women may have antibodies to placental tissue or embryonic tissue. This might explain cases of habitual abortion.

■ ALLERGY AND OTHER DISEASES

What we learn about allergy has applications in many areas. Allergic responses and immune systems are involved in an unbelievable number of diseases. They're involved in tuberculosis, arthritis, multiple sclerosis and rheumatic heart disease. The failure of the immune response may make the body susceptible to cancer.

There may be a tie-in to the unusual susceptibility to infection that some people have. There are children who don't seem to be able to develop resistance or immunity to illnesses. Experts now suspect that many of these children have an inherited immunological weakness. Some of the children have been found to have poorly functioning white blood cells. Transplanting lymph tissue and bone marrow to the children from some member of their family has led to marked clinical improvement.

Dentists suggest that allergies may be the cause of some periodontal disease. And they may also be involved in the sudden infant deaths that occur so mysteriously. A young infant is put to sleep in apparent good health. When the parents look in on him again, he is dead. One theory is that the cause is milk allergy.

And allergy even extends into veterinary medicine. Dogs get hay-fever, and the horse disease called "heaves" is probably a form of respiratory allergy.

ORGAN TRANSPLANTS

One important application of current research in allergy mechanism is in the field of skin grafts and organ transplants. The surgical techniques for transplants are easily done today by competent surgeons, and if it weren't for the fact that the body rejects any foreign organ or tissue, we could replace livers and kidneys like the parts of a car engine, prolonging the lives of millions of people. In fact, to date at least 2,000 kidneys, more than 100 hearts and several liver and lung transplants have been performed on man. But the immune mechanisms of the body—the same mechanisms that are involved in allergy—set up defenses against these transplants.

In fact, many allergists are now working with transplant surgeons and in transplant research and are often called in as consultants on heart or kidney transplant cases.

A French investigator, Professor Bernard Halpern, who in 1942 first discovered synthetic antihistamines, is now experimenting with allergies and rejection of transplant organs. He believes there are two different types of immunoglobulins produced in the body. One is a protective antibody that builds up immunity to viruses or bacteria. The other is a sensitizing body that makes the person hypersensitive to a substance instead of being protected against it, so that he has an allergic reaction when exposed to it in the future.

Some drugs and serums that suppress the immune mechanisms are proving helpful in preserving transplants. The danger is that the drugs also reduce the body's defense mechanisms against various bacteria.

A large pharmaceutical company recently announced that it has succeeded in splitting one of these serums in two. This means that there is a possibility of producing one serum that will prolong skin and organ transplants without reducing the defense mechanisms against inflammation and infection.

Another possible approach is to try to outflank rather than destroy the immune mechanism. If high doses of a protein are injected repeatedly into an animal, its immune mechanism is so overwhelmed it appears to be deprived of its normal means of reacting. Instead of being sensitized, as in the case with moderate doses, it becomes tolerant to the protein. This is known as immunological paralysis. If you stop the injection, the tolerance lasts for another few months or weeks; then the animal gradually recovers its former ability to react against the protein.

During this period if transplants are made, the transplanted tissue is received much better by the animal, and even after the animal regains its ability to react, it does not react to what was transplanted during the paralyzed period.

ALLERGY AND CANCER

Immunology also offers a new approach to the problem of cancer. The structure of cancer tumors is usually quite different from the person's normal cell tissue. Therefore it should theoretically be possible to vaccinate the person against his cancer. Several such attempts have been made. One report cites that a fragment of a cancer was taken from one person and grafted onto a second person who then, reacting against the graft, produced antibodies. These antibodies were injected back into the person with the cancer and the antibodies fought the cancer. Out of twenty cases, there were "one or two spectacular successes, some interesting results and a few failures."

In one research center surgeons made patients allergic to their own tumors by exchanging grafts of tumors between patients who had the same kinds of cancers. The placement of tumor tissues into another person seemed to make that person allergic to their own tumors and helped destroy them. Of twenty-six patients treated who had an extremely serious type of cancer called malignant melanoma, in nearly every case the original cancer disappeared with the transplant technique.

Another technique is being tried in several other centers. Surgeons remove the patient's cancer by surgery so that there is little or none left, but there is still a high probability that the person will have a recurrence of the cancer. A vaccine is prepared from the patient's removed tumor, and the patient is treated with this. It's too early to tell whether this approach has any value.

The body's defense mechanism to breast cancer is being studied at Stanford University School of Medicine. Doctors have long wondered why some patients with widespread cancer are able to survive for long periods while others with smaller tumors have died quickly. This research indicates that the people who have survived a long time have a defense mechanism that slows down the growth of the cancer cells, that their immune system is stimulated, and that their white blood cell and lymph nodes grow and tend to surround and destroy the cancer cells. If ways could be found to stimulate this system, it would enhance the body's defense against cancer.

There is not going to be an overnight cure for cancer, but the possibility exists that we might be able in the future to isolate the specific antigens of a tumor and then work with these antigens to build up resistance in the person.

So far there has not been much convincing evidence of the clinical effectiveness of cancer vaccines. But, on the other hand, the tumor vaccines that have been tested have almost all been tried in very advanced disease where it might be too late to expect any response.

AUTOIMMUNE DISEASES

There is one form of allergy where certain of the body's cells suddenly begin to form antibodies against other components of the body. The organism is actually fighting against its own tissues. No one really knows what brings about the appearance of these self-destroying antibodies known as autoantibodies. Scientists don't know whether it is a result of aging, injury, the action of enzymes or even the action of viruses or bacteria.

No matter what the origin of these autoantibodies, the results are devastating as the body attacks its own tissues. The autoimmune processes occur in a wide variety of places: in the gastrointestinal tract, in the muscles, the joints, the blood, the nervous system, the glands, the eyes.

Every year physicians attribute more and more diseases to the autoimmune reaction. They include arthritis, some kinds of anemia and other blood disorders, encephalomyelitis, nephritis, thyroiditis, rheumatic heart disease, myasthenia gravis and systemic lupus erythematosus (a gradually developing fatal affliction that especially affects young women).

One of the diseases newly labeled as an autoimmune disease is pemphigus, a fatal skin disease that has been one of the mysteries of medicine for centuries. Now it is believed that the disease is caused by antibodies that the patients produce against their own skin.

At Northwestern University scientists have been studying an experimental allergic disease of the nervous system in laboratory animals. Antibodies formed in the animals destroy nerve fibers and produce paralysis and inflammation of the brain and spinal cord. These antibodies appear to be identical with those found in nerve diseases of man, such as multiple sclerosis. The Northwestern investigators have also found a drug called cyclophosphamide that prevents the allergic reaction from occurring and will also cure the paralysis after it has occurred. This is the first time an immunosuppressive drug has reversed the course of an autoimmune disease, and the scientists involved suggest that the drug should be tried in humans who have active multiple sclerosis.

New findings also indicate that Bright's disease (also called glomerulonephritis), an inflammation of the filtering system of the kidneys, is caused by an immune reaction. Studies on laboratory animals show that this kidney disease is caused by an antibody directed against a strain of streptococcus germ. Rats were infected with streptococcus germs isolated from the throat of a twelve-year-old boy with acute kidney disease. The rats soon got the kidney disease, too, and showed large amounts of antibodies to strep germs in their urine.

In this disease, as the kidney loses its filtering efficiency, the patient develops uremic poisoning—indeed may die of it. The disease is a major cause of illness in children, about 10 percent of whom become chronic kidney patients for the rest of their lives, eventually requiring lifelong artificial kidney dialysis treatments or kidney transplants.

Now that the disease is known to be caused by an immune reaction directed at one specific protein, it may be possible to synthesize that protein and use it as a vaccine to stimulate antibody response to prevent the disease.

Another example of how autoimmunity is believed to work is in rheumatic heart disease. Usually a patient who gets a sore throat that is caused by strep germs recovers in a few days without any aftereffects; however, in a small percentage of cases complications follow

—usually rheumatic fever. Sometimes this leads to permanent damage to the heart—rheumatic heart disease.

Strep germs have some structures that are very similar to, in fact almost identical with, structures found in the membranes of the knees and other joints and in the heart valves. When the strep germs invade the body, antibodies are formed in the usual way, but apparently these antibodies act not only against the strep germs but also against the similar structures in the joint membranes and in the heart valve, causing the damage there.

What does the future hold for allergy and for the millions of people who suffer from it?

A decade ago there were only a few investigators working in this field. Now research has been stimulated with support from private individuals, philanthropic and scientific organizations, pharmaceutical companies and government groups. Two national allergy societies for physicians practicing in the field—the American College of Allergists and the American Academy of Allergy—together have formed the Allergy Foundation of America, a national voluntary health agency that has established student scholarships and fellowships for training specialists and researchers. There is also the International Association of Allergology, comprising about thirty national societies and founded with the object of correlating ideas in allergy internationally.

As more and more scientists are attracted to the field, we can expect a pyramiding of discoveries so that there will be greater advances in the future and better methods of prevention and treatment. We can expect further clarification of the basic disease process in allergic reactions. We can hope for more hours devoted to training in allergy in medical schools, and we can hope for more hospitals and institutions to be set up for the study and management of chronic allergy conditions.

And we can hope that, despite the fact that our knowledge of allergy today is far from perfect, the knowledge we do have will be put to more use. The treatments that are available are not being used as fully as possible. There are many misconceptions on the part of both physicians and the general public that are keeping much knowledge from being used. There is a lack of communication between specialties, so that often when an advance is made by an investigator in allergy, physicians in other specialties may not know it for years. There are still far too many allergic sufferers unrecognized and untreated, still far too many parents either scornful or ignorant of what proper treatment can provide their children, still far too many physicians who don't have the latest knowledge or don't have the patience to give the proper allergy care.

For every allergic person who is getting adequate care for his allergy, there are at least ten others who are not being given or are not taking advantage of present knowledge.

Allergy can be relieved by drugs. It can be relieved by injections. It can be relieved by discovering the cause and removing it.

Tens of thousands of suffering people, many of whom don't even know that allergies are the cause of their disturbances, can trade in their miseries today for renewed health. With advances in research the outlook of the person with allergy should be even better.

APPENDIXES

Appendix 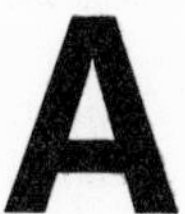

SOME OF THE THINGS YOU CAN BE ALLERGIC TO

The following is a list of the many various things that people have been known to be allergic to. Some of them can affect you when you eat them, some when you touch them, some when you breathe them or their dust or fumes. If you have an allergy and you don't know what is causing it, look over this list and it may give you some ideas as to what your troublemaker might be.

abalone
acacia
Alaskan seal
alder
alfalfa
almond
alternaria
anchovy
angora wool
aniline
anise
antibiotics
ants
apple
apricot
arabic
arbor vitae
arrowroot
artichoke
ash
asparagus
aspen
aspirin (and other salicylates)
aster
aureomycin
avocado
bacon
bacteria
balsam
banana
barley
barn dust
bath powder
bay leaf
beans
beaver
bed bug
bee
beech
beef
beet
beetle
benzocaine
benzoic acid
birch
blackberry
blackcap
black-eyed peas
boric acid
box elder

boysenberry
bran
Brazil nut
broccoli
Brussels sprouts
buckwheat
burlap
cabbage
caddis fly
calves' liver
camel hair
canary feathers
cantaloupe
caracul
caraway seed
carbon paper
cardamom
carrot
cascara
casein
cashew nut
castor bean dust
cattail
cattle hair
cauliflower
cedar
celery
chalk
chamois
cheese
cherry
chestnut
chicken feathers
chicle
chicory
chigger
chili pepper
chives
chocolate
chromium
chrysanthemum
cinnamon
citron
citrus fruit fly
clam
cleansing tissue
clove
clover
cobalt
cocoa
cocobola wood
coconut
cocklebur
cod liver
coffee
cola drinks
copper
cork
corn (food, dust, silk)
cornmeal
corn silk
cornstarch
cosmos
cotton
cotton linters
cottonseed
cottonwood
crab
crabapple
cranberry
crappie
cucumber
currant
curry
cypress
Dacron
daffodil
dahlia
daisy
dandelion
danders of various animals (horses, cats, dogs, rabbits, guinea pigs, bats, gerbils, hamsters)
dates
DDT
deer fly
deer hair
derris root
dill
dock
dogwood
duck
egg
eggplant
elk hair
elm
endive
ermine
eucalyptus
evaporated milk
excelsior
feathers
fern
fiberglass
figs
filbert
fir
firebush (burning bush, kochia)
fish
fish oil
flax
flaxseed
flea
formalin
fox
frog legs
fungus
fur dander
garlic
gelatin
ginger
gladiola
glue
goat (milk, hair)
gold
goldenrod
goose feathers
gooseberry
grain and seed dusts
grain smuts
grapefruit
grapes
grasses
greasewood
guinea pig hair
gum
gum acacia
gum karaya
gum tragacanth
hackberry
hair tonic
hazelnut
hemlock
hemp
henna
herring
hibiscus
hickory
hog hair
honey
honeydew melon
hops
hornet
horsehair
horseradish
horse serum
house dust
housefly
huckleberry
human hair
iceplant
iodine
juniper berry
jute
kale
kapok
karaya gum
kidney bean
Kleenex
kohlrabi
lamb
lanolin
leather
leek
lemon
lentil
lettuce
licorice
lilac
lily
lima bean
lime
linen
linseed oil
liver
llama wool
lobster
loganberry
locust
lycopodium
mahogany
malt
manganese
maple
maple sugar
marigold
marmot

marsh elder
mattress hair
may fly
(Mormon fly)
menthol
mercury
mesquite
milk (cow, goat)
milkweed floss
milldust
mink
mint
mite
mockorange
mohair
molds
mosquito
moths
mugwort
mule dander
mushroom
mushroom fly
muskrat
mustard
mutton
naphthol
nectarine
neomycin
nettle
newspaper
nickel
nutmeg
nuts
nylon
oak
oat
oil of bergamot
oil of cade
oil from flowers,
fruits, trees,
shrubs or vines
okra
olive (green,
ripe)
onion
opossum
orange
Orlon
orris root
ostrich feathers
ox hair
oyster
ozite
pablum
paint
palm
paprika
parakeet feathers
parsley
parsnip
peas
peach
peanut
pear
pecan
penicillin
pepper (black,
green, red)
peppermint
Persian lamb
persimmon
petrolatum
phenol
phenobarbital
pickleweed
pigeon feathers
pigweed
pimento
pine
pineapple
pistachio
plantain
plum (prune)
pomegranate
popcorn
popcorn chaff
poplar
poppy
pork
Postum
potato
poultry dust
powdered food
privet
psyllium seed
pumpkin
pussy willow
pyrethrum
quince seed
quinine
rabbit hair
raccoon
radish
ragweed
raisin
raspberry
rayon
redwood
resorcin
rhubarb
rice
rose
rotenone
rust of wheat
rutabaga
rye
safflower
sage
sagebrush
salicylic acid
sardines
sawdust
scale
scallops
sesame
shadscale
sheep wool
shrimp
silk
silver
sisal
skunk
smut
snapdragon
soybean
spinach
spruce
squash
squirrel
strawberry
stringbean
sugar
sugar beet
sulfathiazole
sulfur
sunflower
sweetbreads
sweet potato
swiss chard
sycamore
tamarack
tangerine
tapioca
tea
teakwood
terramycin
thyme
timothy
tobacco (dust,
smoke)
tomato
tragacanth gum
tree of heaven
trout
tulip
tunafish
turkey
turmeric
turnip
turpentine
twine
upholstery dust
vanilla
varnish
veal
venison
vitamins
walnut
wasp
watercress
water hemp
watermelon
wheat
willow
wood
wormseed
wormwood
yak hair
yams
yeast (baker's or
brewer's)
yellow jacket
youngberry
zinc

Appendix B

INSTRUCTIONS FOR GIVING SELF-INJECTIONS

Many doctors will allow patients to give their own shots, but others feel that injections should be given in a doctor's office. If your doctor allows you to give your own injections, here are directions to follow.

INSTRUCTIONS FOR GIVING DESENSITIZATION INJECTIONS

The injections are to be given *twice* a week for two months and then *once* a week or according to whatever other schedule your doctor gives you. It is absolutely imperative that you always give absolutely the *exact* amount he specifies for each dose.

1. Assemble needle and syringe. We recommend the use of a 1-cc tuberculin syringe and a 26-gauge ⅜-inch needle.
2. Boil for 20 minutes in distilled water.
3. Take pan off fire, gently pour off excess water, and allow to cool.
4. Wipe top of antigen vial with alcohol, express water from syringe, then insert needle and withdraw the specified amount from the treatment vial.
5. Wipe area to be injected with alcohol (upper outer part of either arm).

6. With a quick thrust or jab, holding syringe like a pencil and holding the skin tight, go straight through the skin. The needle should not go in at more than a 45-degree angle, so it will be deep in the tissues and still not in the muscle.
7. Gently draw back on the plunger, and if no blood is seen, inject the entire amount. If any blood is noted, withdraw the needle and use a slightly different area for the injection.
8. Rinse the syringe with water five times and separate the plunger to prevent sticking.
9. Reactions to antigens seldom occur and usually are mild. However, in the event of a reaction, there may be a red, slightly swollen area around the site of the injection. If the reaction is larger than a fifty-cent piece, you should notify your doctor, so that he may advise you concerning the amounts of subsequent injections. If more than a local reaction is noted, take a dose of your antihistamine and notify him immediately.
10. Many physicians prefer disposable syringes.

INSTRUCTIONS FOR GIVING EPINEPHRINE (ADRENALIN)

Some physicians allow asthma patients to give their own injections of epinephrine (Adrenalin).

Obtain from your pharmacy (by prescription):
One 1-cc tuberculin syringe.
Two 26-gauge ⅜-inch needles.
One 30-cc vial of watery epinephrine (Adrenalin), 1:1,000.

1. Assemble needle and syringe.
2. Boil for 20 minutes in distilled water.
3. Take pan off fire, gently pour off excess water, and allow to cool. Then express excess water from syringe.
4. Wipe top of epinephrine vial three times with alcohol, then insert needle and withdraw the amount to be given.
5. Wipe area to be injected with alcohol (upper outer part of either arm.)
6. With a quick thrust or jab, holding syringe like a pencil and holding the skin tight, go straight through the skin. The needle should not go in at more than a 45-degree angle, so that it will be deep in the tissues and still not in the muscle.
7. Gently draw back on the plunger, and if no blood is seen, inject the entire amount. If any blood is noted, withdraw the needle and use a different area for the injection.
8. Rinse the syringe with water five times and remove the plunger to prevent sticking.

If the symptoms are persistent or recur, it is often necessary to repeat the dose one to four times at 30- to 45-minute intervals. You may then wait two hours and repeat injections, if necessary. If there is no improvement after repeated doses, contact your physician.

Appendix **C**

ANTIHISTAMINE PREPARATIONS

Different antihistamines often have different uses and show some variations in properties. We summarize the antihistamines, their properties, uses and occasional side effects here. You will use antihistamines only on your doctor's advice, of course, since most of them are prescription drugs.

The generic name of the drug is given first; then the trade names of the antihistamine as available from the various pharmaceutical manufacturers is given in parenthesis.

We list all forms that the antihistamine drugs are available in; however, we do not recommend the use of antihistamine ointments, creams or lotions for local application to the skin.

CARBINOXAMINE MALEATE (Clistin)

A potent antihistamine producing low incidence of drowsiness. Does not potentiate epinephrine (Adrenalin) or exhibit local anesthetic action. Available in elixir; tablets; and repeat action tablets. (McNeil Laboratories.)

DIPENHYDRAMINE HYDROCHLORIDE (Benadryl Hydrochloride)

Useful antihistamine, but incidence of sedation high. Mild anticough and antinausea effects. May be antihistamine of choice for intravenous use or injection in anaphylactic reaction. Less gastric irritation than other antihistamines. Foot dermatitis has been reported. May have additive effect with sedatives, hypnotics or antianxiety agents administered concomitantly. Caution needed with parenteral use in patients with hypertension or cardiac diseases, since high doses may elevate blood pressure or cause rapid pulse. Capsules; elixir; solution for injection; tablets (delayed action). (Parke Davis & Co.)

DOXYLAMINE SUCCINATE (Decapryn Succinate)
Potent antihistamine, but high incidence of sedation. Vertigo and nervousness occur rarely. Syrup; tablets. (Wm. S. Merrell Co.)

ANTAZOLINE PHOSPHATE (Antistine Phosphate)
Used in eyes for symptomatic relief of tearing, light sensitivity, redness, swelling and itching. Milder and less irritating to tissues than other antihistamines. Except for mild stinging, untoward effects rarely encountered. One or two drops in each eye every three or four hours. (Ciba Pharmaceutical Co.)

CHLOROTHEN CITRATE (Tagathen)
Major untoward effects are sedation and gastrointestinal irritation. Tablets. (Lederle Laboratories.)

METHAPYRILENE HYDROCHLORIDE (Dozar, Histadyl, Semikon Hydrochloride)
Antihistamine with rapid onset, but short duration of action. Moderate sedative effect. Ingredient of many over-the-counter sedative mixtures. Topical preparations not recommended. Capsules; elixir; solution (injection); syrup; tablets; creams; lotions; ointments. (Massengill; Eli Lilly & Co.; A. J. Tutag & Co.)

PYRILAMINE MALEATE (Copsamine, Neo-Antergan Maleate, Paraminyl Maleate, Pyra-Maleate, Pyramal Maleate, Stamine, Stangen Maleate, Statonium Maleate, Thylogen Maleate)
Effective antihistamine with low incidence of sedation. Sometimes causes loss of appetite, nausea and vomiting. Capsules; tablets. (Buffington, Inc.; Van Pelt & Brown, Inc.; Columbus Pharmacol Co.; Paul B. Elder; A. J. Tutag & Co.; Physicians Drug Supply; Bowman Brothers Drug Co.; S. F. Durst & Co.; Merck Sharp & Dohme; Rorer, Inc.)

TRIPELENNAMINE CITRATE AND TRIPELENNAMINE HYDROCHLORIDE (Pyribenzamine)
Potent antihistamine with low incidence of side effects. Major side effect is sedation, but occasionally causes excitation. Mild gastrointestinal effects and mild to moderate dizziness frequent. Sudden deaths have occurred in addicts taking this agent and paregoric concomitantly. Rare instances of anemia and other blood disturbances. Elixir; nasal spray; solution (injection); tablets; delayed action tablets; sustained release tablets; cream; ointment. (Ciba Pharmaceutical Co.)

THONZYLAMINE HYDROCHLORIDE (Neo-hetramine Hydrochloride)

Larger doses necessary to effect antihistaminic response, but more free of sedative and atropinelike properties than many others. Syrup; tablets. (Warner-Chilcott.)

BROMPHENIRAMINE MALEATE (Dimetane)
Effective antihistamine. Principal side effects are drowsiness and skin rash. Elixir; solution (injection); tablets; sustained release tablets. (Robins.)

CHLORCYCLIZINE HYDROCHLORIDE (Di-Paralene Hydrochloride, Perazil)
Effective antihistamine with prolonged action (twelve or more hours) that peaks at three to four hours. Sedation most frequent adverse effect. Tablets. (Abbott Laboratories; Burroughs-Wellcome & Co.)

CHLORPHENIRAMINE MALEATE (Chlor-Trimeton Maleate, Teldrin, Histapan)
Effective antihistamine with low incidence of side effects. Drowsiness most common side effect. Solution (injection); syrup; tablets; repeat action tablets; sustained release capsules. (U.S. Vitamin Corp.; Smith Kline & French; Schering Corp.)

CLEMIZOLE HYDROCHLORIDE (Allecur)
Effective antihistamine with rapid onset of action. Drowsiness occurs in 5 to 10 percent of patients. Weakness, nausea, and burning sensation in chest have occurred rarely. Tablets. (Roerig.)

DESBROMPHENIRAMINE MALEATE (Disomer)
Effective antihistamine for hayfever, dizziness and dermatitis. Most common side effect is drowsiness; a few cases of skin rash have been reported. Syrup; tablets; repeat action tablets. (White Laboratories.)

DEXCHLORPHENIRAMINE MALEATE (Polaramine Maleate)
Effective antihistamine with low incidence of side effects. Most common side effect is drowsiness. Syrup; repeat action tablets. (Schering Corp.)

DIMETHINDENE MALEATE (Forhistal Maleate)
Potent antihistamine. May control itching whether of local, allergic, or systemic origin. Drowsiness frequent. Drops; syrup; tablets; sustained-release tablets. (Ciba Pharmaceutical Co.)

PHENIRAMINE MALEATE (Trimenton Maleate)
Effective antihistamine. Most common side effect is sedation. Elixir; tablets. (Schering Corp.)

PYROBUTAMINE PHOSPHATE (Pyronil)
Effective antihistamine with low incidence of sedation and other side effects. Because of relatively prolonged action, one or two doses daily may be sufficient. Tablets. (Eli Lilly & Co.)

TRIPROLIDINE HYDROCHLORIDE (Actidil)
Effective antihistamine. Action rapid in onset and persists about twelve hours. Low incidence of side effects, most common is sedation. Syrup; tablets. (Burroughs-Wellcome & Co.)

METHDILAZINE AND METHDILAZINE HYDROCHLORIDE (Tacaryl)

Effective antihistamine. Relieves itching and skin rashes of various origins. Drowsiness frequent. Dizziness, nausea, headache, and dry mouth occur infrequently. Syrup; tablets; chewable tablets. (Mead Johnson Co.)

PROMETHAZINE HYDROCHLORIDE (Phenergan Hydrochloride)
Potent antihistamine originally introduced for treatment of allergic conditions, but pronounced depressant effect on central nervous system has led to decrease in such use. Side effects of tremors, spasticity, jaundice, blood upsets, low blood pressure and visual disturbances and dermatitis have been reported. Sedatives, hypnotics, anesthetics and narcotics should be reduced when they are given concomitantly with this agent. Development of photosensitization is contraindication to further treatment. Solution (injection); syrup; suppositories (rectal); tablets. (Wyeth Laboratories.)

TRIMEPRAZINE TARTATE (Temaril)
Similar to promazine. Antihistamine action effective in relieving itching accompanying skin allergies of various origins. Jaundice, blood disorders, tremors and spasticity have occurred rarely. Drowsiness most frequent side effect. Sustained release capsules; syrup; tablets. (Smith, Kline & French Laboratories.)

CYPROHEPTADINE HYDROCHLORIDE (Periactin Hydrochloride)
Antihistaminic agent used to relieve itching associated with skin disorders such as allergic dermatitis, hives and neurodermatitis and to relieve symptoms of hayfever. Drowsiness is most common side effect. Several studies suggest it accelerates weight gain and stimulates growth in children, especially those with asthma. However, most patients lose weight when it is discontinued. Syrup; tablets. (Merck Sharp & Dohme.)

PHENINDAMINE TARTRATE (Thephorin Tartrate)
Unlike other antihistamines, most common side effect is stimulation. Principal symptoms are nausea, palpitation and nervousness; more severe excitation may result in vomiting and insomnia. However, a few patients have experienced sedative effects. Tablets. (Roche Laboratories.)

ACTIFIED
Combines the antihistamine triprolidine hydrochloride and the stimulant pseudoephedrine hydrochloride. Syrup; tablet. (Burroughs-Wellcome & Co.)

CO-PYRONIL
Combines antihistamines methapyrilene hydrochloride (fast-acting, short duration) and pyrrobutamine phosphate (slow-acting, long duration), with a stimulant agent, cyclopentamine hydrochloride, which has nasal decongestant properties. Drowsiness common effect. Suspension; capsules: pediatric capsules. (Eli Lilly Co.)

DEMAZIN
Combines the antihistamine chlorpheniramine maleate and the stimulant phenylephrine hydrochloride. Tablets; syrup. (Schering Corp.)

DIMETANE EXPECTORANT
Contains an antihistamine (brompheniramine maleate), two stimulants

(phenylephrine hydrochloride and phenylpropanolamine hydrochloride) and an expectorant (glyceryl guaiacolate). Dimetane Expectorant-DC also contains codeine. Elixir; tablets; solution (injection). (A. H. Robins Co.)

DIMETAPP
Combines the antihistamine brompheniramine maleate with two stimulants, phenylephrine hydrochloride and phenylpropanolamine hydrochloride. Elixir; tablets. (A. H. Robins Co.)

DISOPHROL
Combines the antihistamine dexbrompheniramine maleate with the stimulant *d*-isoephedrine. Tablets. (White Laboratories.)

NALDECON
Combines antihistamines (phenyltoloxamine citrate and chlorpheniramine maleate) with stimulants (phenylephrine hydrochloride and phenylpropanolamine hydrochloride). Drowsiness reported frequently. Syrup; sustained-release tablets. (Bristol Laboratories.)

NOVAHISTINE
Contains the antihistamine chlorpheniramine maleate and the stimulant phenylephrine hydrochloride. Other ingredients present in certain of the dosage forms include chloroform, menthol, codeine, glyceryl and acetaminophen. Capsules; tablets; elixir. (Pitman-Moore Co.)

ORNADE AND TUSS-ORNADE
Combines antihistaminic agent chlorpheniramine maleate and stimulant phenylpropanolamine hydrochloride and anticholinergic agent isopropamide iodide, which has a drying effect. Tuss-Ornade contains the anticough agent caramiphen edisylate in addition. Delayed release capsules. (Smith, Kline & French Laboratories.)

TRIAMINIC
Combines antihistaminic agents (pheniramine maleate and pyrilamine maleate) with stimulant (phenylpropanolamine hydrochloride). Drowsiness, blurred vision, palpitations of the heart, flushing, nervousness or gastrointestinal upset may occur occasionally. Liquid (expectorant); timed-release tablets; pediatric tablets. (Dorsey Laboratories.)

CORIFORTE
A mixture contains antihistaminic agent (chlorpheniramine maleate), and salicylamide, phenacetin, methamphetamine, caffeine and ascorbic acid. Capsules. (Schering Corp.)

EMPRAZIL
Contains antihistamine (chlorcyclizine hydrochloride), stimulant (pseudoephedrine hydrochloride), and phenacetin, aspirin and caffeine. Tablets. (Burroughs-Wellcome & Co.)

HYCOMINE
Contains stimulant (phenylephrine hydrochloride), anticough agent (hydrocodone bitartrate) and bronchodilator (homatropine methylbromide). In addition, the syrup contains antihistamine (pyrilamine maleate), and ammonium chloride and sodium citrate; and the tablet

contains antihistamine (chlorpheniramine maleate), and acetaminophen and caffeine. (Endo Laboratories.)

SINUTAB

Contains antihistaminic agent (phenyltoloxamine citrate), stimulant (phenylpropanolamine hydrochloride), and acetaminophen and phenacetin. Tablets. (Warner-Chilcott Laboratories.)

TETREX-APC WITH BRISTAMIN

This mixture contains antihistamine (phenyltoloxamine citrate), antibiotic (tetracycline phosphate), aspirin, phenacetin and caffeine.

TRISULFAMINIC

A mixture containing antihistaminic agents (pheniramine maleate and pyrilamine maleate), stimulants (phenylephrine hydrochloride), and trisulfapyrimidines. Suspension; tablets. (Dorsey Laboratories.)

ARISTOMIN

A mixture containing antihistamine (chlorpheniramine maleate), corticosteroid (triamcinolene) and ascorbic acid. As with other adrenal corticosteroids, the dose should be individualized to achieve result with a minimum of side effects, especially in prolonged therapy. Capsules. (Lederle Laboratories.)

DRONACTIN

A mixture containing antihistamine (cyproheptadine hydrochloride) and adrenal corticosteroid (dexamethasone) for various skin allergies. As with other adrenal corticosteroids, the dose should be individualized to achieve the desired result with a minimum of side effects, especially in prolonged therapy. Tablets. (Merck Sharp & Dohme.)

METRETON

A mixture containing antihistamine (chlorpheniramine maleate). The nasal spray also contains adrenal corticosteroid (prednisolone acetate), and the tablet contains prednisone and ascorbic acid. Promoted by various allergic and inflammatory conditions. As with other adrenal corticosteroids, the dose must be individualized to achieve the desired result with a minimum of side effects, especially in prolonged therapy. Nasal spray; tablets; eyedrops. (Schering Corp.)

Appendix D

MANUFACTURERS OF OTHER ALLERGY PRODUCTS

AR-EX PRODUCTS CO.
Chicago, Illinois 60607

Hypoallergenic cosmetics. Safe-Suds, a hypoallergenic household detergent.

ARNAR-STONE LABORATORIES, INC.
Mount Prospect, Illinois 60056

Hazel-Balm—witch hazel and lanolin in aerosol form. Hazel-Balm H-C—witch hazel, lanolin and hydrocortisone for dermatosis accompanied by inflammation. Silicote—a skin protectant containing silicones.

BORCHERDT COMPANY
Chicago, Illinois 60612

Maltsupex, an extract of barley, acts on the intestinal bacteria. Dietary aid for chronic constipation and intractable pruritus ani and bowel upsets following antibiotic therapy.

BREON LABORATORIES
90 Park Avenue
New York, New York 10016

Bronkotabs, tablets for asthma. Bronkosol, a bronchodilator.

BURROUGHS WELLCOME & CO. INC.
Tuckahoe, New York 10707
Mantadil Cream for relief of itching and inflammation.

COOPER LABORATORIES
Mystic, Connecticut 06355
Elixophyllin-Kl, a medicine for asthma, bronchitis and emphysema. Sus-Phrine, a form of epinephrine.

DARA LABORATORIES
Dallas, Texas 75247
Dermatological preparations including Dara Soapless Shampoo, Wibi Lubricating Lotion, Ramel Soap, Gerd Lubricating Lotion, Clesk Cleansing Lotion, Dara Bath Luxuriant, Tropsor, Dy-O-Derm, Ver-Var, and Ver-Acid.

DERMIK LABORATORIES, INC.
Syosset, New York 11791
Tenda-HC and Tenda Creams—protective and therapeutic barrier creams for detergent dermatitis and hand eczema. Steroid creams—Hytone, Vytome, Neo-Hytone, Ze-Tone, Formtone-HC and Ze-Tar-Quin.

DOAK PHARMACAL COMPANY, INC.
Westbury, L.I., New York 11590
Tar distillate "Doak."

DORSEY LABORATORIES, INC.
South Norwalk, Connecticut
Mellobath (bath oil). A protective emollient cream, Aquophor. Nivea Creme, Nivea Skin Oil and Basis Soap.

ELI LILLY AND COMPANY
Indianapolis, Indiana 46206
Cordran, a cream for dermatitis, also available on tape.

KNOLL PHARMACEUTICAL COMPANY
Orange, New Jersey 07051
Quadrinal, a bronchodilator and expectorant.

LAMOND PRODUCTS, INC.
Brooklyn, New York 11225
Dermasorcin Lotion, Dermasul Lotion, Dermastringe, Bentical Shake Lotion, Aquol Bath Oil, Sebanatar and Sebana Shampoos, Lamotane Topical and Sunprotectol.

LEVER BROTHERS
New York, New York
Dove and Phase III, neutral, nonalkaline cleansing bars that help maintain the skin's natural barriers against infection.

MARCELLE
New York, New York 10017
Hypoallergenic cosmetics.

MEAD JOHNSON LABORATORIES
Evansville, Indiana
Pro Sobee, a milk-free soy protein for infants.

MERCK SHARP AND DOHME
West Point, Pennsylvania 19486
Turbinaire Decadron Phosphate, a topical steroid in spray form.

McNEIL LABORATORIES, INC.
Fort Washington, Pennsylvania
Tylenol, a analgesic tablet for people sensitive to aspirin.

NEUTROGENA CORP.
Santa Monica, California 90405
Neutrogenia, a water-soluble soap containing no free alkali.

THE PROCTER AND GAMBLE COMPANY
Cincinnati, Ohio 45201
Safeguard, a non-hexachlorophene, antibacterial bar soap.

REVLON
New York, New York 10019
ZP11, antidandruff hair-dressing with zinc pyrithione for seborrheic dermatitis of the scalp.

RIKER LABORATORIES
Northridge, California 91324
Medihaler-Epi, an aerosol form of epinephrine. Duovent for asthma.

ROSS LABORATORIES
Columbus, Ohio 43216
Similac Isomil, a soy protein formula for infant feeding. Rondee, a decongestant for eustachian tubes.

SARDEAU INC.
Kenilworth, New Jersey 07033
Sardo Bath, Sardoettes, and Sardo Soap for dry, itchy, scaly skin conditions.

SCHERING CORPORATION
Union, New Jersey 07083
Afrin, a nasal spray decongestant. Valisone, an ointment for eczema and other dermatitis.

SCHIEFFELIN & CO.
New York, New York 10017
Almay hypoallergenic cosmetics.

SHEPARD LABORATORIES
Fort Washington, Pennsylvania 19034
Shepard's Cosmetics for care of dry skin. Shepard's Cream Lotion, Hand Cream, Dry Skin Cream and Cold Cream; and mildly scented superfatted Soap.

SYNTEX LABORATORIES, INC.
Palo Alto, California 94304
Synalar (fluocinolone acetonide), topical corticosteroid for skin inflammations.

WARNER-CHILCOTT
Morris Plains, New Jersey 07950

Tedral, a tablet of theophylline, ephedrine and phenobarbital for asthma and bronchitis. Sinubid for sinus problems.

WESTWOOD PHARMACEUTICALS
Buffalo, New York 14213

Dermatological products: Alpha-Keri, Keri Lotion, Fostex Cream, Fostex Cake, Fostril, Sebulex, Lowila Cake, for dandruff, acne, dry and itchy skin and sensitivities to soap.

Appendix E

WHERE TO GO TO ESCAPE RAGWEED

■ RAGWEED POLLEN INDEX FOR INDIVIDUAL CITIES AND TOWNS

(Compiled by Oren C. Durham, secretary, Pollen Survey Committee, American Academy of Allergy, chief botanist, Abbott Laboratories, North Chicago, Ill.)

The index figure for each community is based on three factors which directly affect individual pollen exposure: length of season, maximum aerial concentration of pollen, and total pollen catch on test slides through the season.

Any city or community having an index
above 10 is not recommended
between 5 and 10 is fairly good
below 5 is good
below 1 is excellent

ALABAMA	
Birmingham	(49)
Foley	4
Mobile	8
ALASKA	
Fairbanks	0
Juneau	0
Nome	0
ARIZONA	
Grand Canyon National Park:	
*North Rim (Fall only)	0.15
*South Rim (Fall only)	0.12
Phoenix (Fall only)	0.21
Tucson	
(Spring)	2
(Fall)	3
ARKANSAS	
Gassville	45
Little Rock	62
West Memphis	(81)

Figures in ( ) are calculated from incomplete data.
* Indicates possible exposure to sagebrush pollen.

CALIFORNIA	
Alpine	3
Arcata	3
El Centro	1
Escondido	1
Lassen Volcanic National Park	0.03
Los Angeles (Spring)	0.22
(Fall)	0.8
Monterey	0.24
Oakland	0.2
Pasadena	0.68
Sacramento	0.2
San Diego	1
San Francisco	0.2
Santa Barbara	3
Sequoia National Park	0.03
Tujunga	1.4
*Yosemite National Park	0.3

COLORADO	
Burlington	(23)
Colorado Springs	4
Denver	19
*Glenwood Springs	0.8
Mesa Verde National Park	0.5
Pikes Peak	0.9
Rocky Mountain National Park:	
*Estes Park	1
*Grand Lake	0.2

CONNECTICUT	
Bridgeport	26
Fairfield	26
Hartford	54
New Haven	25
Sherman	13
Stamford	28
Stratford	26
Waterbury	27

DELAWARE	
Wilmington	(54)

DISTRICT OF COLUMBIA	
Washington	42

FLORIDA	
Bradenton	4
Clearwater	7
Coral Gables	2
Daytona Beach	3
Everglades National Park	4
Fort Lauderdale (Beach)	6
Fort Myers	0.19
Fort Pierce	5
Gainesville	20
Jacksonville	6
Key West	0.12
Live Oak	5
Melbourne	21
Miami	2
Miami Beach	0.26
Ocala	13
Orlando	3
Panama City	32
(Sunnyside Beach)	2
Pensacola	10
(Santa Rosa Island)	0.054
St. Petersburg	4
Sebring	3
Tallahassee	6
Tampa	6
West Palm Beach	5
(Morrison Field)	31

GEORGIA	
Atlanta	24
St. Simons Island	77
Valdosta	8

IDAHO	
*Boise	5
Moscow	(0.5)
Pocatello	5
*Sun Valley	0.3

ILLINOIS	
Bloomington	89
Chicago	62
Chicago Water Crib	66
Decatur	114
East St. Louis	(100)
Elgin	73
Evanston	73
Grayslake	63
North Chicago	74
Peoria	122
Quincy	98
Rockford	98
Rock Island	113
Springfield	73
Streator	78
Urbana	80

INDIANA	
Cicero	76
East Chicago	(64)
Evansville	136
Fort Wayne	107
Indianapolis	92
Jeffersonville	(102)

IOWA	
Ames	87
Cedar Rapids	122
Council Bluffs	(148)
Des Moines	69
Iowa City	93
Waterloo	125

KANSAS	
Goodland	23
Kansas City	(101)
Wichita	58

KENTUCKY	
Covington	(122)
Lexington	151
Louisville	99
Trappist	86

LOUISIANA	
New Orleans	43
Tallulah	(33)

MAINE	
Alfred	15
Allagash	1.4
Auburn	13
Augusta	9
Bar Harbor	5
Bethel	1.6
Belfast	1.3
Boothbay Harbor	5
Camden	9

Deblois	1
Eagle Lake	2
Eastport	6
Enfield	1
Grand Lake Stream	1.4
Greenville Junction	0.35
Houlton	3
Jackman	4
Kineo	27
Lincoln	2
Machias	4
Macwahoc	0.46
Millinocket	0.38
Newagen	1
Newport	3.5
New Portland	1
North Augusta	10
Oquossoc	2
Orono	10
Poland Spring	12
Portland	24
Presque Isle	0.44
Quoddy Head	0.6
Rangeley	9
Rockland	8
St. Francis	0.09
Southport	8
Speckle Mt.	2
Stonington	12
Upper Dam	2
York	8

MARYLAND

Annapolis	32
Baltimore	51
Bethesda	65
Frederick	82
Perry Point	65
Takoma Park	(41)

MASSACHUSETTS

Amherst	25
Annisquam	3
Boston	16
Boston, Mass General Hosp.	24
Gloucester (A & G Hosp.)	7
E. Gloucester	5
W. Gloucester	5
Magnolia	5
Nantucket Island	5
Newton Center	44
Northampton	20
Rockport	5
Winchester	19
Worcester	9

MICHIGAN

Alpena	20
Ann Arbor	119
Bad Axe	40
Baldwin	41
Bay City	72
Benton Harbor	110
Big Rapids	57
Blaney	16
Boyne City	35
Cadillac	31
Charlevoix	21
Cheboygan	23
Coldwater	190
Copper Harbor	5
Crystal Falls	14
Detroit	66
East Tawas	75
Escanaba	57
Flint	76
Frankfort	65
Gaylord	54
Gladwin	99
Grand Haven	90
Grand Rapids	126
Grand Traverse	37
Grayling	52
Harbor Bay	61
Hillsdale	78
Houghton	9
Ironwood	17
Isle Royale National Park	0.29
Lake City	33
Lansing	94
Ludington	60
Mackinac Island	19
Mackinaw City	13
Mancelona	39
Manistee	54
Manistique	12
Marquette	12
Menominee	37
Mt. Pleasant	74
Munising	16
Newberry	20
Northport	25
Ontonagon	13
Owasippe	8
Petoskey	30
Port Austin	107
Powers	21
Rogers City	19
Roscommon	21
St. Ignace	8
St. Joseph	103
Sault Ste. Marie	4
Stambaugh	24
Traverse City	39
West Branch	31

MINNESOTA

Duluth	44
Minneapolis	99
Moorhead	125
Rochester	89
Tower	6
Virginia	8
Winona	124

MISSISSIPPI

Biloxi	7
Vicksburg	33

MISSOURI

Kansas City	109
St. Louis	78

MONTANA

Glacier National Park:	
Belton	0.1
Many Glacier	0.1
Miles City	4
*West Yellowstone	0.2

NEBRASKA

Lincoln	63
North Platte	13
Omaha	148
Scottsbluff	38

NEVADA

Lake Mead	
(Hoover Dam)	
(March, April)	4
(Fall)	0.3
Reno	0.1

NEW HAMPSHIRE

Bath	3
Berlin	8
Bethlehem	5
Blue Job Mt.	2
Carrol	0.9
Charlestown	14
Claremont	7
Colebrook	1.4
Concord	7
Conway	3
Crotched Mt.	5
Derby	2
Dixville	3
Dover	5
Errol	0.5
Exeter	26
Federal Hill	7
Franklin	5
Groveton	2
Hampton	4
Hillsboro	5
Hinsdale	11
Holderness	5
Jeremy	18
Keene	7
Laconia	1
Lancaster	0.75
Labanon	17
Lincoln	2
Littleton	3
Manchester	9
Moosilaukee	0.45
Nashua	29
New Ipswich	8
New London	5
North Conway	3
Ossipee	3
Pawtuckaway	0.5
Peterborough	27
Pittsburg	2
Plymouth	4
Rochester	17
Rye	15
Warren	2
Weirs	9
Whitefield	2

NEW JERSEY

Asbury Park	18
Atlantic City	30
Caldwell	88
Dover	36
East Brunswick	38
East Orange	34
Flemington	101
Fort Dix	53
Freehold	72
Haddonfield	74
Highstown	87
Jersey City	5
Linden	58
Madison	62
Maplewood	21
Marlboro	40
New Brunswick	60
Newark	18
Paterson	44
Pitman	51
Red Bank	69
Sandy Hook	39
Sparta	16
Summit	42
Teaneck	31
Trenton	26
Verona	33
Westwood	18
Wildwood	34

NEW MEXICO

Albuquerque	7
Roswell	4

NEW YORK

Metropolitan area:

Battery	27
Bronx	24
Brooklyn	22
Croton	29
Farmingdale	44
Fire Island	
(Ocean Beach)	11
Flushing	30
Garden City	28
Huntington	44
Jamaica	35
Manhattan	25
Northport	31
Pomona	26
Rockaway	40
Staten Island	30
White Plains	32
Yonkers	38

Adirondack area:

Ausable Forks	20
Big Moose	6
Blue Mt. Lake	3
Chateaugay Lake	8
Chilson	6
Elk Lake	4
Ft. Ticonderoga	21
Hague	16
Hudson Falls	37
Indian Lake	6
Inlet	8
Keene	5
Keene Valley	1
Keeseville	26
Lake George	23
Lake Kushaqua	15
Lake Placid	10
Long Lake	6
Loon Lake	5
McColloms	6
McKeever	10
Mt. McGregor	18
Newcomb	9
North Creek	20
Northville	27
Old Forge	22
Owl's Head	9
Paul Smiths	7
Port Henry	14
Raquette Lake	6
Redford	7
Sabattis	8
Santa Clara	15
Saranac Lake	
(Rogers Hosp.)	23
Saranac	19
Schroon Lake	
(Severance)	8
Speculator	12
Ticonderoga	29
Tupper Lake	8
Turin	12

Wanakena	7
Wells	13
Wilmington	16
Catskill area:	
Big Indian	4
Fleischmanns	10
Haines Falls	5
Hunter	29
Phoenicia	13
Pine Hill	5
(Funcrest)	3
Tannersville	11.
Windham	28
Zena	12
Statewide:	
Albany	48
Binghamton	31
Buffalo	54
Celoron	41
Cortland	37
Dannemora	19
East Berne	32
Elmira	43
Elsmere	49
Fairport	32
Forestburg	15
Fremont	38
Geneva	57
Gloversville	29
Hornell	34
Jamestown	65
Jeffersonville	26
Kauneonga Lake	48
Lake Huntington	23
Liberty	16
Lockport	71
Lowville	20
Mamakating	22
Margaretville	15
Minnewaska	20
Montauk	10
Monticello	24
Newburgh	40
Ogdensburg	46
Olean	42
Oneonta	33
Oswego	35
Perry	114
Port Washington	27
Remsen	40
Riverhead	70
Rochester	60
Roscoe	14
St. Regis Falls	33
Schenectady	27
South Fallsburg	47
Springville	49
Syracuse	25
Utica	32
Watertown	43
White Lake	67
Woodridge	21
Eldred (Yulan)	35

NORTH CAROLINA

Asheville	57
Charlotte	42
Great Smoky Mountains National Park: Newfound Gap	(4)
Hatteras	71
Raleigh	28

NORTH DAKOTA

Fargo	(125)

OHIO

Akron	115
Cincinnati	122
Cleveland	56
Columbus	75
Dayton	104
Toledo	122
Youngstown	77

OKLAHOMA

Fort Sill	(73)
Henryetta	(75)
Muskogee	85
Oklahoma City	73
Okmulgee	57
Pawhuska	31
Tulsa	65

OREGON

Coquille	0
Corvallis	0
Crater Lake National Park	0.1
Milton-Freeway	6
Portland	0.55
Turner	2

PENNSYLVANIA

Altoona	52
Broomall	40
Erie	65
Hatboro	48
McKeesport	95
Meadville	75
Philadelphia	55
Pittsburgh	90
Pittsburgh (Brentwood)	74

RHODE ISLAND

Block Island	31
Providence	26

SOUTH CAROLINA

Charleston	11
Columbia	40

SOUTH DAKOTA

Aberdeen	17
Mobridge	10
Pierre	14
Rapid City	12
Sioux Falls	52

TENNESSEE

Great Smoky Mountains National Park:	
Headquarters	13
Newfound Gap	4
Johnson City	51
Knoxville	49
Memphis	73
Nashville	69

TEXAS

Amarillo	41
Big Spring	5
Brownsville	24
Corpus Christi	30
Dallas	115
El Paso	15
Fort Worth	71
Galveston	36
Houston	68
San Antonio	16

UTAH

*Bryce Canyon National Park	0.9
Hurricane	4
Salt Lake City	8
Salt Lake City:	
Airport	2
Canyon Rim	18
Down Town	7
Midvale	37
South Salt Lake	2
Vernal	3
Zion National Park	0.7

VERMONT

Burlington	47

VIRGINIA

Alexandria	(41)
Charlottesville	35
Norfolk	50
Richmond	42
Roanoke	85
Shenandoah National Park:	
Big Meadows	10
Headquarters	35

WASHINGTON

Mt. Rainier National Park:	
Longmire	0
Paradise Valley	0.1
White River	0.04
Olympic National Park	0.1
Seattle	0.02
Seattle-Tacoma Airport	0
Spokane	0.1
Walla Walla	3
Wenatchee	46
Wenatchee Valley Experiment Station	84
Yakima	0.18

WEST VIRGINIA

Charleston	32
White Sulphur Springs	19

WISCONSIN

Eagle River	13
Kenosha	51
Madison	98
Milwaukee	81
Plum Island	40
Sheboygan	90
Superior	(44)

WYOMING

*Grand Teton National Park	0.1
Lander	23
Yellowstone National Park:	
*Mammoth	0.2
*W. Yellowstone (Montana)	0.2

VIRGIN ISLANDS

St. Thomas	0.025

CANADA

ALBERTA

Banff	0
Beaver Lodge	0
Calgary	0.028
Coleman	0.028
Cypress Hills	0.012
Drumheller	1
Edmonton	0
Jasper	0
Lake Louise	0.009
Lethbridge	1
*Manyberries	0.2
*Medicine Hat	7
Vermilion	0
Waterton Lakes Park	0.012

BRITISH COLUMBIA

Saanichton	0.06
*Summerland	0
Vancouver Island	1
Victoria	1.19

MANITOBA

Brandon	2
Dauphin	5
Morden	12
*Pierson	6
Riding Mountain National Park	0.155
Russell	1
The Pas	0.1
Winnipeg	7

NEW BRUNSWICK

Bathurst	0.24
Campbellton	0.06
Chipman	1.44
Dalhousie	0.4
Doaktown	0.71
Edmundston	0.90
Fredericton	0.43
Fundy Nat. Park:	
Haslam Farm	3
Waterside	5
Lakeview	3
Gagetown	11
Grand Manan	1.6
Jemseg	4.39
McAdam	1.5
Moncton	1.43
Newcastle	0.21
Perth-Andover	0.93
Pointe du Chene	9
Sackville	1.7
St. Andrews	1.2
St. George	1.09
St. John	0.9
St. Stephen	14
Shediac Cape	0.8
Sussex	2.93
Tracadie	1.9
Waterside	5
Welsford	1.13
Woodstock	0.68

NEWFOUNDLAND

Corner Brook	0.1
St. John's	0.3

NOVA SCOTIA

Antigonish	0.43
Baddeck	0.44
Cape Breton Highlands Nat. Park	0.36
Chester	0.41
Digby	4
Highlands Nat. Park	0.48
Ingonish Island	2
Kentville	5

Meteghan	3
Middle West Pubnico	0.29
Truro	0.21
Yarmouth	5

ONTARIO

Algonquin Park	16
Bancroft	8
Barry's Bay	2.2
Bellville	30
Black Sturgeon Lake	2
Blind River	3
Cedar Lake	6
Chalk River	2
Cochrane	2
Cornwall	23
Dorset	6
Espanola	3
Fort Francis	1.6
Fort William	0.11
Georgian Bay Islands National Park	16
Gravenhurst	17
Haleburton	3.20
Hamilton	89
Honey Harbor	7
Huntsville	11
Kapuskasing	0.34
Kenora (Cedar Lake)	9
Lake Joseph	4
London	40
Madoc	13
Magnetawan	5
Mallorytown	41
Mindemoya (Manitoulin Island)	8
Muskata Falls	5
New Liskeard	0.26
North Bay	8
Ottawa (district)	17
Parry Sound	19
Peterborough	35
Picton	38
Point Pelee National Park	29
Port Arthur	7
Port Carlings	9
Rosseau	3.3
Sault Ste. Marie	6
Smith Falls	19
St. Lawrence Islands National Park	38
South River	1.74
Sudbury	4
Temagami	3
Tobermory	4
Toronto	45
Metropolitan Toronto areas:	
Toronto Island	29
City Hall	42
Mimico	43
West Toronto	47
S.E. Etobicoke	54
West Scarborough	59
North Scarborough	62
S.W. Etobicoke	62
East Scarborough	65
Weston	65
Willowdale	70
Dufferin-Lawrence	72
Central Etobicoke	77
N. E. Etobicoke	114
Westport	5
Windsor	(59)

PRINCE EDWARD ISLAND

Cavendish	0.5
Charlottetown	2
Mantague	1
O'Leary	2
Prince Edward Island National Park	4
Souris	1
Summerside	1
Tignish	1

QUEBEC

Baie Saint-Paul	4
Berthierville	33
Cap-de-la-Madeleine	45
Carleton	2
Caughnawaga	58
Chandler	0.1
Charlesbourg	2
Dorval	59
Farnham	64
Father Point	1
Gaspé	0.2
Grande Riviere	0.2
Iles-de-la-Madeleine	0.1
Jonquieres (Chicoutimi)	4
Lac-des-Plages	7
Lac-des-Seize-Iles	11
Lennoxville	4
Matane	3
Matapedia	0.1
Mont-Albert Caspesiè	0.1
Mont Joli	0.2
Mont-Laurier	7
Mont Tremblant	8
Montreal	62
New Carlisle	3
Nominingue	7
Normandin	3
Outremont	29
Percé	2
Point au Trembles	36
Pointe-Claire	32
Quebec	18
Rimouski	8
Riviere-du-Loup	8
Ste-Agathe	10
Ste-Anne-de-Bellevue	42
Ste-Anne-de-la Pocatière	9
St-Jovite	6
St-Lambert	5
St-Martin	55

Sherbrooke	**26**
Tadoussac	**2**
Victoriaville	**30**

SASKATCHEWAN

Nelford	**0.1**
Prince Albert	**0.1**
Prince Albert	
National Park	**0**
Regina	**0.3**
Saskatoon	**0.51**
Scott	**0.1**
Swift Current	**1**

BERMUDA

Hamilton	**0**

CUBA

Havana	**0.2**

MEXICO

Juarez	**16**
Matamoros	**(24)**
Mexico City	**4**
Tampico	**4**
Torreon	**4**

TABLE 1

POLLEN SEASONS

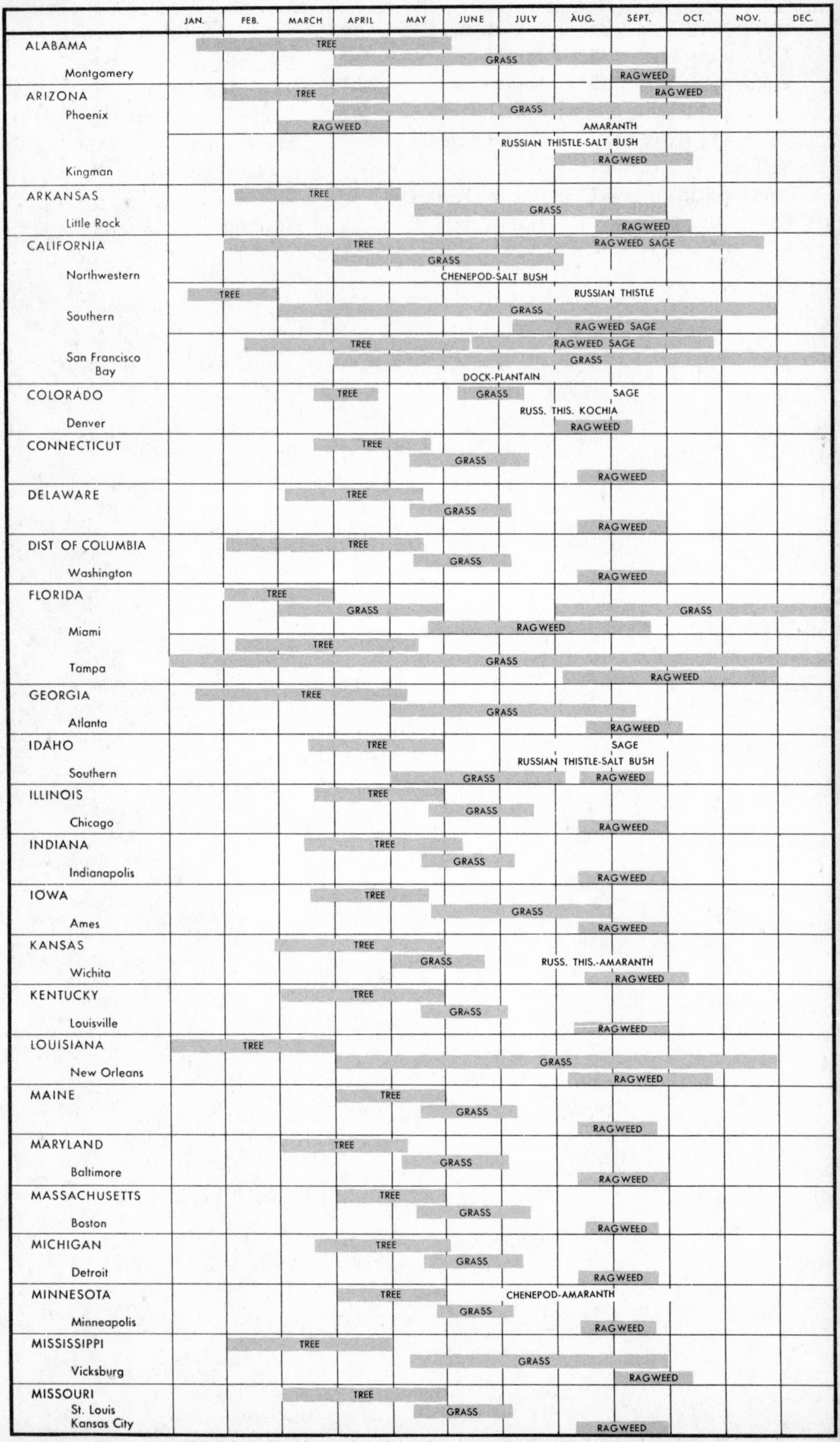

	JAN.	FEB.	MARCH	APRIL	MAY	JUNE	JULY	AUG.	SEPT.	OCT.	NOV.	DEC.
ALABAMA			TREE									
							GRASS					
Montgomery									RAGWEED			
ARIZONA			TREE							RAGWEED		
Phoenix							GRASS					
				RAGWEED				AMARANTH				
								RUSSIAN THISTLE-SALT BUSH				
									RAGWEED			
Kingman												
ARKANSAS			TREE									
							GRASS					
Little Rock									RAGWEED			
CALIFORNIA				TREE					RAGWEED SAGE			
					GRASS							
Northwestern						CHENEPOD-SALT BUSH						
		TREE							RUSSIAN THISTLE			
Southern							GRASS					
									RAGWEED SAGE			
				TREE				RAGWEED SAGE				
San Francisco Bay								GRASS				
							DOCK-PLANTAIN					
COLORADO				TREE		GRASS			SAGE			
								RUSS. THIS. KOCHIA				
Denver								RAGWEED				
CONNECTICUT				TREE								
						GRASS						
									RAGWEED			
DELAWARE				TREE								
						GRASS						
									RAGWEED			
DIST OF COLUMBIA				TREE								
						GRASS						
Washington									RAGWEED			
FLORIDA		TREE										
				GRASS						GRASS		
Miami							RAGWEED					
			TREE									
Tampa							GRASS					
										RAGWEED		
GEORGIA			TREE									
							GRASS					
Atlanta									RAGWEED			
IDAHO				TREE					SAGE			
								RUSSIAN THISTLE-SALT BUSH				
Southern						GRASS			RAGWEED			
ILLINOIS				TREE								
						GRASS						
Chicago									RAGWEED			
INDIANA				TREE								
						GRASS						
Indianapolis									RAGWEED			
IOWA				TREE								
							GRASS					
Ames									RAGWEED			
KANSAS				TREE								
					GRASS			RUSS. THIS.-AMARANTH				
Wichita									RAGWEED			
KENTUCKY				TREE								
						GRASS						
Louisville									RAGWEED			
LOUISIANA		TREE										
							GRASS					
New Orleans									RAGWEED			
MAINE					TREE							
						GRASS						
									RAGWEED			
MARYLAND				TREE								
						GRASS						
Baltimore									RAGWEED			
MASSACHUSETTS					TREE							
						GRASS						
Boston									RAGWEED			
MICHIGAN				TREE								
						GRASS						
Detroit									RAGWEED			
MINNESOTA					TREE			CHENEPOD-AMARANTH				
						GRASS						
Minneapolis									RAGWEED			
MISSISSIPPI			TREE									
							GRASS					
Vicksburg									RAGWEED			
MISSOURI				TREE								
St. Louis						GRASS						
Kansas City									RAGWEED			

TABLE 1

POLLEN SEASONS

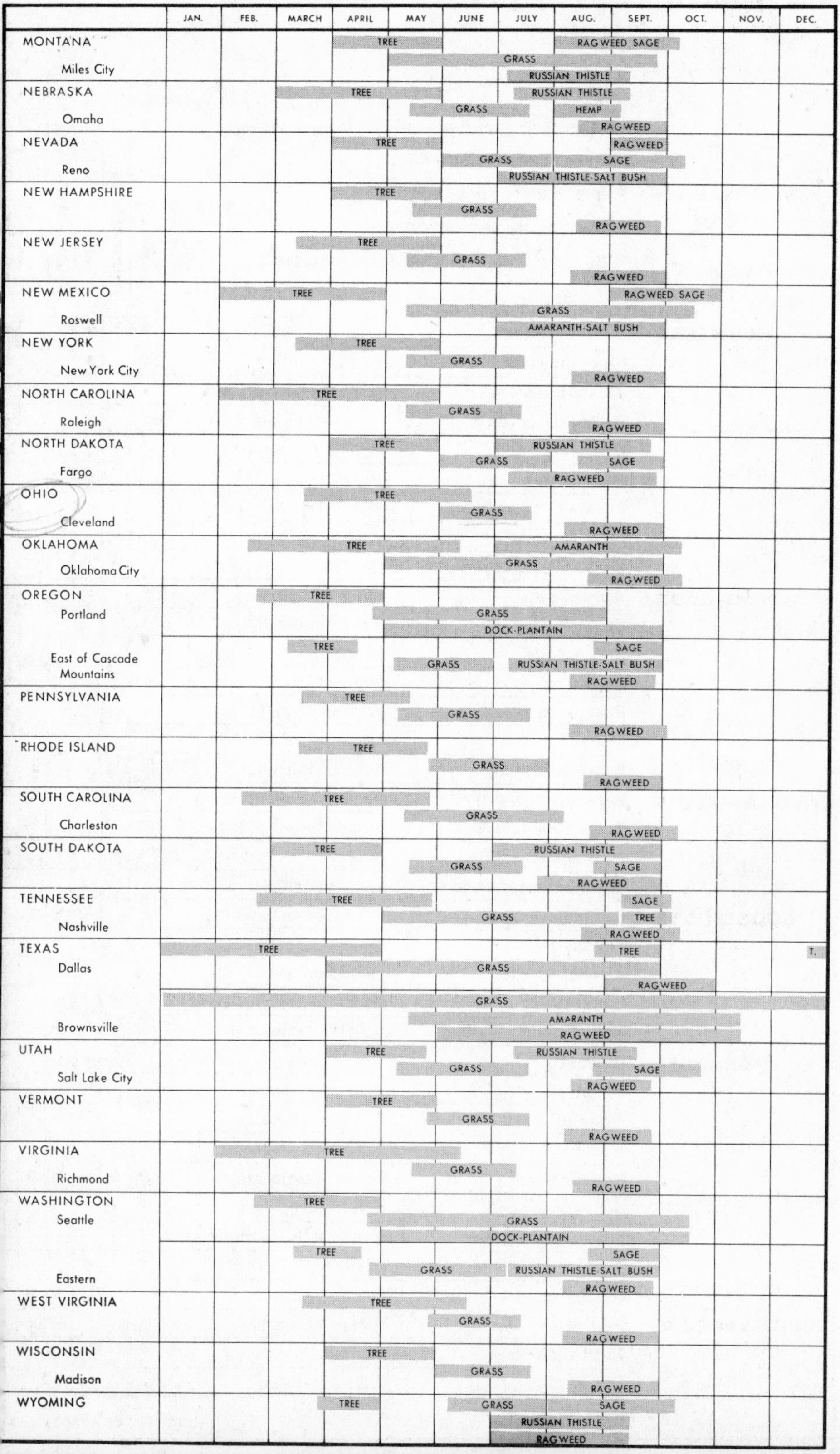

	JAN.	FEB.	MARCH	APRIL	MAY	JUNE	JULY	AUG.	SEPT.	OCT.	NOV.	DEC.
MONTANA				TREE					RAGWEED SAGE			
							GRASS					
Miles City								RUSSIAN THISTLE				
NEBRASKA				TREE				RUSSIAN THISTLE				
						GRASS		HEMP				
Omaha									RAGWEED			
NEVADA				TREE					RAGWEED			
						GRASS			SAGE			
Reno								RUSSIAN THISTLE-SALT BUSH				
NEW HAMPSHIRE				TREE								
						GRASS						
									RAGWEED			
NEW JERSEY				TREE								
						GRASS						
									RAGWEED			
NEW MEXICO			TREE						RAGWEED SAGE			
							GRASS					
Roswell								AMARANTH-SALT BUSH				
NEW YORK				TREE								
						GRASS						
New York City									RAGWEED			
NORTH CAROLINA			TREE									
						GRASS						
Raleigh									RAGWEED			
NORTH DAKOTA				TREE				RUSSIAN THISTLE				
						GRASS			SAGE			
Fargo								RAGWEED				
OHIO				TREE								
						GRASS						
Cleveland									RAGWEED			
OKLAHOMA				TREE				AMARANTH				
							GRASS					
Oklahoma City									RAGWEED			
OREGON			TREE									
Portland						GRASS						
							DOCK-PLANTAIN					
			TREE						SAGE			
East of Cascade Mountains						GRASS		RUSSIAN THISTLE-SALT BUSH				
									RAGWEED			
PENNSYLVANIA				TREE								
						GRASS						
									RAGWEED			
RHODE ISLAND				TREE								
						GRASS						
									RAGWEED			
SOUTH CAROLINA				TREE								
						GRASS						
Charleston									RAGWEED			
SOUTH DAKOTA			TREE					RUSSIAN THISTLE				
						GRASS			SAGE			
								RAGWEED				
TENNESSEE				TREE					SAGE			
							GRASS		TREE			
Nashville									RAGWEED			
TEXAS		TREE							TREE			T.
Dallas						GRASS						
										RAGWEED		
						GRASS						
								AMARANTH				
Brownsville								RAGWEED				
UTAH				TREE				RUSSIAN THISTLE				
Salt Lake City						GRASS			SAGE			
									RAGWEED			
VERMONT					TREE							
						GRASS						
									RAGWEED			
VIRGINIA				TREE								
Richmond						GRASS						
									RAGWEED			
WASHINGTON			TREE									
Seattle							GRASS					
							DOCK-PLANTAIN					
				TREE					SAGE			
					GRASS			RUSSIAN THISTLE-SALT BUSH				
Eastern									RAGWEED			
WEST VIRGINIA				TREE								
						GRASS						
									RAGWEED			
WISCONSIN				TREE								
						GRASS						
Madison									RAGWEED			
WYOMING				TREE			GRASS		SAGE			
								RUSSIAN THISTLE				
								RAGWEED				

TABLE 2

Geographic incidence of the more common weed and grass pollens.

● Important species

○ Species of minor importance

★ Species of local or occasional importance

			Alabama: Birmingham	Arizona: Phoenix	Arkansas: Little Rock	California: Los Angeles	San Francisco	Colorado: Denver
RAGWEEDS	Short ragweed	Ambrosia elatior	●		●			●
	Giant ragweed	Ambrosia trifida	●		●			●
	Western ragweed	Ambrosia psilostachya				★	●	●
	Southern ragweed	Ambrosia bidentata			★			
	Cocklebur	Xanthium commune	○		○		○	○
	Marsh elder	Iva ciliata						
	Burweed marsh elder	Iva xanthifolia						●
	False ragweed	Franseria acanthicarpa				●		
	Slender false ragweed	Franseria tenuifolia		○				
WORMWOODS	Annual sage	Artemisia annua	○					
	Biennial sage	Artemisia biennis						
	Prairie sage	Artemisia ludoviciana						○
	Sagebrush	Artemisia tridentata				★		●
	Pasture sage	Artemisia frigida						●
	Tall wormwood	Artemisia caudata						
	Sand sagebrush	Artemisia filifolia						○
CARELESSWEEDS	Pigweed (redroot)	Amaranthus retroflexus	○		○		○	○
	Spiny amaranth	Amaranthus spinosus	○		○			
	Palmer's amaranth	Amaranthus palmeri		●		●		○
	Western water hemp	Acnida tamariscina						○
GOOSEFOOTS	Lamb's quarters	Chenopodium album	○		○	○	○	○
	Firebush	Kochia scoparia						●
	Russian thistle	Salsola pestifer		★		●		●
	Sugar beet	Beta vulgaris		●				
	Shadscale	Atriplex canescens		★		○		○
GRASSES	Bluegrass	Poa pratensis			●	★	★	●
	Timothy	Phleum pratense			●			●
	Orchard grass	Dactylis glomerata			●		○	★
	Redtop	Agrostis palustris						
	Bermuda grass	Capriola dactylon	●	●	○	●	●	
	Johnson grass	Holcus halepensis	○	○	○	○		
	Sweet vernal grass	Anthoxanthum odoratum						
	Corn	Zea mays	○		○			
	Rye grass	Lolium perenne				●	●	
MISCELLANEOUS	Red sorrel	Rumex acetosella	○		○	○		
	English plantain	Plantago lanceolata	○		○	○	●	
	Hemp	Cannabis sativa						

COURTESY OF ABBOTT LABC

Miami	Tampa	**Georgia:** Atlanta	Savannah	**Idaho:** Boise	**Illinois:** Chicago	Springfield	**Indiana:** Indianapolis	**Iowa:** Des Moines	Sioux City	**Kansas:** Dodge City	Wichita	**Kentucky:** Louisville	**Louisiana:** New Orleans	Shreveport	**Maine:** Portland	**Maryland:** Baltimore	**Massachusetts:** Boston	**Michigan:** Detroit	Sault Ste. Marie	**Minnesota:** Duluth	Minneapolis	Moorhead	**Mississippi:** Jackson	**Missouri:** Joplin	Kansas City	St. Louis	**Montana:** Miles City	**Nebraska:** Lincoln
○	●	●	●		●	●	●	●	●	●	●	●	●	●	●	●	●	●	●	●	●	●	●	●	●	●	○	●
		●			●	●	●	●	●	●	●	●	●	●		●		●		●	●	●	●	●	●	●		●
				○						●	○											○					○	○
						○								○										●	★	○		
○		○	○		○	○	○	○	○	○	○	○	○	○	○	○	○	○		○	○	○	○	○	○	○		
											★		●	○									○	○	○	○		●
				●	●				●	★										○	●	●			○		●	●
				○						○																	○	
		○			○		○					○						○							○			
					○													○	○	○	○							
										○											○	○						○
				●																							●	
																						○						
		○	○	○	○	○	○	○	○	○	○	○	○	○	○	○	○	○	○	○	○	○	○	○	○	○	○	○
		○	○										○	○		○							○		○	○		
					○	○		●	●	●	●										○				●	●		●
		○	○	○	○	○	○	○	○		○	○	○	○	○	○	○	○	○	○	○	○	○	○	○	○	○	○
					★			●	●	●	○							○			○	○			○	○		●
				●	★			○		●	○							○			★	●					●	○
				●																								
				●	●	●	●	●	●	○	●	●			●	●	●	●	●	●	●	●		●	●	●	●	●
				●	●	●	●	●	●	○	●	●			●	●	●	●	●	●	●	●		●	●	●		●
				★	●	●	●	●			○	●			●	●	●	●	○		●	○			●	●	●	●
				★	○	○	○	○			○	○			●	●	●	○	●		●	○			●	●		●
●	●	●	●								○		●	●									●	○				
○	○	○	○										○	○									○	○				
															●	●	●											
		○			○	○	○	○	○	○	○	○		○		○		○			○							○
				○	○	○	○	○	○		○	○			○	○	○	○			○	○		○	○	○		○
			○	○	○	○	○	○	○		○	○			○	○	○	○	○	○	○	○		○	○	○		○
					★		★	●	●												○			○				●

TABLE 2, Continued

Geographic incidence of the more common weed and grass pollens.

● Important species

○ Species of minor importance

★ Species of local or occasional importance

			Nebraska: North Platte	Omaha	Nevada: Reno	New Hampshire: Manchester	New Jersey: Atlantic City	New Mexico: Albuquerque	New York: Buffalo
RAGWEEDS	Short ragweed	Ambrosia elatior	●	●		●	●		●
	Giant ragweed	Ambrosia trifida	○	●			●		●
	Western ragweed	Ambrosia psilostachya	●		○			○	
	Southern ragweed	Ambrosia bidentata							
	Cocklebur	Xanthium commune	○	○		○	○	○	○
	Marsh elder	Iva ciliata							
	Burweed marsh elder	Iva xanthifolia	○	●					
	False ragweed	Franseria acanthicarpa	●		○			●	
	Slender false ragweed	Franseria tenuifolia							
WORMWOODS	Annual sage	Artemisia annua							
	Biennial sage	Artemisia biennis							○
	Prairie sage	Artemisia ludoviciana	○						
	Sagebrush	Artemisia tridentata			○				
	Pasture sage	Artemisia frigida							
	Tall wormwood	Artemisia caudata							
	Sand sagebrush	Artemisia filifolia						●	
CARELESSWEEDS	Pigweed (redroot)	Amaranthus retroflexus	○	○		○	○	○	○
	Spiny amaranth	Amaranthus spinosus							
	Palmer's amaranth	Amaranthus palmeri						●	
	Western water hemp	Acnida tamariscina		●					
GOOSEFOOTS	Lamb's quarters	Chenopodium album	○	○	○	○	○	○	○
	Firebush	Kochia scoparia	●					○	
	Russian thistle	Salsola pestifer	●	○	●			●	
	Sugar beet	Beta vulgaris							
	Shadscale	Atriplex canescens			○			●	
GRASSES	Bluegrass	Poa pratensis	●	●		●	●		●
	Timothy	Phleum pratense		●		●	●		●
	Orchard grass	Dactylis glomerata		●		●	●		●
	Redtop	Agrostis palustris		○		●	○		●
	Bermuda grass	Capriola dactylon						●	
	Johnson grass	Holcus halepensis							
	Sweet vernal grass	Anthoxanthum odoratum							
	Corn	Zea mays	○	○					
	Rye grass	Lolium perenne			●				
MISCELLANEOUS	Red sorrel	Rumex acetosella					○		○
	English plantain	Plantago lanceolata		○		○	○		
	Hemp	Cannabis sativa		●					

Jamestown	**Ohio:** Cincinnati	Cleveland	**Oklahoma:** Oklahoma City	**Oregon:** Pendleton	Portland	**Pennsylvania:** Philadelphia	Pittsburgh	**Rhode Island:** Providence	**South Carolina:** Charleston	**South Dakota:** Pierre	Rapid City	Sioux Falls	**Tennessee:** Memphis	Nashville	**Texas:** Amarillo	Dallas	El Paso	Houston	San Antonio	**Utah:** Salt Lake City	**Vermont:** Burlington	**Virginia:** Richmond	**Washington:** Seattle	**West Virginia:** Charleston	**Wisconsin:** Madison	Milwaukee	**Wyoming:** Cheyenne	Yellowstone Nat'l Park	**Canada:** Toronto	Winnipeg
●	●	●	●			●	●	●	●	●	○	●	●	●		●		●		○	●	●		●	●	●			●	
●	●	●	●			●	●			●	○	●	●	●		●		●	●		○	●		●	●	●				●
○			●	○						○	○				●	○	○	○	●	●							○			●
													○																	
	○	○	○	○		○	○	○	○	○		○	○	○	○	○		○	○	○	○	○		○	○	○	○		○	
			○										○			●		●												
●				●						●	●	●			●					●						○	●			●
				○											●		●			●							○			
																	○		●											
	○					○	○						○	●																
		○																											○	
○				●							●					○				●							○			●
				●																●							●	●		
											●						○			○							●	○		
																					○				○	○				
			○												●		●													
○	○	○	○	○	○	○	○	○	○	○		○	○	○	○	○		○	○	○	○	○	○	○	○	○	○		○	○
			○						○				○			○		○				○								
			○										○			○	○	○	●											
			●													○														
○	○	○	○	○	○	○	○	○	○	○	○	○	○	○	○	○		○	○	○	○		○	○	○	○	○		○	
●										●	●			○	○					○						○	●	○		
●			●	●						●	●				●		○			●						○	●	○		●
																	●													
																	○			●										
●	●	●		●	●	●	●	●	○	●	○	●	●	●						●	●	●	●	●	●	●	●	●	●	●
○	●	●		○	●	●	●	●		●	○	●	○							●	●	●		●	●	●	○		●	●
	●	●	○		●	●	●	●		○			●	●						●	●	●	●	●	●	●			●	
	●	●			○	○	○	●		○			○							○	●	●			●	●	○		●	●
			●						●				●	●	●	●	●	●	●			○								
			○						○				○			○		○	○											
						●		●													●	●		○						
○	○	○	○			○	○		○	○	○		○	○		○						○			○	○				
					●								○	●									●							
	○	○		○	○	○	○	○	○	○		○	○			○		○	○		○	○		○	○	○			○	
	○	○			●	○	○	○		○		○	○	○				○		○	○	○	●	○	○	○			○	○

■ A SUMMARY OF RAGWEED-FREE AREAS BY STATES

(From the American Academy of Allergy.)

ALABAMA—The Gulf Coast at Foley (9 consecutive seasons), good; fairly good at Mobile (3 seasons). Field surveys throughout the remainder of the state reveal wide distribution of ragweeds in waste places and on farms. Birmingham has a very poor record.

ALASKA—No ragweed pollen was found as a result of atmospheric tests made in three places for one season, at Nome, Fairbanks and Juneau.

ARIZONA—Excellent rating for the north and south rims of Grand Canyon. During the fall season in Phoenix conditions are excellent, but there is a spring ragweed season of at least moderate consequence. Our best information for the Tucson area gives it a rating of good for both spring and fall. For other communities in the state there are no atmospheric data.

ARKANSAS—The average exposure to ragweed pollen throughout the state is doubtless very heavy. No refuge areas are known.

CALIFORNIA—*Excellent:* Lassen Volcanic National Park, Sequoia National Park, Oakland, Sacramento, San Francisco, Monterey, Yountville, Yosemite National Park, Los Angeles, Pasadena, El Centro, Escondido, San Diego, Tujunga.

Good: Alpine, Arcata, Santa Barbara.

While air sampling has not been done in the great central valley, it is unlikely that any community there or elsewhere in the state will be found to have an appreciable degree of ragweed pollen pollution.

COLORADO—*Excellent:* Rocky Mountain National Park at Estes Park and Grand Lake, Mesa Verde National Park, Glenwood Springs, the crest of Pikes Peak.

Good: Colorado Springs. Formerly this city's record was not so good. Ragweeds are not common on the west of the slope. Sagebrush is likely to be encountered in this area. Close exposure should be avoided by ragweed sensitive persons.

Denver and the east third of the state constitute an area of moderate to heavy ragweed exposure.

CONNECTICUT—Atmospheric studies have been made in 8 cities. No refuge areas are known.

DELAWARE—Field studies show ragweed to be abundant throughout. Nearest atmospheric studies are those made at Philadelphia and Baltimore. No refuge areas are known.

DISTRICT OF COLUMBIA and adjacent areas of Maryland show heavy ragweed pollen incidence

FLORIDA—*Excellent:* Santa Rosa Island, Key West, Fort Myers, Miami Beach, Coral Gables, Miami, Sunnyside Beach (Panama City).

Good: Daytona Beach, Orlando, Sebring, Bradenton, Everglades National Park, St. Petersburg, Fort Pierce, Live Oak, West Palm Beach.

Fairly good: Fort Lauderdale (Beach), Jacksonville, Tallahassee, Tampa, Clearwater, Pensacola.

Not recommended: Ocala, Gainesville, Melbourne, Panama City. The beaches are almost uniformly desirable; inland areas often not so good.

GEORGIA—Valdosta (only one season), fairly good. Central and northern Georgia and the coastal area, as judged by tests at Atlanta and St. Simons Island and as checked by widely scattered field surveys, have moderately heavy exposure. No recent data.

HAWAII—No significant amounts of any kind of ragweed have been found anywhere on the larger islands except in the area between Schofield Barracks and Pearl Harbor on Oahu. Honolulu is probably ragweed pollen free on account of prevailing northeast tradewinds. No daily atmospheric tests have ever been reported.

IDAHO—*Excellent:* Sun Valley (2 years), Moscow (1 year).

Good: Boise, Pocatello.

All mountainous areas are likely excellent, but exposure to sagebrush pollen is possible throughout most of the state. Close contact with sagebrush should be strictly avoided.

ILLINOIS—No refuge area. Heavy records in 17 cities and towns.

INDIANA—No refuge area. Heavy records in 7 cities and towns.

IOWA—No refuge area. Heavy records in 6 cities and towns.

KANSAS—No refuge area. Atmospheric ragweed pollen incidence diminishes westward.

KENTUCKY—No refuge areas are known, but are barely possible in the Cumberland Mountains.

LOUISIANA—Heavy atmospheric pollution at New Orleans. Air sampling has been carried on only at New Orleans and at Vicksburg, Mississippi, across the river from Tallulah, Louisiana. No recent reports.

MAINE—*Excellent:* St. Francis, Greenville Junction, Millinocket, Presque Isle, Macwahoc, Quoddy Head, New Portland, Newagen, Enfield, Debois, Belfast, Allagash, Grand Lake Stream, Bethel, Eagle Lake, Lincoln, Oquossoc, Speckle Mountain, Upper Dam.

Good: Houlton, Newport, Jackman, Machias, Bar Harbor, Boothbay Harbor.

Fairly good: Eastport, Rockland, Southport, York, Augusta, Camden, Rangeley, North Augusta, Orono.

Not recommended: Stonington, Poland Spring, Auburn, Alfred, Portland, Kinco.

MARYLAND—No refuge area is known. No atmospheric studies have been made in the mountainous parts of western Maryland.

MASSACHUSETTS—*Good:* Annisquam, East Gloucester, West Gloucester, Magnolia, Rockport, Nantucket Island.

Fairly good: Gloucester, Worcester.

Not recommended: Winchester, Boston, Northampton, Amherst, Newton Center.

This is the state, and Boston the chief city, from which ragweed hayfever victims first fled to the mountains and rocky coastal areas of New Hampshire and Maine some 100 years ago. Even so, ragweed pollen is much less abundant in the air in Boston than in most of the larger cities of northeastern U. S. A. Of the 14 communities tested none offers excellent refuge conditions. Neither the Berkshires nor Cape Cod has received attention. Weed destruction seems to be effective on Nantucket Island. Otherwise ragweeds take over all waste areas.

MICHIGAN—*Excellent:* Isle Royale National Park.

Good: Sault Ste. Marie, Copper Harbor.

Fairly good: Houghton.

Fifty years ago much of the area of northern Michigan was doubtless entirely free from ragweeds and ragweed pollen, but sampling done in 57 systematically selected communities during the past 25 years has shown that no effective refuges remain in the lower peninsula, and that those of the northern peninsula are few, as listed above. The following list does not include any city of the lower peninsula. Those toward the beginning of the list are much better than those toward the end and might be suitable for persons with moderate sensitivity.

Not recommended (upper peninsula only): Saint Ignace, Blaney, Munising, Ironwood, Mackinac Island, Newberry, Powers, Menominee, Escanaba.

MINNESOTA—*Fairly good:* Tower, Virginia. Other places as good as or better than Tower and Virginia could likely be found in other parts of the Arrowhead County (northeastern corner of the state).

Not recommended: Duluth, Rochester, Minneapolis, Winona, Moorhead. The state has been inadequately covered.

MISSISSIPPI—Biloxi, on the coast, is fairly good. Field studies reveal an abundance of ragweed on farms throughout, so except for the immediate coast no refuge areas are likely to be found.

MISSOURI—No refuge areas.

MONTANA—*Excellent:* Glacier National Park at Belton and Many Glacier, West Yellowstone. Judging by the excellent records for more than 20 cities and towns in the adjacent parts of Alberta and Saskatchewan and at Yellowstone National Park, most of Montana is practically free of ragweed.

Good: Miles City.

Very meager data and no recent studies for this state. Sagebrush is widely distributed and should be avoided by persons known to be ragweed sensitive.

NEBRASKA—No refuge areas, but considerably less ragweed is found in the western third of the state than in the eastern part.

NEVADA—Very meager data, and no recent air sampling. Ragweeds are rare along the principal highways. Reno, excellent. Lake Mead, excellent in the fall, good in the spring ragweed season. Sagebrush is a possible factor.

NEW HAMPSHIRE—*Excellent:* Moosilaukee, Pawtuckaway, Errol, Lancaster, Carrol, Laconia, Colebrook, Blue Job Mountain, Derby, Groveton, Lincoln, Pittsburg, Warren, Whitefield.

Good: Bath, Conway, Dixville, Littleton, North Conway, Ossipee, Hampton, Plymouth, Bethlehem, Crotched Mountain, Dover, Franklin, Hillsboro, Holderness, New London.

Fairly good: Claremont, Concord, Federal Hill, Keene, Berlin, New Ipswich, Manchester, Weirs.

Not recommended: Hinsdale, Charlestown, Rye, Rochester, Lebanon, Jeremy, Exeter, Peterborough, Nashua.

NEW JERSEY—No refuge areas are known. Those places along the northern shore where relief is sometimes found are subject to high counts when the wind blows from the west. Studies have been made in 29 cities.

NEW MEXICO—Very meager atmospheric data. Ragweeds are probably comparatively rare throughout the state. Roswell is good, and Albuquerque fairly good.

NEW YORK—The reports on Long Island have produced variable records. Fire Island at Ocean Beach is sometimes fairly good, and Montauk likewise fairly good. No other records are available for the Island, except in Brooklyn which is not recommended.

Adirondack area. *Excellent:* Keene Valley.

Good: Blue Mountain Lake, Elk Lake, Keene, Loon Lake.

Fairly good: Big Moose, Chilson, Indian Lake, Long Lake, McColloms, Raquette Lake, Paul Smiths, Redford, Wanakena, Chateaugay Lake, Inlet, Sabattis, Schroon Lake (Severance), Tupper Lake, Newcomb, Owl's Head, Lake Placid, McKeever.

Catskill area. *Good:* Big Indian, Haines Falls, Pine Hill.

Fairly good: Fleischmanns.

Studies have been made in 85 other communities, including all of the larger cities, none of which can be recommended.

NORTH CAROLINA—No refuge areas are known, but air tests at Newfound Gap, Tennessee, on the crest of the Great Smoky Mountains prove the immediate area to be good. Likely there are other places equally good at similar or higher elevations in North Carolina. There are records of heavy concentration of ragweed pollen for four of the large cities of the state.

NORTH DAKOTA—No atmospheric data are available except in the narrow Red River Valley at Margo. No refuge areas are known, but conditions are likely much the same in the southern half of the state as in South Dakota. Judging from data from adjacent areas in Canada, there might be some good places found along the north edge of the state.

OHIO—No refuge areas. Adequate sampling has been done in seven large cities.

OKLAHOMA—No refuge areas. Adequate sampling has been done in seven large cities.

OREGON—No atmospheric studies have been made in eastern Oregon except at Milton-Freewater which is good.

Excellent: Coquille, Corvallis, Eugene, Crater Lake National Park, Portland, Turner.

PENNSYLVANIA—No refuge areas are known. Claims for mountain resorts have never been proved. Sampling has been carried on in ten large cities for many years.

PUERTO RICO—No atmospheric studies have ever been reported, but recent careful field examination failed to disclose any ragweeds on the Island.

RHODE ISLAND—No refuge areas.

SOUTH CAROLINA—No refuge areas are known, but our data are very meager. Nothing recent.

SOUTH DAKOTA—There are no refuge areas better than fairly good.

Fairly good: Rapid City, Mobridge.

TENNESSEE—No refuge areas are known. Along the crest of the Great Smoky Mountains at Newfound Gap conditions are found to be good. There are no accommodations at this point, but there might be places with similar conditions at similar or higher elevations.

TEXAS—Big Spring is the only community out of the ten where studies have been made which has a rating of good. Most of Texas is badly infested with ragweeds. However, they diminish considerably toward the west corner of the state, for example in El Paso.

UTAH—*Excellent:* Zion National Park, Bryce Canyon National Park.

Fairly good: Vernal in the extreme northeast corner of the state and Hurricane in the extreme southwest corner of the state. The average for metropolitan Salt Lake City is fairly good, except for the Canyon Rim area.

VERMONT—Very meager data. Conditions on the east side of the state are probably comparable to adjacent areas of New Hampshire. Heavy atmospheric contamination is found in the upper Lake Champlain area.

VIRGINIA—No excellent or good refuges are known.

VIRGIN ISLANDS—*Excellent:* The island of St. John (Virgin Islands National Park), the island of St. Thomas.

WASHINGTON—*Excellent:* Seattle-Tacoma Airport, Mt. Rainier National Park (Longmire, White River, Paradise Valley), Seattle, Olympic National Park, Spokane, Yakima.

Good: Walla Walla.

Except for the badly ragweed contaminated orchards in the immediate vicinity of Wenatchee, all but one place among the ten tested in the state are excellent or good.

WEST VIRGINIA—No refuge areas are known.

WISCONSIN—No refuge areas are known, but no adequate investigation has been made in the vast lake region of the northern part of the state.

WYOMING—Very meager data except at the national parks.

Excellent: Grand Teton National Park, Yellowstone National Park. Lander is not recommended.

■ REFUGES IN CANADA AND OTHER AREAS ADJACENT TO THE U.S.

CANADA

ALBERTA—With atmospheric tests in 14 communities, we have the following to report:

Excellent: Banff, Beaver Lodge, Edmonton, Jasper, Vermilion, Lake Louise, Cypress Hills, Waterton Lakes Park, Calgary, Coleman, Manyberries, Drumheller, Lethbridge.

Fairly good: Medicine Hat.

Sagebrush pollen is a possible irritant to ragweed sufferers.

BRITISH COLUMBIA—Meager data.

Excellent: Summerland, Saanichton, Victoria.

MANITOBA—*Excellent:* The Pas, Riding Mountain National Park, Russell, Brandon.

Good: Dauphin.

Fairly good: Pierson, Winnipeg.

Sagebrush pollen is a possible irritant to ragweed sufferers.

NEW BRUNSWICK—*Excellent:* Campbellton, Bathurst, Richibucto, Newcastle-Chatam, Dalhousie, Fredericton, Woodstock, Doaktown, McAdam, Shediac Cape, St. John, Grand Manan, Edmundston, Perth-Andover, St. George, Welsford, St. Andrews, St. Stephen, Chipman, Moncton, Sackville, Tracadie.

Good: Sussex, Haslam Farm (Fundy National Park), Lakeview, Jemseg, Waterside (Fundy National Park).

Fairly good: Pointe du Chene, Gagetown.

No high concentrations were found at any place.

NEWFOUNDLAND—Only two communities on the island have been studied.
Excellent: Corner Brook, St. John's.

NOVA SCOTIA—*Excellent:* Truro, Middle West Pubnico, Cape Breton Highlands National Park, Chester, Antigonish, Baddock, Ingonish Island.
Good: Meteghan, Digby, Yarmouth, Kentville.
No other studies have been reported.

ONTARIO—Systematic atmospheric pollen research has been carried on in Ontario since 1928, gradually increasing in volume until records are now available for at least one season in 70 communities. For some communities there are now continuous annual records for more than 30 years. The well-populated area of southern Ontario from Windsor to Cornwall is about as heavily contaminated with ragweed as are the adjacent areas of U.S.A. But farther northward and northwestward, in areas of less intensive cultivation or none at all, air pollution drops rapidly to insignificant levels.

Excellent: Timmins, Fort William, New Liskeard, Kapuskasing, Port Arthur, Fort Francis, Barry's Bay, Black Sturgeon Lake, Chalk River, Cochrane, South River, Haleburton.

Good: Blind River, Mattawa, Temagami, Lake Joseph, Magnetawan, Rosseau, Sudbury, Espanola, Muskata Falls, Tobermory.

Fairly good: Cedar Lake, Dorset, Pembroke, Renfrew, Sault Ste. Marie, Honey Harbor, Bancroft, Kenora, Mindemoya (Manitoulin Island), North Bay, Westport, Port Carlings.

Not recommended, at least for severe cases, are listed here in order of their degree of air pollution from least to greatest: Huntsville, Smith Falls, Algonquin Park, Georgian Bay Islands National Park, Gravenhurst, Lion's Head, Ottawa, Parry Sound, Madoc, Wiarton, Cornwall, Kincardine, Point Pelee National Park, Bellville, Peterborough, Picton, St. Lawrence Islands National Park, London, Mallorytown, Toronto and metropolitan area, Windsor, Hamilton.

PRINCE EDWARD ISLAND—*Excellent:* Cavendish, Mantague, Souris, Summerside, Tignish, Charlottetown, O'Leary.
Good: Prince Edward Island National Park.
No other studies have been reported.

QUEBEC—*Excellent:* Chandler, Iles-de-la-Madeleine, Matapedia, Mont-Albert Caspesie, Gaspé, Grande Riviere, Mont Joli, Father Point, Carleton, Charlesbourg, Percé, Tadoussac.

Good: Matane, New Carlisle, Normandin, Baie Saint-Paul, Jonquieres (Chicoutimi), Lennoxville, St-Lambert.

Fairly good: St-Jovite, Lac-des-Plages, Mont-Laurier, Nominingue, Mont Tremblant, Rimouski, Riviere-du-Loup, Ste-Anne-de-la-Pocatiére, Ste-Agathe, Lac-des-Seize-Iles.

In the southwest tip of the province, adjacent to New York and New Hampshire, air contamination is bad. North of the Ottawa and St. Lawrence Rivers, and in the Gaspé country, conditions are good to excellent.

SASKATCHEWAN—*Excellent:* Prince Albert National Park, Nelford, Prince Albert, Scott, Regina, Saskatoon, Swift Current.

BERMUDA

Atmospheric tests have been made only at Hamilton where no ragweed pollen was detected.

CUBA

Field inspection reveals a number of areas where common ragweed grows along the roadsides, but the atmospheric tests reported from Havana give the city a rating of excellent.

MEXICO

Good: Mexico City, Tampico, Torreon.
Not recommended: Ciudad Juarez, Matamoros.
Slender false ragweed and western ragweed are found in small amounts in all states as far south as Mexico City. Our best information is that ragweed pollen concentrations are very low in most parts and absent in the southern states.

Appendix F

GLOSSARY OF TERMS

ABSCESS—Collection of pus in any part of the body. A boil is an abscess.

ACETYLSALICYLIC ACID—Aspirin.

ACANTHOSIS—Thickening of the skin, often with warty growths.

ACHALASIA—Spasm of the esophagus.

ACNE—Pimples and blackheads on the skin, usually of the face, chest and back.

ACUTE—Having a sudden onset and a short and relatively severe course, as an acute illness.

ADENITIS—Inflammation of a gland, especially a lymph node.

ADENOID—Lymph tissue in the throat behind the nose that often enlarges and obstructs breathing.

ADRENALIN—A brand name for epinephrine, a hormone secreted by the adrenal gland.

AEROALLERGENS—Allergens carried in the air, such as pollen.

AEROTITIS—Inflammation of the middle ear caused by changes in pressure in high-altitude flights.

AEROSOL—Particles of solid or liquid matter suspended in a gas because of their small size. Particulates under one micron in diameter are generally called aerosols.

AGGLUTINATION—Gathering of cells or other particles in a fluid into clumps.

AGRANULOCYTOSIS—Not enough white blood cells in the blood, usually caused by poison or by sensitivity to certain drugs.

AIRWAY RESISTANCE—Narrowing of the air passages of the respiratory system in response to the presence of some irritating substance or substances.

ALLERGEN—A substance capable of causing an allergic reaction.

ALLERGIC COUGH SYNDROME—A persistent, repetitive coughing that is believed to be caused by irritation from allergy of the membranes that line the trachea, or windpipe, and which is made worse by postnasal drip.

ALLERGIC REACTION—A reaction when the allergen and antibody combine in the cells of a body organ or tissue to produce a spasm of involuntary muscles, an increased amount of fluid released from the cells, and an increase in eosinophils, or other allergic phenomena.

ALLERGIC RHINITIS—Allergic reaction in the nose with swelling, itching and watery discharge.

ALVEOLI—Tiny air spaces at the end of the terminal bronchioles of the lungs where the exchange of oxygen and carbon dioxide takes place.

AMYLOIDOSIS—Extensive deposits of the protein substance amyloid in many organs of the body.

ANALGESIA—Relief of pain.

ANAPHYLAXIS—Without protection. Immediate severe allergic reaction in humans which results in sudden collapse and occasionally death.

ANGIOEDEMA—An allergic reaction in the skin and underlying tissue. Giant hives.

ANGIONEUROTIC EDEMA—Swelling, usually of the face, caused by an allergic reaction or emotional factors.

ANGIOSPASM—Contraction of a blood vessel.

ANOREXIA—Loss of appetite for food.

ANTIBODY—Any substance in the bloodstream or other body fluid which exerts restrictive or destructive action on bacteria or other body poisons, or neutralizes their toxins. A skin sensitizing antibody is sometimes called a reagin.

ANTICOAGULANT—A chemical agent that reduces or prevents coagulation of blood.

ANTIGEN—Substance, usually protein in nature, that is capable of producing protective antibodies.

ANTIHISTAMINE—A drug that tends to neutralize histamine.

ARRHYTHMIA—Lack of regular rhythm. Irregularity of the heartbeat.

ARTERIOLE—A small artery.

ASTHMA—Disease characterized by difficulty of breathing, accompanied by a wheezing sound and a sense of tightness in the chest.

ASTHMATIC BRONCHITIS—Basically the same as bronchial asthma.

AUTONOMIC NERVOUS SYSTEM—The nervous system in the body that is automatic and self-governing.

BARBITURATES—A group of drugs to calm nerves and induce sleep. They may become habit forming.

BLOOD GROUPS—Blood types. Classifications of blood according to clumping substances in them. Most important groups are O, A, B, AB and Rh.

BLOOD TYPING—Test to discover one's blood group.

BRONCHIAL ASTHMA—An attack consists of narrowing of the bronchioles by muscle spasm, swelling of the mucous membrane, and thickening and increase of mucous secretions, accompanied by wheezing, gasping and sometimes coughing.

BRONCHIOLES—Small bronchial tubes in the lungs leading to the air cells.

BRONCHITIS—Inflammation of the bronchial tubes.

BRONCHOSPASM—Constriction of the bronchial tubes due to contraction of the muscles surrounding them.

BRONCHUS—A major airway of the respiratory system.

BUFFER—Substance that helps maintain balance of acidity and alkalinity of a solution.

CAFFEINE—Stimulating drug found in coffee, tea and other substances.

CALAMINE SOLUTION—Medication containing zinc oxide and mercuric oxide used to treat skin conditions.

CANKER SORE—An ulceration, often found on the tongue or gums.

CARDIOSPASM—Constriction of the lower end of the esophagus at the entrance of the stomach.

CENTRAL NERVOUS SYSTEM—The part of the nervous system containing the brain, spinal cord and the nerves from the spinal cord.

CHEILOSIS—Creasing and splitting of the skin at the corners of the mouth.

CHEMOSIS—Swelling of the conjunctival membrane of the eye.

CHRONIC—Marked by long duration or frequent recurrence, as a chronic disease.

CILIA—Hairlike cells that line the airways and by their sweeping movement propel the dirt and germ-filled mucus out of the respiratory tract.

CLINICAL STUDY—One that concerns itself with a disease process in a living subject.

COLITIS—Inflammation of the colon, or large bowel.

COLLAGEN—An albuminoid present in connective tissue, bone or cartilage.

COLLAGEN DISEASE—Any disease associated with disturbances in the connective tissues, such as around joints.

COLON—The large bowel, extending from the cecum to the anus, approximately five to seven feet long.

CONJUNCTIVAL TEST—A test in which a small amount of an allergen is placed in the eye.

CONJUNCTIVITIS—Inflammation of the membrane of the eye.

CONNECTIVE TISSUE—Fibrous tissue that connects and holds together, as between muscles, bones and blood vessels.

CONTACT DERMATITIS—An irritation of the skin produced by direct contact with some material to which the skin is sensitive.

CONTACTANT ALLERGENS (CONTACTANTS)—Allergens that produce skin allergy by touching or being applied to the skin; e.g., poison ivy, cosmetics.

CORTICOSTEROID—Chemical substance derived from the cortex layer of the adrenal gland.

CORTISONE—A compound isolated from the adrenal gland or made synthetically. Used in the treatment of various allergies when other means fail.

CORYZA—The common cold; acute rhinitis.

CROUP—An inflammation of the larynx with coughing and difficulty in breathing.

CYSTITIS—Inflammation of the bladder with pain and frequency of urination.

DERMATITIS—Inflammation of the skin.

DESENSITIZATION—Attempt to increase the patient's tolerance to his allergens by a series of injections.

DROPSY—Edema. Swelling of the ankles and legs, often due to heart insufficiency.

DUODENUM—The beginning of the small intestine just after the stomach, that receives bile from the liver, food from the stomach, and juices from the pancreas.

DUST COUNT—The number of dust particles in the air.

DYSPNEA—Shortness of breath.

DYSURIA—Impaired ability to excrete urine; also painful urination.

ECZEMA—An acute or chronic, noncontagious, itching, inflammatory disease of the skin that can be wet or dry and is associated with the development of scales and crusts.

ELECTROENCEPHALOGRAPHY (EEG)—Process of recording the brain waves.

ELIMINATION DIET—A trial diet is designed to find and eliminate allergenic foods.

EMPHYSEMA—A chronic lung disease characterized by an anatomical change in the lungs associated with a breakdown of the walls of the alveoli. These alveoli can enlarge, lose their resilience and subsequently disintegrate.

ENDOTOXIN—A toxic substance or poison formed within bacteria that is released when the bacteria die.

ENTERITIS—Inflammation of the intestinal tract.

ENVIRONMENT—Surroundings in the home, at work, at school or in the area where you live.

EPIDERMIS—The outer layer of the skin.

EPINEPHRINE—A hormone secreted by the adrenal gland.

EPITHELIUM—Skin. Also the linings of the passages of the hollow organs of the digestive, respiratory and urinary systems.

ESTROGEN—The female sex hormone manufactured by the ovaries.

ETHMOIDITIS—Inflammation of the ethmoid sinus.

ETHMOID SINUS—A sinus or cavity in the skull behind the bridge of the nose.

EUSTACHIAN TUBE—The tube leading from the back of the throat to the ear.

EXCHANGE TRANSFUSION—A method of removing most of a newborn infant's blood and substituting a transfused donor blood to correct Rh sensitivity.

EXTRASYSTOLE—A heartbeat occurring out of turn and thus producing a skipped beat and irregular rhythm.

FIBRILLATION—Uncoordinated, irregular heartbeat.

GAMMA GLOBULIN—The part of the blood containing antibodies.

GASTRITIS—Inflammation of the lining of the stomach.

GASTROENTERITIS—Inflammation of both the stomach and intestines.

GENE—One of the units responsible for inheritance that are present in the sperm cells of the male and egg cells of the female.

HAYFEVER—An allergic condition characterized by acute inflammation of the mucous membranes of the eyes, nose, throat and respiratory tract, accompanied by sneezing, running nose and watery eyes and itching of the eyes, nose and throat.

HEAT RASH—Pink and red spots on the skin due to inflammation of the sweat glands.

HEPATITIS—Inflammation of the liver.

HEREDITY—The inheritance of physical and mental qualities or of diseases from ancestry.

HERPES—Inflammation of the skin caused by a virus. Herpes simplex is a cold sore. Herpes zoster is shingles.

HISTAMINE—A chemical released by the interaction of the allergen and antibody and considered the cause of swelling and itching of allergic skin manifestations.

HIVES—A skin condition of smooth, slightly elevated wheals, which are redder or paler white than the surrounding skin and are accompanied by severe itching.

HORMONE—A chemical produced by a gland and secreted into the bloodstream that affects function of distant organs.

HYPERSENSITIVITY—An exaggerated reaction to any substance.

HYPERVENTILATION—Excessive deep breathing that may lead to dizziness. Overbreathing.

HYPOSENSITIZATION—The treatment of the patient by injections of small, increasing concentrations of allergenic extract in order to stimulate the production of protective antibodies. Immunization.

IATROGENIC—Caused by a physician.

IMMUNE—Free from the effects of allergy or infection by either having already had the disease or being protected by an inoculation of an antigen in a small dose.

IMMUNITY—A state, natural or acquired, in which the body is resistant to an allergy or a disease.

IMMUNIZATION—The process of rendering immune.

IMMUNOLOGY—The science and study of the nature and causation of protection against infections and allergenic substances.

IMPETIGO—A contagious, inflammatory skin disease characterized by pustules.

INDUCE—To bring on or about; to cause.

INFECTIOUS DISEASE—A disease transmitted by bacteria, viruses, fungi or protozoa.

INFLAMED—Condition of tissues being red, swollen and painful.

INGESTANT ALLERGENS (INGESTANTS)—Substances that are swallowed to which a person is sensitive; e.g., foods or drugs.

INHALANT ALLERGENS (INHALANTS)—Allergens that enter the body through the nose and respiratory tract. Usually pollens, mold spores, house dust and animal dander.

INJECTANT ALLERGENS (INJECTANTS)—Substances injected into the body to which a person is allergic.

INTERTRIGO—A skin inflammation in the folds of the skin, such as in the crook of the elbow or under the breast.

INTRACTABLE ASTHMA—Asthma that continues over a long period of time despite adequate specific treatment.

INTRADERMAL TEST—A diagnostic skin test in which a small amount of an allergen is injected between the layers of the skin.

INTRAVENOUS TEST—A test in which a substance or material is placed within a vein.

INTRINSIC ASTHMA—An old term used to denote that the basis of the allergic symptoms is found in the patient's own body; i.e., the patient is hypersensitive to allergens originating in his own body.

ISCHEMIA—Temporary restriction of blood flow, usually due to a spasm of an artery.

JAUNDICE—Yellow discoloration of the skin and eyes due to bile pigments in the blood.

JEJUNUM—The upper portion of the small intestine.

KERATINIZATION—Process of skin taking on a horny consistency, as in corns.

LARYNGOSPASM—Spasm and closure of the larynx.

METABOLISM—The normal building up and breaking down of cells and tissues in the body, the physical and chemical changes that are constantly taking place in the cells, the burning of oxygen and transformation of food for heat, energy and growth.

MIGRAINE—Severe headache often associated with nausea, vomiting and other symptoms.

MOLD—A large group of microscopic plants reproduced by spores.

MOLD SPORES—The microscopic reproductive elements of fungus plants.

NASAL TEST—A test in which a small amount of an allergen is placed in the nostril.

NEPHRITIS—Inflammation of the kidneys.

OBJECTIVE SIGNS—Conditions that can be seen or felt or measured by the examiner, as opposed to subjective signs that only the patient experiences.

OTITIS MEDIA—Inflammation of the middle ear.

PALPITATION—Unduly rapid beating of the heart that is felt by the patient; pounding of the heart.

PARTICULATE—A particle of solid or liquid matter.

PATCH TEST—A test in which a small amount of a suspected allergen is placed under a patch on the skin.

PERENNIAL HAYFEVER—Year-round nonseasonal allergic rhinitis.

PHARYNGITIS—Sore throat. Inflammation of the mucous membrane of the pharynx.

PHOTOCHEMICAL PROCESS—The chemical changes brought about by the radiant energy of the sun acting upon various substances.

PICA—The craving for odd foods.

PLACEBO—A pill with no active medicine, such as a sugar pill.

PLATELET—Thrombocyte. One of the small particles that circulate in the blood and aid in blood clotting.

PNEUMOTHORAX—Condition of air being in the chest cavity surrounding the lung.

POLLEN—The fine yellow dust in seed plants.

POLYARTHRITIS—Inflammation of several joints.

POLYNEURITIS—Inflammation of many nerves.

PRECIPITATOR—Any of a number of devices using mechanical, electrical or chemical means to collect particulates. Used for measurement, analysis, or control.

PSORIASIS—A noncontagious chronic skin disease characterized by reddish silvery patches on the chest, knees and elbows.

PSYCHONEUROSIS—Mental disorder which is of psychogenic origin and is associated with anxiety state, but not with loss of insight or loss of reality perception.

PSYCHOSIS—A deep, far-reaching, extreme mental disorder.

PSYCHOSOMATIC—Pertaining to the relationship of the mind and body.

PULMONARY FUNCTION—The adequacy of the lung's performance.

RAGWEED—The weed *Ambrosia* whose pollen causes hayfever.

RASH—Multiple bumps or spots on the skin.

REAGIN—An antibody that will react with an antigen to cause an allergic reaction in a sensitive person.

REHABILITATION—Restoring to a useful life people who have had a severe, prolonged, crippling illness.

RESPIRATORY ORGANS—The lungs, nose, throat, sinuses and their accessory structures.

RESTRICTED—Limited or removed from the diet.

RH FACTOR—A component of the blood that may cause blood transfusion reaction or may cause destruction of red blood cells in a newborn infant when a mother is Rh negative and the baby is Rh positive.

SCLERODERMA—A skin disease involving hardened patches and color changes. It can also affect other organs in the body.

SCLEROSIS—Hardening of tissues with deposits of fibrous tissue to replace the original structure.

SCRATCH TEST—An allergy skin test performed by scratching the skin and then applying an allergen to the scratch.

SEASONAL CATARRH—Hayfever.

SEBORRHEIC DERMATITIS—A skin disease due to oversecretion of the sebaceous gland.

SEDATIVE—A drug or other agent to induce calmness and relieve pain.

SENSITIVITY (HYPERSENSITIVITY)—An increased reactivity to specific substances that are harmless to nonallergic individuals.

SENSITIZED—Having developed a sensitivity to a certain substance, such as to pollen, animal dander or dust.

SEROUS OTITIS MEDIA—Exudation of serum and mucus into the inner ear, causing hearing disturbances.

SERUM—The fluid portion of the blood or a clear watery fluid of any serous membrane.

SHOCK—A drop in blood pressure caused by inadequate amounts of blood circulating in the bloodstream. It can be caused by loss of blood, systemic reaction from an allergy injection, severe infection, severe injury to tissues, or rarely emotional factors.

SHOCK ORGAN—The organ or tissue in which an allergic reaction takes place.

SINUSES—Air cavities in the head lined by mucous membrane, in connection with the nasal passages.

SINUSITIS—Inflammation of one of the sinuses in the head.

SKIN TEST—A test to detect substances responsible for allergic disease; performed by applying the suspected allergen to the skin by patch test, scratch test, or injection into the skin.

SMOG—The irritating haze resulting from the sun's effect on certain pollutants in the air. Also a mixture of fog and smoke.

SPECULUM—Any instrument inserted into a body opening to see inside the body.

SPIROMETER—An instrument that measures the flow of air in and out of the lungs.

SPORES—The microscopic "seeds" of molds.

SQUAMOUS—Scaly or platelike, as in squamous cells of the skin.

STATUS ASTHMATICUS—An attack of asthma that persists for more than forty-eight hours despite repeated medication.

STEROID—A class of compounds with a carbon-ring structure and including certain drugs of hormone origin, such as cortisone or ACTH.

SUSCEPTIBLE—Easily affected by substances causing allergy.

SYNERGISM—The working together of two agents to produce something that neither could accomplish alone, as in the action of the mixtures of certain drugs.

TACHYCARDIA—Rapid heartbeat of more than 100 beats per minute.

THRESHOLD—A level of resistance of the body which fluctuates according to internal and external stimuli.

TOLERANCE—Endurance or ability to live with allergens.

TOXEMIA—A condition of poisons circulating in the blood causing illness. Toxemia of pregnancy is often caused by inadequate kidney function.

TRACHEA—Windpipe; the main section of the tubes taking air to and from the lungs.

TRACHEITIS—Inflammation of the trachea, or windpipe.

TRACHEOTOMY—Surgical incision into the trachea, often done to relieve suffocation.

TRANQUILIZER DRUG—Any drug given to calm the nerves and allay apprehension.

TYMPANIC MEMBRANE—The eardrum.

UREMIA—Accumulation of waste products in the blood because of the inability of the kidneys to function properly.

URTICARIA—Hives; an allergic condition of the skin characterized by small or large blotches or welts and itching.

UVEITIS—Inflammation of uvea of the eye, which is the part that contains the iris.

VACCINATE—To immunize against a disease by inoculation with a substance made of weakened germs.

VACCINE—A preparation containing specific allergens, used to help develop tolerance.

VASOSPASM—Marked contraction and spasm of a blood vessel.

VERTIGO—Dizziness; the feeling that the surroundings are spinning around.

VISCOUS—Sticky; semifluid.

XERODERMA—Excessively dry skin that often has the appearance of scaly fish skin.

INDEX

INDEX

Abdomen
bloating of, 320, 335
pain of, 25, 66, 68
See also Gastrointestinal allergies.
Abdominal belt, 154, 155
Abdominal breathing, 82, 150
Abscess, 417
Acanthosis, 417
Acetylsalicylic acid. *See* Aspirin.
Achalasia, 417
Acidosis, 144, 157
ACTH, 115, 139–140
Actinomycetes, 101
Activities for asthmatic children, 61, 62, 78, 85
Adenitis, 417
Adenoids, 417
See also Tonsils and adenoids.
Adrenalin, 61, 417
Aeroallergens, 417
See also Airborne allergens.
Aerosol spray, 114, 137, 140–141, 417
Aerotitis, 417
Agglutination, 417
Aging, 20
Agranulocytosis, 417
Airborne allergens, 36–38, 87–117, 122, 417
determining causes of symptoms, 37
in year-round allergy, 55
See also Hayfever.
Air conditioning, 38, 109–110
Air pollution, 59, 111
asthma and, 122, 124, 127–130
bronchitis and emphysema and, 165, 166
ranking of cities, 112
research on effects, 364–365
symptoms caused by, 128–129
Alcohol, 156, 200
Algae, sensitivity to, 55, 92, 101, 102
Alginate colloid injections, 351
Allergens, 19, 20, 104, 122, 134, 418
isolated from pollen, 364
list of, 381–383
Allergic Index, 332–333

Allergic look, 49, 67, 69
Allergic mechanism, 357, 418
  theories, 358–361, 363, 372
Allergic rhinitis, 418
  See also Hayfever.
Allergic salute, 49–50 *ill.*, 54
Allergic shiner, 49
Allergic tension-fatigue syndrome, 67–70
Allergic threshold, 242
Allergist, allergists
  attitudes of, 27, 46
  first trip to, 332–335
  going to, 331–352
  how to find, 331–332
  knowledge and training, 15, 16, 132, 133
  number of, 15
Allergoid, 367–368
Allergy
  causes of, 18–20, 21, 34–38, 70–71, 92–93, 99–102, 108
  in children, 44–86
  costs of, 14
  deaths from, 45, 119
  effects on children's lives, 45–46, 48, 119
  incidence of, 13, 14, 44–45
  in infants, 24–43
  mechanisms, 20–21, 357, 358–361, 363, 372, 418
  not contagious, 64
  origin of name, 356
  progressive patterns, 26–27, 47
  symptoms caused by, 19, 20, 48, 55–56, 87
  to anesthetics, 290
  to bacteria, 62–64, 127
  to drugs, 278–310
  to insects, 258–277
  to vaccines and transfusions, 290–291
Allergy Foundation of America, 376
Allergy-proofing your house, 38
  See also Housecleaning.
Allergy survey questionnaire, 52
Allpyral, injections of, 351–352
Almay Cosmetics, 245
Alternaria, 96
Alveoli, 120, 418
American Academy of Allergy, 376
American College of Allergists, 376
Aminophylline, 139
Aminopyrine, 122
Amphetamine, 113
Amyloidosis, 418
Anaphylaxis, 280–281, 418
  discovery of, 356
  from penicillin reaction, 284
Anderson, Capt. William R., 365
Anemia, 374
Anesthetics
  allergy to, 244, 290
  use of in allergic persons, 86
Angioedema, 219, 418
  See also Hives; Swelling.
Angiospasm, 418
Animals
  causing allergy, 36–37, 39, 43, 48, 83, 92, 101, 108, 109, 122, 125, 135, 143, 291
  for research, 361–362
  having allergy, 362, 372
Anorexia, 418
  See also Appetite, loss of.
Antibiotics, 63, 114, 144–145, 251
  in foods, 210
  mold infections after use, 287
  sensitivity to, 278–279, 286–287
  side effects from, 287, 324
Antibodies, 21, 358, 359, 418
  to cancer, 373
  theory of kinds, 372–373
Anticoagulant, 148
Antigens, 21, 357, 363, 418
Antihistamines, 113, 114, 343–345, 418
  allergy to, 113
  list of preparations, their uses and side effects, 386–391
  side effects, 344
Antiseptics, and sun sensitivity, 296
Ants, 266–267
Appetite, loss of, 28, 68, 418
Apple, allergy to, 32
Applied research, 357
Arbeiter, Dr. Herbert, 48
Aretaeus, 119
Ar-Ex Products Company, 245, 392

Arnar-Stone Laboratories, 392
Arrhythmia, 418
due to allergy, 322–323
Arteriole, 418
Arthritis, 20, 374
and allergic mechanisms, 371
Artificial coloring. *See* Food additives.
Artists, causes of dermatitis, 234
Aspergillus, 97
Aspirin, 114, 122
sensitivity to, 146, 281–282, 287–290
related foods to avoid, 205
other substances to avoid, 289–290
substitutes, 288
Assassin bug, 271–272
Asthma, 22, 111, 114, 115, 118–158, 161, 418
acute attack, 135
and alcohol, 156
from aspirin and hormones, 282, 287–288
causes of, 133, 136
in children, 48, 56–57, 59–62, 78, 85
from cockroaches, 276
deaths from, 45, 61–62, 119
epidemic areas, 361
and food allergies, 29
heparin to treat attack, 252
hereditary factor, 26
and hormones, 47–48
incidence of, 14, 59, 119
in infants, 38–39
from mold, 96
outlook, 157–158
prevention of attacks, 155–156
recurring attacks, 142–144
school days lost, 44–45
symptoms, 118
tests for diagnosis, 366–367
time of attacks, 23
treatment, 132–155, 368
and weather, 103
Asthmatic children, 61, 62, 78, 85
Asthmatic Children's Foundation Residential Treatment Center, 80
Astronaut, wash-out from allergy, 287–288
Autoantibodies, 374–376
Autoimmune diseases, 374–376
Auto mechanics, possible causes of dermatitis of, 235
Aviators, possible causes of dermatitis of, 234

Bacterial allergy, 62–64, 127
Bacterial vaccines, 63, 117, 146
Bad breath, 73, 163
Bagassosis, 319
Baker's dermatitis, 233, 234
Band-aid, allergy to, 292
Barber's dermatitis, 234
Barbiturates, 86, 418
allergy to, 293, 294
Barometric pressure, 103
Barrel chest, 150
Basic research, 357
Bass, Dr. Harry, 175
Bayless, Dr. Theodore M., 209
Beans, 30
Beautician's dermatitis, 234
Bedding, 105, 108, 125
Bed-wetting, 66–67, 68
Bee stings, 259–260
See also Insects.
Behavior problems, 56, 65, 67–70, 71–76
due to allergy, 211–212
Belinkoff, Dr. Stanton, 171
Benaim-Pinto, Dr. Carlos, 100
Benson, Dr. John A., 279
Berman, Dr. Bernard A., 5, 38–39, 125
Bernton, Dr. Harry S., 277
Berries, 204
Berry, Dr. Franklyn, 171
Beta-adrenergic receptors, 361
Bierman, Dr. C. Warren, 285
Biological rhythms
effects on allergies, 23
factor in treatment effectiveness, 370
Birds. *See* Animals.
Black widow spider, 269–270
Blackley, Dr. Charles H., 93, 355
Blazer, Philip, 244

Blisters, due to drug reaction, 232
Blood
  count, 335
  groups, 418
  in stools, 28
  tests, 341–342, 366
  transfusions
    reactions to, 291, 360
    transferring allergy, 359
  typing, 418
Blood vessel reactions due to allergy, 323
Bookbinders, causes of dermatitis of, 234
"Booze and snooze," 34–35
Borcherdt Company, 392
Borden Company, 245
Boric acid, 40
Bostock, Dr. John, 92, 355
Breast feeding, 33–35
Breathing exercises, 145, 149–155
  for breaking smoking habit, 191–192
Breathlessness. *See* Shortness of breath.
Breon Laboratories, 392
Bright's disease, 375
Bronchi, 120–122, 160–163
Bronchial asthma, 418
  See also Asthma.
Bronchial obstruction, 60, 122
Bronchiectasis, 163
Bronchioles, 120, 418
Bronchitis, 49, 121, 127, 129, 158, 159–176, 419
  days lost because of, 88
  definition, 161–162
  heparin to treat, 252
  screening programs, 170–171
Bronchodilators, 61, 137–139, 143, 144
Broncho Junction, 84–85
Bronchoscopy, 167
Bronchospasm, 419
Bronchus, 419
Broom-manufacturing workers, causes of dermatitis of, 234
Brown, Dr. Halla, 277
Brown recluse spider, 269–270
Bryan, Dr. William, T. K., 202
Bryan, Mrs. Marian, 202
Burroughs Wellcome & Co., 393
Butchers, cause of dermatitis of, 234
Buttercup, 241
Button-manufacturing workers, causes of dermatitis of, 234

Caffeine, 113
Calamine lotion, 419
Camps, 82–85
Cancer
  and allergic mechanisms, 373–374
  and immune response, 371
  research on vaccines, 373–374
Candy-manufacturing workers, causes of dermatitis of, 234
Canker sores, 324, 419
  in infants, 25, 49
Canning-industry workers, possible causes of dermatitis of, 234
Capillaries, 21, 71
Caplin, Dr. Irvin, 5, 136, 138
Cardiac asthma, 122
Cardiospasm, 419
Carotid body, 147–148
Carpeting, 38
Carrington, Dr. Charles B., 157
Cashew allergy, 241
Castor bean allergy, 101, 233
Cataracts due to allergy, 325
Catarrh. *See* Hayfever.
Caterpillars, allergy from touching, 276
Cats, allergy to, 23, 36, 101
Causes of allergy, 18, 20, 21, 34–38, 70–71, 92–93, 99–102, 108
  of asthma, 133
  in infants, 24–43
  list of, 381–383
Cauterization, 115
Cavanaugh, Dr. James, 38–39, 125
Caverly Child Health Center, 80
Celiac disease, 48
Cement workers, possible causes of dermatitis of, 234
Cephalothin test, 366
Cereal allergy, 35
Cheilosis, 419

Chemosis, 419
See also Eye disorders.
Cherovinsky, Dr. Paul, 171
Chicken allergy, 320
Chigger, 270–271
Childhood allergies, 44–86
deaths from, 45
effects on children's lives, 45–46
incidence of, 44–45
patterns, 46–48
symptoms, 46–47
Children, and parents, 16
Children's Asthma Research Institute and Hospital, 78, 80
Children's Convalescent Hospital Asthma Unit, 80
Children's Heart Hospital Asthma Unit, 80
Chocolate allergy, 18, 30, 31, 69, 203, 208–209
Chromate allergy, 229–230
Chronic obstructive lung disease, 159–176
Chrysanthemum allergy, 241
Cigarettes. *See* Smoking.
Cilia, 120–121, 419
Cinnamon allergy, what to avoid, 32
Circulation problems due to allergy, 323
Citrus fruits, as allergy cause, 30
Climate, 22, 61, 79, 96, 98, 111, 134–135, 136
Coal tar medicines
reactions to, 292, 298
sun reaction, 41
Cobalt itch, 233
Cockroach allergy, 101, 276–277
Cohen, Dr. Sumner, 174
Cola, 202
C.O.L.D. (Chronic obstructive lung disease), 159–176
questionnaire, 172–174
screening program, 170–171
treatment, 171–176
Cold, allergy to, 83, 103, 144–146, 326–327
Colds, 127, 165
how to tell if you have cold or hayfever, 48–49, 54–55, 90, 91
summer colds, 90
Cold turkey, 190
Colic, 18, 25, 48
following skin rashes, 26
reaction to hot milk, 27
sign of allergy, 28
Colitis, 419
Collagen disease, 419
Coloring agents, allergy to, 297–298
Conditioning, 70–71
Congenital laryngeal stridor, 39
Conjunctival test, 419
Conjunctivitis, 419
See also Eye disorders.
Connell, Dr. John T., 364
Constipation, in infants, 25
Construction workers, causes of dermatitis of, 234
Contactant, 419
Contact dermatitis, 116, 419
caused by drugs, 281
possible causes, 252–257
See also Dermatitis.
Controlled environment, 365, 367
Convalescent Hospital for Crippled Children of the Cincinnati Orphan Asylum, 80
Convulsions, 48
due to allergy, 321–322
Cooking, effect on allergenicity, 200
Cooks, possible causes of dermatitis of, 236
Cooper Laboratories, 393
Cooperman, Dr. Jack, 265
Coral, 273
Corn allergy, 69, 207–208
foods to avoid, 31, 212–213
other things to avoid, 254
rash due to, 233
Corn itch, 233
Corticosteroids, 61, 419
and asthma, 139–140
reducing side effects, 140
Corticotropin. *See* ACTH.
Cortisone, 115, 419
Coryza, 419
See also Colds.
Cosmetics, 101, 133
allergy to, 241–248
common allergens in, 245–248
hypoallergenic, 244–245

Cosmetics (*cont.*)
and sun sensitivity, 295–296
Cosmos allergy, 93
Costs of allergies, 14
Cottonseed allergy, 101, 207
things to avoid, 254
Cough, 51, 56–57, 114, 119, 142, 161, 162, 164, 166–168
from allergy, 28, 320, 418
diagnosis of, 335–337
in infants, 25
treatment, 175
See also Croup.
Cough reflex, 167
Cradle cap, 40
Creams. *See* Medicines; Drugs.
Cromolyn sodium, 139
Crook, Dr. William G., 69
Cross-sensitivities, 203–205
Croup, 49, 65–66, 127, 419
Crying, 28, 68
Cushing's syndrome, 61
Cyclopropane, 86
Cystic fibrosis, 60, 141
Cystitis, 419
Cysts, on lungs, 175

Dairy workers, possible causes of dermatitis of, 235
Daisy allergy, 241
Dampness, 89, 94, 98, 107–108
Dara Laboratories, 393
da Vinci, Leonardo, 315
DDT. *See* Pesticides.
Declomycin and sun reaction, 295
Dehydration, 144
Delayed reaction, 199, 279–280
to penicillin, 284
to skin tests, 338
Dental plates, reaction to, 324
Dentists, possible causes of dermatitis of, 235
de Pavie, Botallus, 92
Depression, 72
Dermatitis, 219–257, 282, 332, 419
and cataracts, 323
caused by drugs, 309
caused by insects, 276–277
Dermatitis (*cont.*)
diagnosis of cause, 220–237, 337
incidence of, 14
in infants, 39–42
patterns on body, 224–228
possible causes, 252–257
of scalp, 242
treatment, 249–252
Dermik Laboratories, 393
Dermographia, 329–330
Desensitization, 419, 351–352
injections for, 58, 90, 99, 100–101
to insect stings, 275–276
new methods, 367–369
to poison ivy, 240
stronger doses, 368
Detergent burn, 220
Deviated septum, 92
Diagnosis of allergy, 332–342
in infants, 24–31
research on new methods, 366–367
Diaper rash, 40
Diaphragmatic breathing, 149–150, 154
Diarrhea, 28, 51
effects on allergy, 31
in infants, 25
treatment for rash, 40
Diet, 133
See also individual food items.
Diet chart, 203
Diphtheria antitoxin, reactions from, 290–291
Disinfectant industry workers, possible causes of dermatitis of, 235
Disobedience, 56, 65
Disodium cromoglycate, 368
Diving, 83
Dizziness, due to allergy, 320
Doak Pharmacal Company, 393
Dogs
as cause of allergy, 36
having hayfever and asthma, 362
See also Pets.
Doctor
choosing, 53–54
explaining to child, 53

Doctor (*cont.*)
going to, 51–54, 331–352
See also Allergist.
Dolowitz, Dr. David, 252
Donora, 128
Dorsey Laboratories, 393
Draft rejections, 14
Drainage of bronchi, 142–143
Drinking, of fluids, 61
See also Alcohol.
Driving, 109, 110
Dropsy, 420
Drowsiness, due to allergy, 324
Drugs, 61, 115, 139–140, 417
allergies to, 29, 122, 143, 145, 219, 231–232, 243, 251, 278–310
diagnosis of, 281–283
from additives, 297–298
list of products containing allergy-producing drugs, 300–310
new tests for, 366
symptoms of, 280–281
aminophylline, 139
aminopyrine, 122
amphetamine, 113
anesthetics, 86, 244, 290
antibiotics, 63, 114, 144–145, 210, 251, 278–279, 286–287, 418
anticoagulants, 148
antihistamines, 113, 114, 343–345, 386–391, 418
antiseptics, 296
aspirin, 114, 122, 146, 205, 281–282, 287–290
for asthma, 132–155, 368
barbiturates, 86, 293, 294, 418
boric acid, 40
bronchodilators, 61, 137–139, 143, 144
calamine lotion, 419
coal tar medicines, 41, 292, 298
corticosteroids, 61, 139–140, 419
cortisone, 43, 115, 419
cromolyn sodium, 139
cyclopropane, 86
declomycin, 295
decongestants, 51, 112, 114, 115
delayed reactions, 279–280, 284
Drugs (*cont.*)
for dermatitis, 40–42, 251
disodium cromoglycate, 368
for emphysema, 171–176
ephedrine, 114
epinephrine, 114, 139, 146, 420
expectorants, 136–137
eyedrops, 114
for eye symptoms, 50–51, 114
fixed drug reaction, 231, 294, 309
glucagon, 368
heparin, 252, 368
high blood pressure medicine, 92
hormones, 102, 115, 139–140, 143, 371, 421
hydrocortisone, 114
imipramine, 67
interactions of, 282–283
iodide salts, 136
iodine, 293, 305–307
laxatives, 292
lobeline, 194
manufacturers, 392–395
morphine, 86
narcotics, 86
nebulizers, 138–139, 141
neomycin, 286
nose drops, 58, 114
nose spray, 114
paraben, 243–251
penicillin, 6, 14, 48, 63, 101, 122, 145, 233, 278, 283–288, 299, 300–301, 312, 366
photosensitivity, 232, 294–297, 329
placebo, 422
prednisone, 115
pyramidon, 122
quinine, 122, 293
reactions, 279, 308–309
salicylates, 288–290
sedatives, 61, 293–294
side effects, 280, 287, 324, 344
steroids, 57, 424
streptomycin, 286
sulfonamide, 286, 301–305
sulfones, 292
sun sensitivity and, 294–297
tetracycline, 305

Drugs (*cont.*)
tranquilizers, 114, 141–142, 424
See also Medicines.
Dry-cleaning workers, possible causes of dermatitis of, 235
Duodenum, 420
Dust
allergy to, 38, 48, 92, 99, 101, 104–108, 135, 364
caused by house-dust mite, 101, 110
desensitization against, 116, 122
collecting for injections, 347–348
dust-proofing your house. *See* Housecleaning.
insect dust. *See* Insect allergy.
Dust count, 420
Dye, allergy to, 230, 297
Dyspnea, 420
Dysuria, 420

Ear disorders, 317–319, 320
infections, 48, 55–56, 114, 127
Eczema, 83, 219, 420
caused by cod liver oil, 29
caused by drugs, 231, 309
caused by milk, 33
caused by mold, 96
caused by sensitivity to light, 328–329
exposure to fever blisters, chickenpox, or shingles, 43
housewife eczema, 249
in infants, 26, 39–42
in pregnancy, 370
treatment, 41–42
vaccination during, 42–43, 250
Egg allergy, 30, 31–32, 206
foods to avoid, 31–32, 213–214
vaccinations and, 291
Eisen, Dr. A., 146
Eisenstadt, Dr. W. Sawyer, 5, 138
Electrical-manufacturing workers, possible causes of dermatitis of, 235
Electroencephalography (EEG), 420
Electronic air cleaner, 107, 109
Electrosleep therapy, 147
Eli Lilly and Company, 393
Elliotson, Dr. John, 355
Ellis, Dr. Elliott, 62
Emotions, 65, 70–79, 82–86, 143, 155–156, 369
allergic tension-fatigue syndrome, 67–71
asthma and, 59, 62, 69, 130–132, 141–142
effects of allergies on, 45–46
effects on allergies, 22, 29, 61, 92, 102
on first trip to doctor, 53
skin allergy and, 218, 252
smoking and, 193–194
special needs during allergy attack, 42
Emphysema, 121, 129, 158, 159–176, 420
definition, 162
screening programs, 170–171
test for, 171
treatment, 171–176
Emphysema-bronchitis syndrome, 162
See also Emphysema.
Encephalomyelitis, 374
Endotoxin, 420
Energy, lack of as sign of allergy, 28, 67–70, 73
Enteritis, 420
Environmental factors, in causing allergies, 361
Eosinophils, 91, 359
Ephedrine, 114
Epidemic areas of allergy, 361
Epilepsy, due to allergy, 322
Epinephrine, 114, 139, 146, 420
Epstein, Dr. John H., 5
Erythema, 219
caused by drugs, 309
Estrogen, 420. *See also* Hormones.
Ethmoiditis, 420
Eustachian tube, 55, 65, 127, 420
Exanthematosis, caused by drugs, 310
Exchange transfusion, 420
Exercise
in asthma, 62, 79, 81–82, 148–155
for emphysema, 175–176
Exertion, effect on allergy, 22, 61, 102

Exfoliative dermatitis, 219
caused by drugs, 232, 310
Expectorants, 136–137
Exterminators, possible cause of dermatitis of, 235
Extrasystole, 420
Eye disorders, 48, 49, 242, 243, 323–324
cataracts and allergy, 323
dark circles, 49, 67–69, 129
eyelid reactions, 324
eye symptoms, 49–50
treatment of symptoms, 50–51, 114
Eyedrops, 114
Eye test, 338

Facial tissues, 58
Facies, 49
Falliers, Dr. Constantine, 334
Farmer's lung disease, 124, 319
Fatigue, 102
effect on allergy, 22, 31
as sign of allergy, 28, 67–70
Feathers, 38, 48, 92, 108, 125
Feather workers, possible cause of dermatitis of, 235
Feeding problems, 73
Feet, dermatitis of, 231
Fein, Dr. Bernard T., 5, 149, 322
Feinberg, Dr. Alan, 100
Feinberg, Dr. Samuel, 15, 100, 284
Feingold, Dr. Ben, 5, 210
Fenspiride, 139
Fever blisters, 324
in infants, 25
Fiberglass fabric, 230–231
Fibrillation, 420
Fire ants, 267
Fireproofing workers, possible causes of dermatitis of, 235
Fish allergy, 204
Fishermen, possible cause of dermatitis of, 235
Fixed drug reaction, 231, 294, 309
Flavoring agents, allergy to, 297–298
Flax allergy
flaxseed, 220
things to avoid, 254
Fleas, 268
Flies, 267–268
Florists, possible causes of dermatitis of, 235
Flour and grain workers, possible causes of dermatitis of, 235
Floyer, Sir John, 119
Fluids, 144
in asthma, 136
Fluorides, allergy to, 293
Flu vaccine, 43, 146
Food additives, 200–201, 210–212
allergy to, 282
Food allergy, 110, 122, 197–216
asthma from, 60, 198
bed-wetting from, 67
caused by insects, 277
in children, 27–36
dizziness from, 320
hayfever from, 198
headaches from, 198, 199, 312, 314
hearing difficulties from, 320
hives from, 198
major troublemakers, 29–34, 206–210
outgrowing, 27
prevention and treatment, 35
related foods to avoid, 31–33, 203–206
symptoms, 28–29, 198–199, 211
tension-fatigue syndrome from, 68–69
tests for, 30–31, 201–202
Food coloring
allergy to, 282
foods to avoid if allergic to, 32
Food diaries, 30–31, 202
Food intolerance, 27–28
Food substitutes, 212
Formaldehyde allergy, 230
Formula, infant, 25
Frazier, Dr. Claude, 5, 259
Fredrickson, Dr. Donald, 193
Fries, Dr. Joseph H., 208
Fumes, 155
effect on allergy, 22, 92, 106–107, 110, 123, 127–128
of popcorn, 207

Fungus, 101, 124
Furniture, 105–108, 125
Furriers, possible causes of dermatitis of, 235
Fusarium, 97

Gaillardia, allergy to, 241
Galen, 355
Gamma globulin, 115, 143, 358, 360, 420
  gamma E, 360
  globulin A, 360
  reactions to, 291
Gardeners, causes of dermatitis of, 234
Garment-industry workers, possible causes of dermatitis of, 235
Gas, and food allergy, 320
Gastroenteritis, 420
Gastrointestinal allergies, 66
Gerrard, Dr. John, 209
Glaser, Dr. Jerome, 62
Glazer, Dr. Israel, 147
Globulin A, 360
Glomectomy, 147–148
Glucagon, 368
Glue-industry workers, possible causes of dermatitis of, 235
Gnats, 267–268
Goddard, Dr. Roy F., 60
Golden glow, 93
Goldenrod, 93
Goldman, Dr. Stanley L., 82
Gordon, Dr. William, 355
Grass pollen seasons, 95–96, 111
  See also Pollen.
Grocerymen, possible causes of dermatitis of, 235
Guilt feelings, 73–74, 76–77

H substance, 20–21, 60
Hair, allergy to, 92
Hair products, 243, 244
  See also Cosmetics.
Halpern, Prof. Bernard, 372
Harkang, Dr. Joseph, 322
Hayfever, 87–117, 420
Hayfever (*cont.*)
  after the season, 90
  age of onset, 89
  causes of, 36–37
    insect dust, 277
  in children, 48–49
  complications, 89
  incidence of, 13, 14, 88
  kinds, 88
  origin of term, 92
  perennial, 88, 422
  respiratory infections and, 63–64
  school and work days lost because of, 88
  seasonal, 88
  symptoms, 46, 88–89
    first described, 92
Haywood, Dr. Theodore, 5
Headache, 48, 49, 68
  due to allergy, 211, 311–315
  due to food allergy, 198, 199
  histamine cephalalgia, 314
  tension headache, 314
  treatment, 315
Health Hill Hospital for Convalescent Children, 80
Hearing impairment, 48, 55–56, 64–65, 318
  from food allergy, 320
Heartburn, 51
Heart disease, 60, 122, 138, 163, 418
  due to allergy, 322–323
  emphysema and, 160
  pain, 68
Heat allergy, 327–328
Heating, 105–107
Heat rash, 420
Helminthosporium, 97
Heparin, 368
Hepatitis, 420
Heredity, 25–26, 49, 361
  in sensitivity to cold, 326–327
  in skin allergy, 218
Herpes, 421
  simplex, 324
High blood pressure medicine, 92
Hippocrates, 70, 118, 355
Histamine, 21, 60, 421
  air pollution and, 127
Histamine cephalalgia, 314

History of allergy, 70, 92–93, 118–119, 128, 197, 258, 315, 355–357
  food allergy, 197–198
  inoculations, 345
  insect allergy, 258
  sinus cavities, 315
  skin allergy, 217
Hives, 21, 49, 421
  due to cold allergy, 326–327
  in dogs, 242
  due to drugs, 231, 309
  in infants, 26
  due to infection, 219
  of insects, 265–266
Holmes, Dr. Oliver Wendell, 111
Home environment, 78
Homes for allergic children, 77–81
Honey, as treatment for hayfever, 369
Hormodendrum, 96
Hormones, 102, 115, 139–140, 143, 421
  allergy to, 371
  asthma and, 23
  changes during allergy, 72
  effects on allergy, 22, 47–48, 103
  emphysema and, 165
  mosquitoes and, 269
  See also Corticosteroids; Adrenalin.
Horn, Dr. Daniel, 178
Hornets, 18
  allergy to sting, 262
  how to destroy hives, 266
Horse allergy
  horsehair, 108–109
  reactions to vaccines and, 43, 291
Hospitals for allergic children, 77–81
Housecleaning, 38, 98, 99, 104–108
House-dust mite, 101
Humidity, 103, 104, 107, 155, 250
  See also Dampness.
Hydrocortisone, 114
Hydrops of the middle ear, 65
Hypoallergenic cosmetics, 244–245
Hypersensitivity, 421
Hyperventilation, 421
Hypnosis treatment, 146–147, 369
  for smoking, 192
Hyposensitization injections, 115–117, 345–352, 421
  for asthma, 134
  effectiveness, 348–349
  repository immunization, 349–351
  See also Desensitization.

Iatrogenic disease, 279, 421
Ice-cream makers, possible causes of dermatitis of, 236
Imipramine, 67
Immune mechanism, 372–373
Immunity, 3, 358, 359, 421
  second immune system, 359–360
  See also Desensitization.
Immunization, 42–43, 359–360, 421
Immunological paralysis, 373
Immunological reaction, 359–360
Immunological weakness, 371
Impetigo, 421
Incidence of allergies, 13, 14, 88
  in children, 44–45
Infants with allergy, 24–43, 358
  asthma, 38–39
  how to tell if symptoms are allergic, 25
  removing allergy causes, 38
  skin rashes, 39–42
Infection, 102, 143, 155
  abscess, 417
  asthma and, 122, 123, 126–127, 133, 139
  cause of skin rash, 282
  complicating allergy, 55, 62–64, 90, 121
  cough after, 117
  of ear, 318
  effect on allergy, 22, 31, 47, 59, 62–64
  following insect sting, 263
  of sinuses, 315–317
  vaccines and, 117
Infertility
  due to allergy, 370
  test for, 370

Influenza vaccine
and asthma, 43
and egg sensitivity, 43
Information gap, 15, 16
Ingestant, 421
See also Foods; Medicines.
Inhalants, 421
See also Airborne allergens.
Inhalation therapy, 137
Injectants, 421
Injections, 53
coseasonal, 346–347
perennial, 346, 347
preseasonal, 346, 347
schedules, 346–347
self-injections, 384–385
See also Desensitization; Hyposensitization.
Ink manufacturers, possible causes of dermatitis of, 236
Insect allergy, 55, 83, 92, 258–277
asthma caused by cockroaches, 276
as cause of death, 259, 260
caused by eating insect debris, 277
caused by insect dust, 99–101, 277
dermatitis from contact, 276–277
desensitization for, 275–276
fleas, 268
flies, 267–268
kissing bug, 271–272
mites, 271
mosquitoes, 268–269
scorpion, 272–273
spider, 269–270
stinging insects, 259–266
ants, 266–267
complications after stings, 263
cross sensitivities, 262
destroying hives, 265–266
preventing stings, 264–265
reactions to, 262–263
ticks, 271
wheel bug, 271
Insecticide, 110, 269
allergy to, 233
Insomnia, 68
International Association of Allergology, 376
Intertrigo, 421
Intractable allergies, 77, 79–80
in asthma, 421
Intradermal test, 201, 338, 421
Intravenous test, 421
Intrinsic asthma, 421
Iodide salts, 136
Iodine allergy, 293
products to avoid, 305–307
Irritability, as sign of allergy, 28, 67–71
Ischemia, 422
Ishizaka, Dr. Kimishige, 360
Ishizaka, Dr. Teruko, 360
Isomil, 34
Itching, 89, 250, 251, 335

Janitors, possible causes of dermatitis of, 236
Jaundice, 422
Jejunum, 422
Jellyfish, 273
Jewelry workers, possible causes of dermatitis of, 236
Johnson, Dr. Kenneth J., 207

Kamin, Dr. Peter B., 322
Kapok, 38
Karaya gum allergy, 123, 243
things to avoid, 255
Katsh, Dr. Seymour, 371
Kaufman, Dr. Herbert, 340
Keighley, Dr. John F., 137
Keratinization, 422
Kerosene, 110
K.I.C.H., 194
Kidney disease, 374, 375
Kilfeher, Dr. John, 174
Kimball, Dr. E. Robbins, 34
Kinins, 360
Kissing bug, 271, 272
Knoll Pharmaceutical Company, 393
Krameria, 241

Laboratory tests, 341–342
Labyrinthitis, 127

Lacquer allergy, 241
Lamond Products, 393
Lanolin allergy, 243, 251
  things to avoid, 255
Larson, Dr. Donald, 101
Laryngitis, 127
Laryngospasm, 422
La Scola, Dr. Raymond L., 147
Laundry workers, possible causes of dermatitis of, 236
Lavage, 142
Laxatives
  allergy to, 292
  effect on allergies, 29
Learning difficulties, 45
Lecks, Dr. Harold, 82
Lever Brothers, 393
Licorice allergy, 283
Light sensitivity, 297, 328–329
Lipstick allergy, 18, 242–243
  See also Cosmetics.
Lip symptoms, 241, 242, 324
  blisters, 221–222
  dry lips, 51
Lobeline, 194
Lockey, Dr. Stephen D., 5, 211, 300, 308
Lotions. *See* Medicines.
Loveless, Dr. Mary Hewitt, 350
Lowance, Dr. Mason, 5
Lower respiratory tract, 120–121
Lozenges, 145
Lucretius, 355
Lung tests, 342
Lung washout. *See* Lavage.
Lupus erythematosus, 375
Lyons, Dr. Harold S., 131

Machine workers, possible causes of dermatitis of, 236
Make-up. *See* Cosmetics.
Mallen, Dr. P. Mario Salazar, 285
Mango allergy, 241
Manufacturers, of allergy products, 392–395
Maple bark strippers' disease, 319
Marcelle Hypo-Allergenic Cosmetics, 245, 393
Marijuana, 115
Marks, Dr. Meyer B., 50
Marph, Charles, 15
Match-industry workers, possible causes of dermatitis of, 236
May apple allergy, 241
Mead Johnson Laboratories, 393
Meals, frequency for hayfever, 114
  See also Food.
Measles vaccine
  egg sensitivity and, 43
  when taking cortisone, 43
Meat packers, causes of dermatitis of, 234
Mechanical pressure, allergy to, 329–330
Medical profession, possible causes of dermatitis of, 236
Medicines, 392–395
  antihistamines and properties, 386–391
  for asthma, 136, 139–140
  as cause of allergy, 29, 122, 143, 243, 251, 278–310
  cod liver oil, 29
  cost of, 14
  decongestants, 51, 112, 114, 115
  for dermatitis, 40, 251
  gamma globulins, 115, 143, 291, 358, 360, 420
  merthiolate, allergy to, 292
  metaphen, allergy to, 292
  new experimental drugs, 367–368
  side effects, 280
  to relieve symptoms, 46, 113, 114, 343–345
  See also Drugs.
Medina, Dr. Ambrosio, 174
Ménière's syndrome, 320
Menopause, 103
Menstruation, 103
Mental problems, due to allergy, 211–212
Merck, Sharp and Dohme, 394
Mercury allergy, 292
  products to avoid, 307–308
Merthiolate, allergy to, 292
Mesquite, 95
Metal workers, possible causes of dermatitis of, 237
Metaphen, allergy to, 292

Mexican firebrush, 95
Microstatic precipitator, 109
Midges, 268
Migraine headache, 28, 313–314, 422
    See also Headache.
Mildew, 97
    See also Mold.
Military rejections, 14
Milk allergy, 29, 33–34, 68, 209–210
    due to additives, 200–201
    foods to avoid, 31, 214–215
    prevention by breast feeding, 33–34
    withholding, 31
Milk intolerance, 27–28, 209–210
Milk substitutes, 34, 212
Mirror-manufacturing workers, possible causes of dermatitis of, 236
Mist, 140–141
Mites, 270–271, 364
Mold allergy, 92, 96–98, 107–108, 124, 422
    desensitization against, 116
    destruction of, 98, 122
    where found, 96–97
        in foods, 97
Money allergy, 18
Morphine, 86
Mosquitoes, 268–269
Moths, allergy from touching, 276–277
Mount, Dr. Frank, 174
Mouth breathing, 49, 51, 56
Moving, 134–135
Mucorales, 97
Mucus, 136, 142, 161, 162
Mueller, Dr. Harry, 146
Mull-soy, 34
Multiple sclerosis, and allergic mechanisms, 371, 375
Muscle and joint soreness, 69
Mushroom pickers' disease, 319
Musicians, possible causes of dermatitis of, 236
Myasthenia gravis, 375
Myxomycetes, 101
McElhenney, Dr. Thomas R., 101
McGovern, Dr. John P., 6, 101, 284, 394
McNeil Laboratories, 394

Narcotics, 86
Nasal polyps, 56–57, 90, 114, 122
Nasal symptoms, 21, 67, 88–89, 90–92
    as sign of food allergy, 28
    streptococcal infections and, 29
    due to underactive thyroid, 92
    year-round symptoms, 54–59, 113, 114
Nasal test, 422
Nash, Ogden, 217
National Asthma Camp, 85
National Foundation for Asthmatic Children, 81
National Hayfever Relief Camp, 85
National Jewish Hospital, 78–79, 81
Nebulizer, 138–139, 141
    See also Bronchodilator.
"Nebulizer clutchers," 138–139
Neomycin allergy, 286
Nephritis, 422
    See also Kidney disease.
Nervousness. *See* Irritability.
Neuritis, 48
Neutrogena Corp., 394
Newborn, 358
New Orleans epidemic asthma, 124
Nickel allergy, 228–229
Night cough, 25
    See also Cough.
Nosebleed, 48
Nose drops, 58, 114
Nose spray, 114
Nutramigen, 34
Nutrition, 102
    balanced diet, 32
    effect on allergy, 22, 29
Nuts, 204

Occupational dermatitis, 232–237
    prevention of, 233–234
    See also Dermatitis.
Ochsner, Dr. Alton, 192
Odors, 200
    effect on allergy, 22, 92, 123
Office workers, possible causes of dermatitis of, 234

One-shot hayfever treatment, 116–117, 349, 351
Orange allergy, 241
  to juice, 32
  See also Citrus fruit.
Organ transplants, 372–373
Orris root allergy, 243
Otitis media. *See* Serous otitis media.
Outgrowing allergies, 26–27, 46, 121
Overdependence, 72
Overholt, Dr. Richard H., 148
Overprotection, 73, 74, 76–77, 131–132

Pain on urination, as food allergy, 199
Paleness, 67–69
Paley, Dr. Aaron, 131
Palpitation, 422
Paper-manufacturing workers, possible causes of dermatitis of, 236
Paraben, 243, 251
Paracusis, allergic, 64–65
  See also Hearing impairment.
Parasites, 123
Parentectomy, 78
Parents, 252
  attitudes toward allergy, 45–46, 62, 71–76, 83–84, 131–132
  cuddling, 42
  diagnosing child's allergy, 24–31
    hidden allergies, 45
  ignoring advice, 16
Particulate, 422
Pass, Dr. Franklin, 5
Passive transfer test, 338
Patch test, 221, 224, 232, 338, 422
  for hair dye, 244
Patterson, Dr. Roy, 362
Pavlovian conditioned reflex, 70–71
Peanuts, 18, 30, 31
Pemphigus, 375
Pencil-manufacturing workers, possible causes of dermatitis of, 236
Penicillin allergy, 63, 101, 122, 145, 278, 283–288
  headaches due to, 312
Penicillin allergy (*cont.*)
  incidence of, 6, 14, 48
  in laboratory workers, 233
  less allergenic forms, 299
  due to milk, 284, 286
  products to avoid, 300–301
  tests for, 283, 366
Penicillium, 97
Penicilloyl polylysine (PPL), 283
Perennial allergic rhinitis, 54–59, 88
  See also Hayfever.
Perfume. *See* Cosmetics.
Periodontal disease, and allergy, 372
Perkins, Dr. Herbert, 360
Peroxide allergy, 244
Persistent positive reactor, 232
Personality disturbances, 68
  See also Behavior; Emotions.
Perspiration, 229, 231, 249
  attracting insects, 264
Peshkin, Dr. M. Murray, 77
Pesticides, 243
  in foods, 210
Peterson, Dr. William, 369
Pets, as cause of allergy, 36–37, 48
  See also Animals.
Pharmaceutical companies, 386–391, 392–395
Pharyngitis, 422
Phenolphthalein, allergy to, 292
Philodendron allergy, 241
Photographers, possible causes of dermatitis of, 234
Photosensitivity, 232, 294–297, 329
  with drugs and cosmetics, 294–296
  with plants, 296
Physical allergies, 325–330
  to cold, 326–327
  to heat, 327–328
  to light, 328–329
  to mechanical pressure, 329–330
Pica, 422
Pigeon-breast, 49
Pigeon breeders' disease, 319
Pill dispensers, 370
Pimples, 127
Pine allergy, 241
Placebo, 422
Plantain, 95

Plants
as cause of allergy, 93, 95, 237–240, 241
sun sensitivity and, 296
Plasma cell, 358
Plastic, allergy to, 294
Platelets, 422
Plumbers, possible causes of dermatitis of, 236
Pneumonia, caused by allergy, 157, 319–320
Pneumothorax, 422
Poi, 35, 212
Poinsettia allergy, 241
Poison ivy, 237–240
Poison oak, 237–240
Poison sumac, 237–240
Pollen, 92–96, 110–111, 122, 422
age of child at usual allergy onset, 47
how gathered to prepare injections, 347–348
kinds, 90
predictions about, 363
research on, 362–366
seasons, 90, 95–96
sensitivity to, 47–48
symptoms, time of, 37
treatment of allergy to, 38, 116
See also Ragweed.
Pollen counts, 102, 103–104
by city and state, 396–403
research on, 365
Pollen theory, 93
Pollen-free areas, summaries by state and city, 404–416
Pollination, 93–94
Pollinosis. *See* Hayfever.
Polyarthritis, 422
Polyneuritis, 422
Polypeptides, 21
Portuguese man-of-war, 273
Positive pressure breathing, 140–141
Postnasal drip, 57
Postural drainage. *See* Drainage.
Posture exercises, 153
Pottery workers, possible causes of dermatitis of, 236
Powder. *See* Cosmetics.
Precipitator, 422
Prednisone, 115
Pregnancy, 103, 242, 357–358, 370
asthma and, 156
preventing allergy in the unborn baby, 35–36
Pressure, allergy to, 330
Prickly heat, 40
Priming by pollen, 364
Primrose allergy, 241
Printers, possible causes of dermatitis of, 236
Procter and Gamble Company, 394
Prodromal symptoms, 47, 136
of headaches, 313
Provocative food test, 201, 342
Psoriasis, 422
Psychiatric problems, due to allergy, 211–212
Psychogenic factors. *See* Emotions.
Psychogenic theories, 75–76
Psychosomatic, 422
Puberty, 103
Pulmonary function, 423
Purpura, 219
due to drug reaction, 232, 309
Pursed-lip breathing, 153–154
Putty-manufacturing workers, possible causes of dermatitis of, 236
Pyramidon, 122
Pythagoras, 197

Q Day, 190–191
Queen Alexandra Solarium for Crippled Children, 81
Quinine, allergy to, 122, 293

Ragweed Index
by city and state, 396–403
ragweed-free areas, 404–416
Ragweed pollen, 92–110
destruction of, 94–95
isolating fractions, 368–369
pollination, 90, 93
prevalence, 93, 94
research on, 362–366
sensitivity to, 93
size of, 93
in spring, 90
Rain, effect on allergy, 103

Rapid remitters, 79
Rash, 219
See also Dermatitis; Skin.
Reagin, 423
Rebound phenomenon, 58, 114
Rectal itch, 334
See also Antibiotic side effects.
Redness, 219
due to drug reactions, 232
around the mouth, 220
Redwood Glen Camp, 85
Redwood trees, 124
Referred pain, 312
Rejection of organs, 74, 76, 372
Remodeling, 107
Repository injections, 116–117, 349–351
Research, 353–377
Residential treatment centers. *See* Homes and hospitals.
Resistance
and allergic mechanisms, 371
See also Desensitization.
Restaurant workers, possible causes of dermatitis of, 236
Restlessness, 28, 67–71, 73
Revlon, 394
Rh babies, 358, 423
prevention, 358
Rheumatic fever, 20
Rheumatic heart disease, 375–376
allergic mechanisms, 371
Richet, Dr. Charles, 355
Riker Laboratories, 394
Rinkel, Dr. H., 201
Rope workers, possible causes of dermatitis of, 237
Rose fever, 95
See also Hayfever.
Roses, 93
Ross Laboratories, 394
Rubber allergy, 229
Russian thistle, 95

Sahuaro School, 81
Saint Mary's Hospital for Children, 81
Salicylates, in food and other substances, 288–290
Samter, Dr. Max, 288
Sardeau Inc., 394
Scapegoating, 76
Schering Corporation, 394
Scherr, Dr. Merle, 5, 84
Schick, Professor Bela, 356
Schieffelin & Co., 394
Schorr, Dr. William, 5, 243
Scleroderma, 423
Sclerosis, 423
Scorpions, 272–273
Scratching, 51, 250
restraints to prevent, 41–42
Scratch test, 201, 291, 337–340, 423
Sea anemones, 273
Sea squirts, 123–124
Seborrheic dermatitis, 423
Secondary gains, 72–73
Secretary otitis media. *See* Serous otitis media.
Sedative drugs, 61
reactions to, 293–294
Self-injections, 384–385
Self-medication, 142
Sensitivity, 423
Sensitization, 20
Serous otitis media, 65, 317–319, 422, 423
Serum, 423
Serum sickness, 281, 291
penicillin as cause of, 284
Shen Nung, 355
Shepard Laboratories, 394
Shock, 423
Shock organ, 423
Shoes, allergy to, 231
Shoe-manufacturing workers, causes of dermatitis of, 234
Shortness of breath, 119, 122, 161, 162, 163, 164, 168–169
Shots. *See* Desensitization.
Side effects
of antihistamines, 386–391
See also Medicines.
Silk
allergy to, 294
cause of reactions to medicines, 294
Sinus, 423

Sinusitis, 56–57, 113, 114, 120, 123, 127, 315–317, 423
- caused by allergy, 89
- days lost because of, 88
- diagnosis of, 91
- factors affecting, 316
- headaches and, 312
- symptoms of, 91
- treatment of, 317

Skin allergies, 217–257
- causes, 218–248
- and respiratory allergy, 26
- symptoms, 219–220
- *See also* Dermatitis.

Skin grafts, 372

Skin rashes
- caused by drugs, 309
- in infants, 39–42
- infection and, 63

Skin tests, 37, 47, 90, 95, 98, 337–341, 423
- in asthma, 39, 102, 115, 125
- in contact dermatitis, 221
- in drug sensitivity, 283
- in food allergy, 201
- positive reactions (*ill.*), 339

Skin windows, 359

Slater, Dr. Hyde, 355

Sleep, lack of, 102

Sleepiness, due to allergy, 324

Slime mold, 101

Slow learning, 56, 65, 67–70

Smallpox vaccination
- eczema and, 250
- exposure to people with rashes, 42–43
- when taking cortisone drugs, 43

Smell, loss of, 56–57, 89, 316

Smith, Sydney, 88

Smog, 135, 423

Smoke, allergy to, 92, 177

Smoker type, quiz, 178–190

Smoking, 138–139, 155, 163, 165, 175
- action on lungs, 166
- asthma and, 138–139
- how to stop, 177–196
- sex and, 195
- withdrawal clinics, 192–194
- withdrawal symptoms, 195

Snuff takers' disease, 319

Soap allergy, 249, 250, 251
- sun sensitivity and, 232, 295–296

Sobee, 34

Sore throat, 58, 127

Soybean allergy
- foods to avoid, 215
- products to avoid, 256

Speculum, 423

Speer, Dr. Frederick, 5, 28, 68

Spice workers, possible causes of dermatitis of, 237

Spiders, 269–270

Spirometer, 423

Spitting up, 27, 28

Spore, 423

Sporting-goods workers, possible causes of dermatitis of, 237

Squamous cell, 423

Stanford Convalescent Home, 81

Status asthmaticus, 156–157, 424

Steam therapy, 61, 64, 141

Stein, Dr. Myron, 171

Steroids, 424
- for polyps, 57
- *See also* Asthma; Dermatitis.

Stings and bites
- treatment for local reaction, 273–274
- treatment for systematic reactions, 274–275
- *See also* Insects.

Stomachache, 49
- *See also* Abdomen, pain of.

Stone workers, possible causes of dermatitis of, 237

Strawberries, 21, 22–23

Streptococcal infection, 29

Streptomycin allergy, 286

Stroh, Dr. James E., 209

Sulfonamide allergy, 286
- products to avoid, 301–305

Sulfones, allergy to, 292

Sulzberger, Dr. Marion, 340

Summation effect, in food allergy, 200

Sun allergy, 83, 232, 296–297, 328–329
- sensitivity from cosmetics or drugs, 294–297

Sun allergy (*cont.*)
See also Photosensitivity.
Sun lotions, 329
Sunair Home and Hospital for Asthmatic Children, 81
Sunny Hill Hospital for Children, 81
Surgery, 85–86
anesthetics and allergy, 86, 244, 290
Sweating, 28, 68
See also Perspiration.
Swelling, 219
Swimming, 83
Symptoms of allergies, 19–22, 73, 114
in children, 48–50, 55–56
determining the cause, 37, 51–53
in infants, 25
of disorders resembling hayfever, 91, 92
of dust allergy, 99
early descriptions, 88
of food allergy, 28
of hayfever, 89–91
of mold allergy, 97–98
variations in, 22–23
Synergism, 424
of drugs, 282–283
Syntex Laboratories, 394
Synthetics, allergy to, 230
Szanton, Dr. Victor, 64
Szentivanyi, Dr. Ando, 361

Tachycardia, 424
Tanners, possible causes of dermatitis of, 237
Taste, loss of, 57
Taxidermists, possible causes of dermatitis of, 237
Teeth deformities, 49, 56
Temperature, 135, 136, 155, 250
causing allergic reactions, 326–328
causing cough, 167
effect on allergy, 22, 31, 61, 103, 109, 124
Tension, as symptom of allergy, 67–71
Tests
for food allergy, 29, 30–31
research on, 366–367
skin tests, 37, 39, 47, 90, 95, 98, 102, 115, 125, 201, 221, 283, 337–341, 423
Tetanus immunizations, 43, 83–84, 108–109, 291
reactions, 290–291
Tetracycline allergy, products to avoid, 305
Theatrical profession, possible causes of dermatitis of, 237
Theophylline. *See* Aminophylline.
Threshold concept, 22, 23, 71, 102, 200, 424
Thymus gland, 48, 359
Thyroiditis, 374
Thyroid nodules, 122
Ticks, 271
Tics, 68
Tokyo-Yokohama asthma, 128
Tolerance, 424
to drugs, 113
Tomatine, 368
Tongue fissures, 28
Tonsils and adenoids, 57, 58–59, 86, 114, 123, 127, 417
Toys, 105
possible causes of dermatitis in toy-manufacturing workers, 235
Toxemia, 424
Trachea, 120, 424
Tracheitis, 127, 424
Tracheotomy, 285, 424
Tranquilizer, 114, 141–142, 424
Transfusions, reactions to, 291
Transillumination, 91
Transplantation, and allergy, 372–373
Treatment, 38, 46–47, 54, 343–352
of allergic tension-fatigue syndrome, 70
of allergy and infections, 63–64
of asthma, 60–62
of bed-wetting, 66–67
of croup, 65–66
of facial deformities, 50–51

Treatment (*cont.*)
failure to follow directions, 369–370
of hayfever, 112–119
research on new methods, 367–371
of year-round allergy, 58–59
Tree pollen, 110
seasons, 95–96
See also Pollen.
Triatoma, 271–272
Troches, 145
Tuberculosis and allergic mechanisms, 371
Tubotympanic catarrh, 65
Tulip allergy, 241
Tullis, Dr. David C. H., 123
Tumbleweed, 241
Tympanic membrane, 424

Ulcerative colitis, 48
Undertakers, possible causes of dermatitis of, 237
Unger, Dr. Donald, 312, 370
Upper respiratory tract, 120–121
Uremia, 424
Urination, pain on, 199
Urticaria, 424
Uveitis, 424

Vaccinations, 42–43, 424
eczema and, 250
Vaccines
allergies to, 290–291
bacterial, 117
Vaccinia, 250
Van Arsdel, Jr., Dr. Paul T., 285
Vaporizers, 141
See also Steam.
Vaseline, 114
Vasospasm, 424
Vertigo, 424
Villa Santa Cruz, 81
Viral vaccines, 63
Virus, allergy to, 62–64
Vitamin C, 145
and prickly heat, 40
Vitamin E, 208–209
Vitamins, 145
as cause of allergies, 29
lack of, causing symptoms, 29
Voice, loud, as indication of hearing loss, 56
Vomiting, 28
Von Pirquet, Professor Clemens, 356

Waldbott, Dr. George L., 128
Warner-Chilcott, 395
Wash-and-wear clothes, allergy to, 230
Wasps, 260
how to destroy hives, 266
King Menes' death, 258
See also Insects.
Weather, 59, 98, 103, 104, 122, 124, 155, 363
asthma and, 135
See also Climate, Temperature.
Weight loss, 89
Westwood Pharmaceuticals, 395
Wheat allergy, 205, 206
foods to avoid, 32, 215–216
substitutes for, 212
See also Cereal allergy.
Wheel bug, 271
Wheezing, 51, 59, 114, 119, 120, 161, 335
See also Asthma.
White blood cells, 359
Wilson, Dr. William, 5, 320
Wind, 114
Winter itch, 250
Wittich, Dr. Fred W., 320
Wolf, Dr. A. Ford, 5
Wood, Dr. H. Curtis, 145
Woodworkers, possible causes of dermatitis of, 236
Wool allergy, 108, 249
in wool workers, 237
Worms, intestinal, and asthma, 123

Xeroderma, 424
X-ray treatment, 115

Year-round allergy. *See* Perennial allergic rhinitis.

Yeast allergy, foods to avoid, 216
Yellow jackets
how to destroy hives, 266
sting reactions, 259, 262
Yellow jackets (*cont.*)
See also Insects.
Yoga, 51

Zinnias, allergy to, 93